LONG-TERM RESULTS IN
VASCULAR
SURGERY

Edited by

James S.T. Yao, MD, PhD
Magerstadt Professor of Surgery
Division of Vascular Surgery
Department of Surgery
Northwestern University Medical School
Chicago, Illinois

William H. Pearce, MD
Associate Professor of Surgery
Division of Vascular Surgery
Department of Surgery
Northwestern University Medical School
Chicago, Illinois

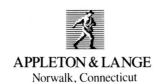

APPLETON & LANGE
Norwalk, Connecticut

Copyright © 1993 by Appleton & Lange
Simon & Schuster Business and Professional Group

93 94 95 96 97 / 10 9 8 7 6 5 4 3 2 1

Prentice Hall International (UK) Limited, *London*
Prentice Hall of Australia Pty. Limited, *Sydney*
Prentice Hall Canada, Inc., *Toronto*
Prentice Hall Hispanoamericana, S.A., *Mexico*
Prentice Hall of India Private Limited, *New Delhi*
Prentice Hall of Japan, Inc., *Tokyo*
Simon & Schuster Asia Pte. Ltd., *Singapore*
Editora Prentice Hall do Brasil Ltda., *Rio de Janeiro*
Prentice Hall, *Englewood Cliffs, New Jersey*

Library of Congress Cataloging-in-Publication Data

Long-term results in vascular surgery/edited by James S.T. Yao, William H. Pearce; with associate authors.
    p. cm.
   ISBN 0-8385-9385-2
   1. Blood-vessels—Surgery—Longitudinal studies.   I. Yao, James S. T.   II. Pearce, William H.
   [DNLM: 1. Follow-Up Studies.   2. Vascular Surgery.   WG 170 L857]
  RD598.5.L65   1993
  617.4′13059—dc20
  DNLM/DLC
  for Library of Congress   92-48800
                                                  CIP

ISBN 0-8385-9385-2

90000

9 780838 593851

Acquisitions Editor: Jane Licht
Production Editor: Sondra Greenfield
Designer: Janice Bielawa

PRINTED IN THE UNITED STATES OF AMERICA

Contents

Contributors

William M. Abbott, MD
Professor of Surgery,
Harvard Medical School
Chief of Vascular Surgery
Department of Vascular Surgery
Massachusetts General Hospital
Boston, Massachusetts

Joseph Alpert, MD
Clinical Professor of Surgery
University of Medicine and Dentistry
Department of Surgery
Newark Beth Israel Medical Center
Newark, New Jersey

George Andros, MD
Medical Director
Vascular Laboratory
Saint Joseph Medical Center
Burbank, California

B. Timothy Baxter, MD
Assistant Professor, Section of Vascular
 Surgery
University of Nebraska Medical Center
Omaha, Nebraska

Ramon Berguer, MD, PhD
Professor of Vascular Surgery
Chief, Division of Vascular Surgery
Wayne State University
Harper Hospital
Detroit, Michigan

F. William Blaisdell, MD
Professor of Surgery
Chairman, Department of Surgery
University of California, Davis
Sacramento, California

Bruce J. Brener, MD
Clinical Professor of Surgery
University of Medicine and Dentistry
Director of Vascular Surgery
Newark Beth Israel Medical Center
Newark, New Jersey

David C. Brewster, MD
Associate Clinical Professor of Surgery
Harvard Medical School
Massachusetts General Hospital
Boston, Massachusetts

Donald K. Brief, MD
Clinical Professor of Surgery
University of Medicine and Dentistry
Chief of General Surgery
Newark Beth Israel Medical Center
Newark, New Jersey

Allan D. Callow, MD, PhD
Research Professor of Surgery
Department of Surgery
Washington University School of
 Medicine
St. Louis, Missouri

Benjamin B. Chang, MD
Associate Professor
Vascular Surgery Section
Albany Medical College
Albany, New York

Alexander W. Clowes, MD
Professor
Department of Surgery
University of Washington School of
  Medicine
Seattle, Washington

Michael D. Colburn, MD
Resident in General Surgery
UCLA School of Medicine
Los Angeles, California

Jeffrey C. Cooke, MD
Resident in General Vascular Surgery
Massachusetts General Hospital and
  Harvard Medical School
Boston, Massachusetts

Denton A. Cooley, MD
Surgeon and Chief
Texas Heart Institute
Houston, Texas

Joseph S. Coselli, MD
Associate Professor of Surgery
Department of Surgery
Baylor College of Medicine
The Methodist Hospital
Houston, Texas

E. Stanley Crawford, MD
Professor of Surgery
Department of Surgery
Baylor College of Medicine
The Methodist Hospital
Houston, Texas

Debra Creighton, BA
Department of Surgery
Newark Beth Israel Medical Center
Newark, New Jersey

Jack L. Cronenwett, MD
Professor of Surgery
Section of Vascular Surgery
Dartmouth-Hitchcock Medical Center
Lebanon, New Hampshire

Frances Cross, MD
Department of Surgery
Newark Beth Israel Medical Center
Newark, New Jersey

**Christopher G. Cunningham, LCDR,
  MC, USNR**
Head, Section of Vascular Surgery
Nation Naval Medical Center
Bethesda, Maryland

Simon G. Darke, MS, FRCS
Honorary Lecturer
Southampton Medical School
Consultant Surgeon
Bournemouth General Hospital
Dorsett, England

Richard H. Dean, MD
Professor and Chairman
Division of Surgical Sciences
Bowman Gray School of Medicine of
  Wake Forest University
Winston-Salem, North Carolina

James A. DeWeese, MD
Chief of Vascular Surgery Emeritus
Department of Surgery
University of Rochester Medical Center
Rochester, New York

Magruder C. Donaldson, MD
Assistant Professor of Surgery
Harvard Medical School
Department of Surgery
Division of Vascular Surgery
Brigham and Women's Hospital
Boston, Massachusetts

Donald B. Doty, MD
Chairman, Division of Cardiovascular
  and Thoracic Surgery
Department of Surgery
University of Utah School of Medicine
Salt Lake City, Utah

Leopoldo B. Dulawa, MD
Vascular Laboratory
Saint Joseph Medical Center
Burbank, California

James M. Edwards, MD
Assistant Professor of Surgery
Division of Vascular Surgery
Oregon Health Sciences University
Portland, Oregon

David E. Eisenbud, MD
Department of Surgery
Newark Beth Israel Medical Center
Newark, New Jersey

William R. Flinn, MD
Associate Professor of Surgery
Division of Vascular Surgery
Department of Surgery
Northwestern University Medical
  School
Chicago, Illinois

Robert J. Goldenkranz, MD
Assistant Clinical Professor
University of Medicine and Dentistry
Department of Surgery
Newark Beth Israel Medical Center
Newark, New Jersey

Richard M. Green, MD
Chief, Section of Vascular Surgery
University of Rochester School of
  Medicine and Dentistry
Rochester, New York

Lazar J. Greenfield, MD
Chairman, Department of Surgery
The University of Michigan Hospitals
Ann Arbor, Michigan

Roger M. Greenhalgh, MD
Professor of Surgery and Chairman
Department of Surgery
Charing Cross and Westminster Medical
  School
London, England

Igor D. Gregoric, MD
Resident
Department of Surgery
The University of Texas Medical School
  at Houston
Houston, Texas

Sushil K. Gupta, MD
Chief of Surgery
Metrowest Medical Center
Framingham, Massachusetts

George E. Hajjar, MD
Post-Doctoral Scholar
UCLA School of Medicine
Los Angeles, California

John W. Hallett, Jr, MD
Associate Professor of Surgery
Mayo Medical School
Mayo Clinic
Rochester, Minnesota

Robert W. Harris, MD
Vascular Laboratory
Saint Joseph Medical Center
Burbank, California

D. Higman, FRCS
Lecturer in Surgery
Charing Cross and Westminster
  Medical School
London, England

Kim J. Hodgson, MD
Assistant Professor of Surgery
Southern Illinois University School
  of Medicine
Springfield, Illinois

Jan Huston, MD
Department of Surgery
Newark Beth Israel Medical
  Center
Newark, New Jersey

Toshio Inahara, MD
Clinical Professor of Surgery
Division of Vascular Surgery
Oregon Health Sciences University
Portland, Oregon

Michael J.H.M. Jacobs, MD, PhD
Vascular Surgeon
Department of Surgery
Academis Hospital
Maastricht, Netherlands

K. Wayne Johnston, MD, FRCSC
Professor of Surgery
Division of Vascular Surgery
University of Toronto
Toronto Hospital (General Division)
Toronto, Ontario, Canada

Peter G. Kalman, MD, FRCSC
Vascular Surgery Division
University of Toronto
Toronto Hospital (General Division)
Toronto, Ontario, Canada

Robert L. Kistner, MD
Clinical Professor of Surgery
University of Hawaii
John A. Burns School of Medicine
Honolulu, Hawaii

Robert P. Leather, MD
Professor
Vascular Surgery Section
Albany Medical College
Albany, New York

Jere W. Lord, Jr, MD
Professor of Clinical Surgery (Retired)
New York University—Bellevue Medical
  Center
New York, New York

John A. Mannick, MD
Moseley Professor of Surgery
Harvard Medical School
Surgeon-in-Chief
Brigham and Women's Hospital
Boston, Massachusetts

Mark A. Mattos, MD
Assistant Professor of Surgery
Southern Illinois University School of
  Medicine
Springfield, Illinois

Walter J. McCarthy, MD
Assistant Professor of Surgery
Division of Vascular Surgery
Department of Surgery
Northwestern University Medical School
Chicago, Illinois

W.D. McMillan, MD
Division of Vascular Surgery
Department of Surgery
Northwestern University Medical School
Chicago, Illinois

Charles L. Mesh, MD
Assistant Professor of Surgery
Case Western Reserve University
  School of Medicine
Cleveland, Ohio

D. Craig Miller, MD
Professor of Cardiovascular and
  Thoracic Surgery
Stanford University School of
  Medicine
Falk Cardiovascular Research Center
Stanford, California

Wesley S. Moore, MD
Professor of Surgery
Chief, Section of Vascular Surgery
UCLA School of Medicine
Los Angeles, California

Timothy J. Nypaver, MD
Clinical Fellow
Division of Vascular Surgery
Henry Ford Hospital
Detroit, Michigan

Robert W. Oblath, MD
Vascular Laboratory
Saint Joseph Medical Center
Burbank, California

Kenneth Ouriel, MD
Associate Professor of Surgery
Department of Surgery
University of Rochester School of
  Medicine and Dentistry
Rochester, New York

Victor Parsonnet, MD
Clinical Professor of Surgery
University of Medicine and Dentistry
Director of Surgery
Newark Beth Israel Medical Center
Newark, New Jersey

William H. Pearce, MD
Associate Professor of Surgery
Division of Vascular Surgery
Department of Surgery
Northwestern University Medical
  School
Chicago, Illinois

William C. Pevec, MD
Assistant Professor
University of California, Davis
Sacramento, California

John M. Porter, MD
Professor of Surgery
Head, Division of Vascular Surgery
Oregon Health Sciences University
Portland, Oregon

Janet T. Powell, MD, PhD
Reader in Cardiovascular Biology
Charing Cross and Westminster Medical
  School
London, England

Mary C. Proctor, MS
Department of Surgery
University of Michigan
Ann Arbor, Michigan

William J. Quiñones-Baldrich, MD
Associate Professor of Surgery
Vascular Surgery Section
UCLA School of Medicine
Los Angeles, California

George J. Reul, MD
Clinical Professor,
Division of Thoracic and Cardiac
  Surgery
Department of Surgery
The University of Texas Medical School
  at Houston
Associate Chief of Surgery
Texas Heart Institute
Houston, Texas

Robert B. Rutherford, MD
Professor of Surgery
University of Colorado Health Sciences Center
Denver, Colorado

Sergio X. Salles-Cunha, PhD
Vascular Laboratory
Saint Joseph Medical Center
Burbank, California

George E. Sarris, MD
Senior Fellow
Department of Cardiovascular and
  Thoracic Surgery
Stanford University School of Medicine
Stanford, California

Peter A. Schneider, MD
Vascular Surgery
Saint Joseph Medical Center
Burbank, California

James J. Schuler, MD
Chief, Division of Vascular Surgery
University of Illinois Hospital
Chicago, Illinois

Elizabeth Scott, MD
Division of Vascular Surgery
Department of Surgery
Northwestern University Medical School
Chicago, Illinois

Cynthia Shortell, MD
Instructor, Chief Resident
Department of Surgery
University of Rochester School of
  Medicine and Dentistry
Rochester, New York

Ken W. Sniderman, MD, FRCPC
Radiology Division
University of Toronto
Toronto General Hospital
Toronto, Ontario, Canada

James C. Stanley, MD
Professor of Surgery
Head, Section of Vascular Surgery
University of Michigan
Ann Arbor, Michigan

Ronald J. Stoney, MD
Professor
Division of Vascular Surgery
University of California
San Francisco, California

David S. Sumner, MD
Professor of Surgery
Chief, Section of Peripheral
Vascular Surgery
Southern Illinois University School of
 Medicine
Springfield, Illinois

Jonathan B. Towne, MD
Professor of Surgery
Department of Vascular Surgery
Medical College of Wisconsin
Milwaukee County Medical Complex
Milwaukee, Wisconsin

Frank J. Veith, MD
Professor of Surgery
Albert Einstein College of Medicine
Chief of Vascular Surgical Services
Montefiore Medical Center
New York, New York

Roger Wang, BA
Northwestern University Medical School
Chicago, Illinois

Kurt R. Wengerter, MD
Assistant Professor of Surgery
Department of Surgery
Albert Einstein College of Medicine
Montefiore Medical Center
New York, New York

Anthony D. Whittemore, MD
Associate Professor of Surgery
Harvard Medical School
Chief, Division of Vascular Surgery
Brigham and Women's Hospital
Boston, Massachusetts

James S.T. Yao, MD, PhD
Magerstadt Professor of Surgery
Division of Vascular Surgery
Department of Surgery
Northwestern University Medical School
Chicago, Illinois

Nobuya Zempo, MD
Visiting Scientist
Department of Surgery
University of Washington School of
 Medicine
Seattle, Washington

Preface

As Charles G. Rob rightly stated in the introduction of *The Classics of Vascular Surgery,* "We do not know when arterial surgery began; it developed slowly during many centuries. The pace gradually increased from about 1900 to 1945 and accelerated dramatically for the next 35 years, from the end of World War II to the present day."[1] Indeed there has been further dramatic development since his statement. Since 1980, vascular surgery has emerged as a specialty in the field of surgery. Not only have surgical techniques been perfected to provide optimal care for patients, but we have also witnessed an explosion of technology in both diagnostic and therapeutic procedures. The objective of this book is to examine the long-term results of these procedures.

Long-term results of vascular surgery must be reported in a uniform way, and Robert Rutherford, chairman of many committees on reporting standards of the joint Society for Vascular Surgery and the North American chapter, International Society for Cardiovascular Surgery, describes the current reporting standards for long-term results for vascular surgical procedures. Not infrequently, the longevity of a vascular procedure is undermined by a patient's continuing smoking habit or by restenosis. Roger Greenhalgh and Alexander Clowes, both experts in these fields, offer up-to-date knowledge about these two important factors. The introduction of ultrasound now provides surgeons with a noninvasive technique for monitoring the results of surgery. David Sumner, a pioneer in noninvasive testing, outlines a concise surveillance program for various vascular reconstructive procedures.

Nearly three decades after Eastcott and colleagues[2] reported successful reconstruction of the internal carotid artery in a patient with intermittent attacks of hemiplegia, the role of the carotid endarterectomy in the prevention of stroke has finally been clarified by the North American Symptomatic Carotid Endarterectomy Trial (NASCET). Allan Callow's report on the durability of carotid endarterectomy reconfirms the validity of this procedure. Surgical procedures of equal importance in the treatment of cerebral ischemia, such as vertebral artery reconstruction, carotid-subclavian bypass, and innominate artery bypass, are critically reviewed by Ramon Berguer, Wesley Moore, and George Reul.

Clearly, one of the major advances in vascular surgery is infrainguinal bypass for limb salvage. With procedures ranging from femoropopliteal vein graft to femorotibial and the *in situ* vein graft, many patients with limb-threatening ischemia are now returned to full function. The development of various prosthetic grafts has extended bypass grafting to many patients. Unless long-term patency of these grafts is achieved, however, patients will again revert to an ischemic state. Experts in this field, such as William Quiñones-Baldrich, Anthony Whittemore, George Andros, Robert Leather, Walter McCarthy, and William Abbott, give succinct reviews of their experience with different types of infrainguinal bypass. Planning with regard to limb ischemia is often difficult, and Frank Veith gives his experience in treatment strategies for patients with severe ischemia. In order to extend graft patency, antithrombotic drugs may be needed. William Flinn reviews the experience in our group on the use of warfarin therapy to extend prosthetic graft patency.

Since 1906, when Goyanes of Madrid[3] first reported the use of vein graft to restore arterial flow in a patient with a popliteal aneurysm, extensive follow-up of these patients has been relatively unknown. The 25-year follow-up by James DeWeese is unique and further supports the surgical treatment of popliteal aneurysm. The importance of the profunda femoral artery in revascularization, first recognized by Frank Leeds and R.S. Gilfillan,[4] needs further examination. Jonathan Towne provides us with an up-to-date review on this important artery.

Dissection and thoracoabdominal aortic aneurysm continue to offer challenges to vascular surgeons. The Stanford experience reported by Craig Miller is a standout in this field. For management of thoracoabdominal aneurysm, no one can surpass the collective experience of Stanley Crawford and Joseph Coselli. Bypass graft is now a standard surgical procedure for managing aneurysm or occlusive disease of the abdominal aorta. The long-term results of these procedures detailed by David Brewster, John Hallett, and Jack Cronenwett leave little doubt about the value of aortic reconstruction. Endarterectomy, the first procedure for direct arterial surgery pioneered by E.J. Wylie,[5] now has a lesser role in the treatment of major arterial occlusion. In selected cases, however, endarterectomy remains a viable procedure. This point of view is nicely illustrated by the chapter on this subject by Toshio Inahara.

Other than direct reconstructive procedures, indirect procedures, such as percutaneous transluminal angioplasty and extra-anatomical bypass, also play an important role in the relief of arterial ischemia. Many of these procedures have now been performed for a decade or more. The chapter by Peter Kalman, Ken Sniderman, and Wayne Johnston of Toronto on percutaneous balloon dilation, the chapter by Bruce Brener on femorofemoral bypass, and the one by William Blaisdell on axillofemoral bypass represent the longest experience with these procedures.

Unlike the long-term results for procedures for lower extremity ischemia, those for upper extremity procedures for patients with Raynaud's syndrome are less known. John Porter and the Northwestern group provide information on medical and surgical care of these patients. One of the most difficult problems to manage is thoracic outlet syndrome, and many factors may influence the result. The chapter by Richard Green analyzes factors determining the success of thoracic outlet decompression. Although somewhat uncommon, arteriovenous malformation continues to present a therapeutic challenge for vascular surgeons. Recurrence is always a possibility. William Pearce of the Northwestern group provides data on the natural history and long-term follow-up of these patients.

Visceral artery reconstruction is now a standard procedure for renovascular hypertension or for mesenteric ischemia. In the pediatric population, treatment of renal artery stenosis offers a technical challenge. Three experts in this field, Ronald Stoney, Richard Dean, and James Stanley, provide a complete review of their long-term surgical experience.

Perhaps, of all vascular reconstructive procedures, the longevity of venous reconstruction remains the most enigmatic. Although vein stripping is frequently performed, there is a need to determine its longevity. Simon Darke of Southampton Medical School, Dorsett, England, gives a five- to ten-year follow-up of this common surgical procedure. Vena cava reconstruction and spiral vein graft are now acceptable procedures, and Donald Doty describes his unique experience with these procedures. Lazar Greenfield presents the authoritative experience of the fate of the filter, a necessity in the prevention of pulmonary embolism. Robert Kistner, a pioneer in venous valve repair, provides us with the long-term results of this technique in the treatment of chronic venous insufficiency. Finally, every vascular surgeon has been involved in the repair of an injured vein. James Schuler describes his extensive experience and clarifies the role of surgical repair in such an injury.

The collection of articles in this book firmly establishes that many vascular surgical procedures have stood the test of time. Revascularization procedures, if done appropriately and properly, will yield long and lasting results.

James S.T. Yao, MD, PhD
William H. Pearce, MD

REFERENCES

1. Rob CG. *The Classics of Vascular Surgery.* Medford, NJ: Apollo Press; 1981.
2. Eastcott HHG, Pickering GW, Rob CG. Reconstruction of internal carotid artery in a patient with intermittent attacks of hemiplegia. *Lancet.* 1954;2:994–996.
3. Goyanes J. Nuevos trabajos de cisrugia vascular substiticion plastica de las venlas o arterioplastia venosa applicada como nuevo metodo al tratamiento de los aneurismos. *Siglo Med.* 1906;53:546–561.
4. Leeds FH, Gilfillan RS. Revascularization of the lower limb: importance of profunda femoris artery. *Arch Surg.* 1961;82:25–31.
5. Wylie EJ. Thromoendarterectomy for atherosclerotic thrombosis of major arteries. *Surgery.* 1952;32:275–292.

I

Basic Considerations

1

Reporting Standards
for Long-Term Results
of Vascular Surgery

Robert B. Rutherford, MD

Standards for reporting the results of the treatment of vascular disease have been suggested by the ad hoc committees of the Joint Council of the Society of Vascular Surgery and the North American Chapter of the International Society for Cardiovascular Surgery and have been published in the *Journal of Vascular Surgery* for reports on lower extremity ischemia,[1] venous disease,[2] extracranial arterial disease,[3] and aneurysms.[4] In addition, the author has published recommendations for reports on complications following vascular surgery.[5] The original report of the ad hoc committee[1] was subsequently adopted and published by the Society for Cardiovascular International Radiology in their journal.[6] These, and other reports still in preparation, are not meant to be the conclusive statement on reporting standards, rather they represent our initial attempts to determine some uniform reporting practices. There have been criticisms,[7,8] as one would expect when arbitrary positions are taken. Some are valid and these will be accommodated and residual problems addressed in a supplemental issue of the *Journal of Vascular Surgery* in the not too distant future. It is not the intent of this contribution to reiterate all of the pertinent details of these reports. Space does not permit this. However, there are a number of important aspects that apply particularly to reports containing long-term results of vascular procedures, as well as certain generic aspects that deserve emphasis, and these will be the focus of this report. Finally, even though the author is still the chairman of the Ad Hoc Committee on Reporting Standards and many of the recommendations here paraphrase the committees' reports, the choice of those recommendations presented here along with some other suggestions represent the author's personal views.

THE EFFECT OF THE EXCLUSION OF INITIAL FAILURES ON LONG-TERM RESULTS

It is axiomatic that long-term results appear better if calculated on the basis of initial successes only, that is, with initial deaths, and technical, symptomatic, and hemodynamic failures eliminated. For example, a "cumulative long-term patency" of 66% that ignores 25% of cases who failed because of an inability to complete the procedure, early thrombosis, hemodynamic failure, or death, actually represents an extended benefit in less than half of those in whom the procedure was undertaken.

Disagreement persists over what should constitute a reportable failure, with most claims for exemption relating to minor events that either had little effect on long-term outcome or caused little inconvenience. At the other extreme the purists feel that, much like randomization to a treatment group in a prospective trial, "intent to treat" is enough for inclusion. Several examples serve to illustrate the difficulty with this criterion. A distal tibial bypass is attempted for limb salvage, but exploration of the sole tibial artery visualized on arteriogram shows that it is not suitable and the procedure is abandoned. Exploratory surgery is performed on a patient in refractory shock with a ruptured aneurysm, but she succumbs just as proximal control is obtained, so the repair is not carried out. A patient is taken to the angiography suite for balloon angioplasty, but the guide wire cannot be passed, or, as another example, attempted passage produces a small dissection and the procedure is abandoned with no adverse consequences. A prosthetic femoropopliteal bypass thromboses 20 hours after operation during a hypotensive episode, but patency is readily restored by immediate thrombectomy, and completion angiography demonstrates no technical flaws. These and other similar scenarios are a common problem in our literature. In the past they were usually discounted out of hand, and this practice undoubtedly persists to some extent in current publications on vascular surgery, even though the now accepted standard is that *if any intervention is actually undertaken,* even if it cannot be successfully completed, it must be counted, and no failure from that point on can be arbitrarily eliminated.[1] However, it is permissible to report initial failures and then calculate the long-term success rate of initial successes, but *only if the overall success rate is also prominently stated.* For example, if patency is the measure of success being used, then it should be made clear throughout the article whether *overall* or *selective* patency is being referred to, that is, the patency of initial successes only. The principle here is one of full and open disclosure, rather than one of allowing a "cumulative" patency rate to be cited that readers only realize is actually a selective patency rate based on the elimination of a significant number of initial failures because they catch a sentence buried in the materials and methods section.

APPROPRIATE CRITERIA OF LONG-TERM SUCCESS

Patency is obviously an important criterion for success of vascular reconstructive procedures, and, as will be discussed later, it is important that it be properly defined and estimated. But should patency be the ultimate criterion? Are there other criteria that add a valuable dimension? Patency alone provides a reliable index of success for extremity bypasses performed for arterial occlusive disease, although even there it does not always reflect initial success or long-term benefit: both the limb salvage rate and the hemodynamic failure rate add additional dimensions. However, the patency rate alone is an insufficient measure of success in operations for carotid, aneurysmal, or venous disease. Let us consider these different areas separately.

Carotid Disease

Carotid endarterectomy is rarely performed to treat complete occlusion, so although long-term patency can be reported, significant carotid restenosis (arbitrarily 50% or more) or occlusion is a better indicator. It is also valuable to indicate the *symptomatic* restenosis rate as well as the overall restenosis rate, even though the former will also be covered in large part under the most important index of success, freedom from stroke. Although both should be reported, freedom from stroke or symptoms of cerebral ischemia is a more valid index of success than patency without significant restenosis because it represents the main goal of carotid endarterectomy. In this regard, symptoms caused by disease in the other carotid, vertebral, or subclavian artery distributions should be recorded but not counted as a failure of unilateral carotid endarterectomy. Only a cerebrovascular event in the territory of the carotid surgery should be counted against it. Also, the event should not be limited to permanent stroke. Transient ischemic attacks (TIAS) and reversible ischemic neurologic deficits (RINDs) should also be included. Actually, the new nomenclature suggested in the cerebrovascular standards[3] automatically allows for this, because TIAS and RINDs are now considered "brief" and "temporary" strokes, respectively. Nonlateralizing symptoms should also be counted *in the event of carotid restenosis.* Thus, the "ischemia-free interval" specific for that carotid artery should be calculated as the major indicator of success for carotid endarterectomy, and it should be presented in a life table format, just as patency rates are.

In reporting on patients operated on for acute or permanent stroke, one may need to use an additional criterion for judging success, for example, change in neurologic status. A "neurologic event disability scale"[3] could be used to gauge the degree of improvement or worsening, but the long-term result could still be gauged on the basis of events occurring after postoperative neurologic status has stabilized.

Aneurysmal Disease

Graft occlusion is not a major problem after prosthetic repair of major or central arterial aneurysms. Thus, patency after abdominal aortic aneurysm (AAA) repair is not the most valid measure of long-term success. Since the main threat posed by an AAA is death from rupture and that posed by popliteal or other extremity aneurysms is limb loss from thromboembolic events, long-term survival rates in the former group and limb salvage rates in the latter should be documented. By the same token, freedom from stroke is important in assessing the results of surgery for carotid aneurysms. Patency is important primarily in peripheral reconstructions, but for all of these aneurysm locations, freedom from recurrent aneurysm formation and its complications (e.g., aortoenteric fistulas), should be considered a major index of long-term success. In this regard, anastomotic aneurysm, aneurysm in the graft itself, and aneurysm in the immediately adjacent segment should all count as failures, whereas new aneurysms developing elsewhere or in segments that are separated from the graft by a segment of normal artery (or an artery of unchanged caliber) should not count against the original operation but be considered as part of the patient's overall disease.

Venous Disease

Venous hypertension is the final common denominator which determines the severity of the sequelae of venous disease in the lower extremities, whether the underlying cause is valve reflux, obstruction to outflow, or both. Long-term patency of certain procedures, such as venous thrombectomy or thrombolysis, venous bypass, valve segment interposition, or valvuloplasty, is important and should be reported, but control of the sequelae of chronic venous insufficiency (CVI) is the primary goal of all of these procedures, and therefore, this, and not patency, should be the main criterion of long-term success. Furthermore, other venous interventions, such as high ligation and stripping, and perforator interruption (and even elastic support and frequent leg elevation for that matter), are competitive forms of treatment, the effectiveness of which cannot be gauged by patency rates.

A persistent and significant reduction in ambulatory venous pressure (AVP) would seem a valid hemodynamic index of long-term success, but this measure is not always practical and improvement in the AVP short of normalization has been shown to be beneficial, so it is not even clear what level of AVP reduction constitutes success. A prolongation of venous refill time (VRT), as measured by a simple photoplethys-mographic test, has been used as an index in recent years, but it does not appear to be sensitive or accurate enough for this purpose. In addition, changes in the VRT have not correlated well with subjective clinical benefit. Currently, only the avoidance of *severe* stasis dermatitis (i.e., severe enough to require treatment) and the presence or recurrence of venous ulceration are universally accepted as clinical end points. Freedom from these constitute a valid end point for venous operations designed to control the postphlebitic syndrome. In the standards suggested in the report on venous disease,[2] Porter and colleagues recommended a simple but practical gradation of CVI, with severe stasis dermatitis and ulceration as the last, or severe, stage. *Sustained* improvement of one full stage or degree of severity of CVI could be considered a long-term success. However, the committee went one step further and combined this with some objective evidence of hemodynamic improvement (e.g., a reduction in AVP or prolongation of VRT) to provide an outcome scale ranging from −3 to +3 similar to that which had been previously devised for arterial occlusive disease.[1] This would seem to be a more valid index of long-term success. Again, sustained categoric improvement could serve as the criteria for success and be represented on a life table plot.

Another important consideration in assessing the success of treatment of venous disease is what constitutes a valid control for comparison. Many patients still require elastic support and frequent elevation, and it is known that this combination alone controls much if not most chronic venous insufficiency. Therefore, to demonstrate real benefit for a particular venous reconstruction, it seems important either to have *both* the group operated on and control group wear elastic stockings and elevate the limb, or to have the group operated on *not* wear elastic stockings and elevate the limb to demonstrate that the operation is truly superior to conservative management. Similarly, concomitant use of high ligation and stripping and perforator interruption, so often performed along with venous reconstructions, has obscured outcome assessment of the latter procedures. This adjunctive benefit must be controlled in comparative studies before success can be claimed.

Finally, keep in mind that relief of obstruction, such as patency of a previously thrombosed venous segment, may alone confer benefit even if some degree of valvular insufficiency can later be detected. Such a finding of valvular insufficiency has been used to condemn the long-term results of both thrombectomy and thrombolysis for iliofemoral venous thrombosis even though such patients would obviously have done worse if they had unrelieved outflow obstruction *in addition to* the degree of venous reflux observed.

Clearly, judging the long-term results of venous surgery remains the most problematic of all the areas of vascular disease.

Extremity Arterial Occlusive Disease

As stated previously, patency is the main criterion employed in judging the long-term success of arterial reconstructions for lower extremity occlusive disease. This is appropriate since the patency rate is a good means of gauging the merits of long bypasses and the grafts employed. However, again we must consider the goals of intervention and the fact that they differ for different levels of severity of ischemia. In the case of arterial claudication, the goal is the restoration of the ability to walk far enough without muscular ischemic pain to be able to return to work or resume other important activities. For the patient with critical ischemia, the relief of rest pain, healing of ischemic ulcers, or healing of local amputations for gangrene are the goals. These goals are collectively called *limb salvage* but are more appropriately termed *foot salvage* since preservation of a painless functioning foot is the therapeutic goal.

If a bypass relieves claudication only to have it recur later, the revascularization procedure has failed *if* it has occluded or significantly restenosed, whereas if it is functionally patent and the cause of deterioration is progression of disease in the inflow or outflow arteries, the bypass graft cannot be blamed for failure. Again, sustained categoric improvement plus objective evidence of hemodynamic improvement should be required to claim success. The details of this approach are in the original standards.[1]

Limb salvage is a more problematic consideration. First of all, one should not take credit for limb salvage in the first place if the limb was not truly threatened to begin with. Transient ischemic rest pain, blue toe syndrome, or achieving healing without objective evidence of severe forefoot ischemia in the first place, do *not* qualify under the term *limb salvage*. Again, these criteria have been well detailed in the original recommended standards.[1] Furthermore, it is not appropriate to quote a limb salvage rate for mixed series of lower extremity bypasses that include a number of patients with claudication as well as those with true limb threat. More important is the method of calculation of the long-term limb salvage rate for those who were operated on for actual chronic critical ischemia. Preserving a painless, functional foot is the clearly stated goal, so a Syme's amputation, or any presumed lowering of the level of amputation, does not qualify. The main cause for concern here is the observation that in most reported series the limb salvage rates exceed the patency rates by 15–30%. Some of this may result from an initial loose definition of limb threat. However, because healing requires an inflammatory response and therefore needs more perfusion than it takes to simply maintain tissue viability and avoid ischemic rest pain, it is entirely appropriate to claim limb salvage if the bypass was responsible for surmounting this critical period, even if it subsequently thromboses, as long as a viable, pain-free limb is preserved nevertheless. Thus, as long as the original criteria for critical ischemia were valid, the limb salvage rate itself is valid and adds a worthwhile dimension to patency rates for bypasses performed for true limb threat.

PRIMARY VERSUS SECONDARY PATENCY

Considerable confusion has been created in the past by authors quoting patency rates without regard to whether or not additional interventions were employed to maintain or restore that patency. Now it is accepted that patency without intervention be called *primary patency* and that patency achieved with intervention be called *secondary patency*, but more precise definitions are required for the sake of standardized reporting practices. The ad hoc committee has defined primary patency as uninterrupted patency with *no* procedures *ever* being performed on the bypass or reconstructed segments, that is, at or within its margins (anastomoses). Thus, inflow or outflow procedures for progression of disease *beyond* its anastomoses are the only exceptions to the rule. Patent grafts may require intervention for stenoses discovered by surveillance or for aneurysm formation, or in the case of *in situ* bypass, residual arterovenous fistulas at or within its margins. Uninterrupted patency sustained in this manner may be reported as *assisted primary patency,* but it can be reported as such only if the actual primary and secondary patency rates are also quoted.[8] There has also been some confusion regarding just what constitutes secondary patency. Once there is any intervention to maintain or restore patency, primary patency is lost, but secondary patency also requires that after such interventions, flow be restored through most (over half) of the length of the graft and at least one of the original anastomoses. Thus, not all "secondary reconstructions" confer secondary patency.

To some, these rules may seem arbitrary and strict. It is natural for vascular surgeons to want their own results (particularly patency rates) to be as high as possible, but it must be remembered that the vascular surgeon's ego should not rest on the primary patency rate but on secondary patency, which, after all, reflects the ultimate duration of benefit from the surgeon's efforts, including the original procedure, close surveillance, and secondary intervention. In contrast, the purpose of primary patency is to compare the intrinsic durability of the procedure itself. Thus, primary patency is the valid way of comparing bypass grafts, not of comparing surgeons. For a full perspective on the procedure, both primary and secondary patency rates should always be reported.

Patency Criteria

It is no longer acceptable in scientific articles intended to influence and guide the readers' clinical practice for patencies to be based on palpable pulses or subjective improvement. Pulse palpation by housestaff or nurses is notoriously unreliable as is subjective testimony regarding relief of symptoms. Consider the example of a patient with claudication with iliac stenosis who is treated by balloon angioplasty. In one scenario, five years after surgery his femoral pulse may still be palpable (as it was *before* treatment) even though there has been significant restenosis, but because of arthritis or a more sedentary lifestyle with advancing age, he may volunteer that he is not claudicating as much as before treatment. Obviously, palpable pulses and subjective symptomatic improvement are not evidence of continued patency here. In a second scenario, the iliac segment has remained wide open after balloon angioplasty, but the superficial femoral artery distal to it has become occluded in the interim. The patient's ankle/brachial index has dropped and he complains of a return of claudication pain. Would this be considered a failure of percutaneous transluminal angioplasty? Actually, both extremes exist in our current literature on the long-term results of iliac percutaneous transluminal angioplasty. What is needed are objective criteria of patency *and* continuing hemodynamic improvement. These together could constitute what we might term *functional patency.* In this day of noninvasive surveillance and so many vascular imaging options, there is no excuse (if one wishes to contribute data to the scientific literature) not to demonstrate patency by objective criteria. To paraphrase the recommendations of the ad hoc committee,[1] the appropriate segmental limb-pressure index (e.g., thigh or ankle brachial index) must remain at least 0.10 above the preoperative level (if not normalized) and not drop more than 0.10 from the initial postoperative level—without proof of patency by conventional arteriography or some other vascular imaging method (e.g., digital subtraction angiography, Duplex scan, magnetic resonance imaging). Plethysmographic tracings significantly (>50%) greater than preoperative levels are acceptable proof of patency *only* in diabetics or others with incompressible, calcified arteries that preclude evaluation by Doppler-derived segmental limb pressures.

METHOD OF ESTIMATING LONG-TERM PATENCY AND OTHER CRITERIA OF SUCCESS

The life table method[9,10] is generally accepted as the best method of estimating long-term results, be it expressed in terms of patency, limb salvage, freedom from stroke, aneurysm formation, or venous stasis sequelae. However, even this method needs standardization for reporting purposes. This is well covered in the original recommendations by the ad hoc committee,[1] but some of the salient recommendations deserve to be reiterated here:

1. The reporting intervals for patients lost to follow-up or those who died with patent grafts stops at the time of their last *objective* patency evaluation.
2. Patients whose grafts have failed since their last examination are statistically treated as having failure dates halfway between those two examinations (thus the frequency of examination increases the accuracy of the life table).
3. Life table analysis should include the following columns in the table: intervals in months, number at risk at the start of the period, number that failed during the period, number that were withdrawn patent because of death or being lost to follow-up, interval of patency, cumulative patency, and standard error. Such a life patency table should be included for every claim made in the article (e.g., a *better* patency rate). Such life table data should be submitted in table form to allow analysis even if the patency rates are also graphically illustrated (the graphs may be published without the tables at the discretion of journal editors).
4. When patencies determined by life table analysis are presented graphically, either the numbers at risk at the start of each interval must be shown or the standard error of each estimate of patency must be displayed, preferably both. In addition, these lines should be joined in step-wise fashion and not be represented by a continuous line or curve. When the estimate of the standard error of patency exceeds 10%, the line beyond this point should be either omitted or represented by a dotted line to indicate poor reliability of estimates beyond that point.
5. All comparisons of life table estimates must be done using the log rank test of significance, which compares two or more life tables over the *entire* period of data. It is not correct to compare patencies at specific intervals using a comparison of standard errors at these times. Finally, although it is not a prerequisite part of the life table, adding a column with cumulative mortality to this table provides valuable perspective and should be routine practice when reporting operations in which the relative value of the procedure may be influenced by the longevity outlook.

SUMMARY AND CONCLUSIONS

In reporting long-term results of vascular interventions, one should choose outcome criteria that best express the goals of the procedure and reflect its durability. Often multiple criteria give a better perspective than a single one: for example, primary *and* secondary patency, patency *and* limb salvage for lower extremity arterial reconstruction, survival *and* freedom from aneurysm formation for abdominal aortic aneurysm repair, freedom from stroke *and* restenosis for carotid endarterectomy. Historic controls are no longer acceptable, and in parallel comparisons cases should be compared, and preferably be comparable, in regard to risk factors, adjunctive measures, level of severity by clinical categorization (if not completely stratified), hemodynamic status, runoff, or any other factor known to affect outcome, if valid conclusions are to be drawn regarding the superiority of the procedure. Results should not be presented only in the best possible light, for example, with initial failures excluded or with success rates enhanced by reintervention; overall success rate and primary patency should also be reported. Functional assessment should be included in addition to patency and, wherever possible and appropriate, should be combined with objective criteria of hemodynamic improvement so that claims of long-term success can be based on a standardized, graded scale of objective improvement. Disability scales are a valid alternative in certain circumstances. The cumulative incidence of procedure-related major or permanent complications should also be reported. Finally, the main outcome criteria chosen should be calculated by the life table method and graphically plotted against time, following recommended rules.

REFERENCES

1. Rutherford RB, Flanigan DP, Gupta SK, et al. Suggested standards for reports dealing with lower extremity ischemia. *J Vas Surg.* 1986;4:80–94.
2. Porter JM, Rutherford RB, Clagett GP, et al. Reporting standards in venous disease. *J Vasc Surg.* 1988;8:172–181.
3. Baker JD, Rutherford RB, Bernstein EF, et al. Suggested standards for reports dealing with cerebrovascular disease. *J Vasc Surg.* 1988;8:721–729.
4. Johnston KW, Rutherford RB, Tilson MD, et al. Suggested standards for reporting arterial aneurysms. *J Vasc Surg.* 1991;13:452–458.
5. Rutherford RB. Suggested standards for reporting complications in vascular surgery. In: Towne JB, Bernhard WM, eds. *Complications in Vascular Surgery,* 3rd ed. St. Louis, Mo: Quality Medical Publishing, Inc.; 1991:1–10.
6. Rutherford RB, Becker GJ. Standards for evaluating and reporting the results of surgical and percutaneous therapy for peripheral arterial disease. *JVIR.* 1991;2:169–174.
7. Suggested standards for reports dealing with lower extremity ischemia: Letters to the editor by Dardik H, McClurken ME. Reply by Mehta S, Rutherford RB. *J Vasc Surg.* 1987;5:501–503.
8. Suggested standards for reports dealing with lower extremity ischemia: Letter to the editor by Testart J, Watelet J. Reply by Rutherford RB. *J Vasc Surg.* 1988;7:718.
9. Peto R, Pike MC, Armitage P, et al. Design and analysis of randomized trials required prolonged observations of each patient. I. Introduction and design. *Br J Cancer.* 1976;34:585.
10. Peto R, Pike MC, Armitage P, et al. Design and analysis of randomized trials required prolonged observations of each patient. II. Analysis and examples. *Br J Cancer.* 1977;35:1.

2

Smoking and Its Influence on Graft Patency

Janet T. Powell, MD, PhD, D. Higman, FRCS, and
Roger M. Greenhalgh, MD

Vascular reconstruction offers the prospect of limb salvage for patients with critical ischemia and of a welcome relief of symptoms to patients with intermittent claudication. The palpable pulse in or distal to the graft following vascular reconstruction may be relatively short-lived. The attrition rate for femoral distal bypass grafts is highest in the first few months following vascular reconstruction with some 15 to 20% of vein grafts being occluded within the first year (Fig. 2-1)and a similar percentage of above-knee prosthetic grafts becoming occluded within the first year after femoropopliteal reconstruction.[1,2] The attrition rate for the below-knee prosthetic grafts is considerably higher.[2]

For vein grafts, such failures have been attributed to discrete stenoses within the grafts, generalised intimal hyperplasia, thrombosis of the graft, or the progression of proximal or distal arterial disease. For prosthetic grafts the occlusion is often attributed to thrombosis rather than to the progression of proximal or distal disease, with the compliance mismatch at the distal anastomosis and the physical stresses to below-knee grafts potentiating such thrombosis. The introduction of antiplatelet therapy, using aspirin and dipyridamole, has improved the patency rates of prosthetic grafts.[3] Similar antiplatelet therapy has failed to improve the patency rates of vein grafts.[1] Considerable effort has therefore been devoted to trying to identify other factors that influence the outcome of arterial reconstruction, particularly those factors that could be subject to therapeutic intervention.

Smoking is a potent risk factor for the development and progression of peripheral arterial disease.[4] The influence of smoking on the outcome of vascular reconstruction has been a matter of long debate. Before 1985, only a single study, which did not distinguish between aortic and distal grafts or between vein grafts and prosthetic grafts, used an objective assessment of smoking: carboxyhemogloblin with a half-life of $t\frac{1}{2} \approx 5$ hours[5]: This study showed that smoking had an adverse effect on graft patency. Studies based on the patient's history of smoking have given less conclusive results, although in one study of femorodistal vein grafts, graft patency at 2 years was 60% in nonsmokers compared with only 30% in smokers.[6] The ability of patients to deceive the clinician about their continuing smoking habits is well recognized.[7]

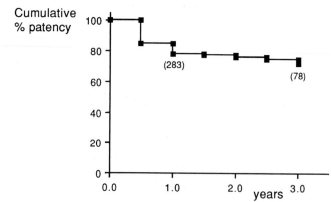

Figure 2-1 The patency of 293 femoropopliteal vein bypass grafts. The number of patients with patent grafts is given in parentheses.

The establishment in 1985 of a multicenter trial of antiplatelet drugs in patients undergoing saphenous vein bypass and of prosthetic materials in femoropopliteal bypass, provided an independently monitored group of patients in whom blood risk factors associated with atherosclerosis or thrombosis could be studied. We were particularly concerned to try and resolve the dilemma about the effect that smoking may have on success of arterial reconstruction. It was therefore appropriate to investigate objective markers of smoking (carboxyhemoglobin t½ ≈ 5 hours, thiocyanate t½ ≈ 6 days) in addition to the other plasma risk factors, such as fibrinogen, that are influenced by smoking.[8]

THE FEMOROPOPLITEAL BYPASS TRIAL

Study design, patients, and methods

The study was coordinated from two centers in England, one in London and one in Birmingham, where the two trial coordinators were based. Patients entered into the trial were visited by the trial coordinator every 3 months during the first year following vascular reconstruction and every 6 months thereafter, and the patency of the graft was assessed at each visit. Patients were admitted into the trial where femoropopliteal reconstruction was performed either to relieve intermittent claudication or for critical ischemia. If the saphenous vein was considered suitable as a bypass conduit, patients were randomized to receive either antiplatelet therapy or placebo following arterial reconstruction. If the saphenous vein was either unavailable or unsuitable, a prosthetic graft was used, the patients being randomized either to human unbilical vein or to a polytetrafluoroethylene graft.

Blood samples taken both preoperatively and at 6 months following vascular reconstruction were available from 157 patients undergoing vein bypass, mean age 66.7 years, and 93 patients undergoing prosthetic bypass, mean age 67.5 years. Although 293 patients had entered the vein arm of the trial during this study, fasting blood samples were available on 157 patients only: the demographic details of those 157 patients showed them to be representative of the total patient group.[9] The blood samples were used for the measurement of two smoking markers, carboxyhemoglobin and thiocyanate, together with lipids, lipoproteins, apoproteins, and fibrinogen. Individual results were compared by nonparametric Mann-Whitney U tests. Life table analysis was used to calculate patency of the grafts. Multivariate discriminate function analysis was carried out on the total data sets. In the life table analysis the P values were obtained from the Lee-Desu statistic.

TABLE 2-1. CHARACTERISTICS OF PATIENTS UNDERGOING FEMOROPOPLITEAL BYPASS

	Vein graft (1 y)		Prosthetic graft (1, y)	
	Patent	*Occluded*	*Patent*	*Occluded*
n	113	44	70	23
Mean age (y)	67.0	65.5	67.8	66.6
Men (%)	79 (70)	33 (75)	49 (70)	15 (65)
Diabetes (%)	22 (19)	7 (16)	13 (19)	5 (22)
Claudication (%)	41 (36)	18 (41)	23 (33)	12 (52)
Rest pain or gangrene (%)	72 (64)	26 (59)	47 (67)	11 (48)

Smoking and plasma variables

The demographic data for the patients undergoing both vein and prosthetic bypass are presented in Table 2-1, including the indication for surgery and the incidence of diabetes. One hundred forty-four of the 157 patients undergoing vein bypass and 87 of the 93 patients undergoing prosthetic bypass had a smoking history of more than 20 years. On direct questioning, only 31 of 157 patients with vein bypass admitted to continuing smoking 6 months following their bypass surgery. Analysis of smoking markers, serum thiocyanate concentration greater than 70 µmol/L or blood carboxy-hemoglobin concentration greater than 2% or both, suggested that 71 of 157 patients (45%) continued to smoke after bypass grafting. For the patients with prosthetic grafts, 24 admitted to continuing smoking after bypass, although analysis of smoking markers indicated that 59 of the 93 patients (63%) continued to smoke 6 months following arterial reconstruction. Thus, about one-quarter of the patients appeared to be untruthful about their smoking habits. Median concentrations of both carboxyhe-moglobin and thiocyanate were significantly higher in patients with both vein and prosthetic grafts that had failed (Table 2-2). When the patients were divided into groups, one in which the serum thiocyanate concentration was less than 70 µmol/L and the other in which it was greater than 70 µmol/L, life table analysis clearly showed the significantly improved patency of both vein and prosthetic grafts at 1 year in the groups with the lower thiocyanate concentrations.

For vein grafts, 84% of the patients who were nonsmokers had patent grafts at 1 year compared with only 63% of the smokers, $P<0.02$ (Fig. 2-2). For prosthetic grafts,

TABLE 2-2. PLASMA RISK FACTORS AND FEMOROPOPLITEAL GRAFT PATENCY AT 1 YEAR[a]

	Vein graft		Prosthetic graft	
	Patent	*Occluded*	*Patent*	*Occluded*
n	113	44	70	23
Cholesterol (µmol/L)	6.04[b]	5.30	6.8	6.2
LDL cholesterol (µmol/L)	3.30	2.97	3.7	2.97[c]
Carboxyhemoglobin (%)	1.5	1.7[c]	1.2	2.4[c]
Thiocyanate (µmol/L)	56	83[c]	60	92[c]
Fibrinogen (g/L)	3.90	4.80[d]	3.92	4.98[c]
Apolipoprotein (a) (mg/L)	10.7	11.8[c]	nd[e]	nd[e]
Apolipoprotein A1 (g/L)	1.19[c]	1.23		

[a] The results are given as medians, footnote letters indicate the significance of the differences attributed to the most at-risk group.
[b] Significant difference $P < 0.005$
[c] Significant difference $P < 0.05$
[d] Significant difference $P < 0.001$
[e] Not determined

Figure 2-2 The patency of femoropopliteal vein bypass grafts. For smokers (•) the serum thiocyanate concentration is greater than 70 μmol/L, and for nonsmokers (■) the serum thiocyanate concentration is less than 70 μmol/L. The number of patients with patent grafts is given in parentheses. (*Reprinted with permission from: Wiseman S, Kenchington G, Dain R., et al. Influence of smoking and plasma factors on patency of femoropopliteal vein grafts. Br Med J. 1989; 299:643–646.*)

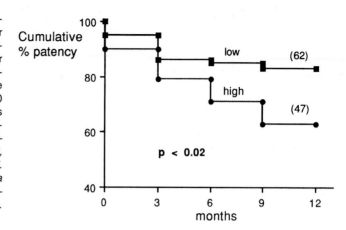

of the nonsmokers, 87% had a patent graft 12 months after bypass compared with only 68% of the smokers, $P<0.05$ (Fig. 2-3).

Median plasma fibrinogen concentration was also significantly higher in patients with occluded grafts than in those with patent grafts 1 year after bypass: these differences are again clearly shown by life table analysis. For patients with vein grafts, the patency at 1 year was 90% when the plasma fibrinogen concentration was below the median, compared with 57% in patients with higher fibrinogen concentrations, $P<0.0002$ (Fig. 2-4). For patients with prosthetic grafts, patency at 1 year was 90% when the plasma fibrinogen concentration was below the median, compared with only 63% in patients with higher concentrations, $P<0.025$ (data not shown).

Apart from smoking markers and fibrinogen, plasma cholesterol; triglycerides; high-density lipoproteins; low-density lipoproteins; very low-density lipoproteins; apolipoproteins A, BI, and (a); D-dimer; and the type I inhibitor of plasminogen activator were measured in these patients. For vein grafts, discriminant-function analysis selected the fibrinogen and the smoker marker thiocyanate as the two most powerful predictors of graft patency. Together these two variables correctly predicted outcome in 82% of grafts, 95 out of 113 patent grafts and 34 out of 44 occluded grafts.

Histologic examination of some of the occluded vein grafts showed no evidence of atherosclerosis within the graft. Smoking may have other structural effects on the maturing vein graft. An electron microscopic study showed that the saphenous veins of smokers and nonsmokers can be readily distinguished. One characteristic differ-

Figure 2-3 The patency of prosthetic femoropopliteal grafts. For smokers, (•) the serum thiocyanate concentration is greater than 70 μmol/L, and for nonsmokers (■) the serum thiocyanate concentration is less than 70 μmol/L. The number of patients with patent grafts is given in parentheses. (*Reprinted with permission from: Wiseman S, Powell JT, Greenhalgh RM, et al. The influence of smoking and plasma factors on prosthetic graft patency. Eur J Vasc Surg 1990; 4:57–61.*)

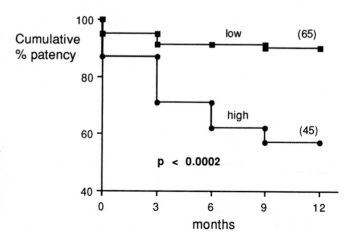

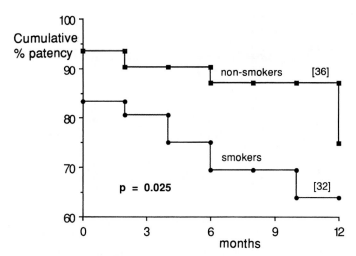

Figure 2-4 The relation of patency of vein grafts to plasma fibrinogen concentration. Patients with concentrations above the median are shown by the round symbols (•), and the patients with the concentrations below the median are shown with the square symbols (■). The number of patients with patent grafts is given in parentheses. (*Reprinted with permission from: Wiseman S, Kenchington G, Dain R, et al. Influence of smoking and plasma factors on patency of femoropopliteal vein grafts. Br Med J. 1989; 299:643–646.*)

ence is that in smokers the subendothelial basement membrane is markedly thickened (Fig. 2-5). The endothelium of the saphenous vein of a continuing smoker also may suffer greater damage during preparation for grafting than the saphenous vein of a nonsmoker.

INTERPRETING RESULTS AND IMPROVING GRAFT PATENCY

These studies have identified two important variables associated with the failure of arterial reconstruction: continuation of the smoking habit and increased levels of plasma fibrinogen. Smoking has been clearly identified as the most important risk factor for the development of peripheral arterial disease.[4] It is also possible that smoking is the most important risk factor associated with the accelerated progression of peripheral arterial disease. The structural changes observed in the saphenous veins of smokers may constitute an unrecognized risk factor for the development of stenosis, thrombosis, or intimal hyperplasia in vein grafts. One of the most useful pieces of advice that the vascular surgeon gives the patient is to stop smoking.[10] Stopping smoking is a cheap and effective form of therapy. Nicotine, however, is powerfully addictive, and many patients find it very difficult to stop smoking. When they are further advised that any vascular reconstruction will only be considered after they have stopped smoking, it must become hard for them not to deceive the clinician if they should continue to smoke. It is for these reasons that all previous studies have failed clearly to demonstrate the adverse effects of smoking on the outcome of vascular reconstruction. Even within the same femoropopiteal bypass, smoking habits, as obtained from direct questioning, had no influence on the graft patency rates.[1]

Carboxyhemoglobin and Thiocyanate Levels and Patency

We used two smoking markers: carboxyhemoglobin, which has a relatively short half-life of only a few hours, and thiocyanate, whose half-life is almost 1 week. It was this latter smoking marker with the longer half-life that showed the stronger effect on graft patency. Perhaps many of the patients refrained from smoking in the few hours before they were seen by the coordinator for their follow-up visit. Even a few hours of

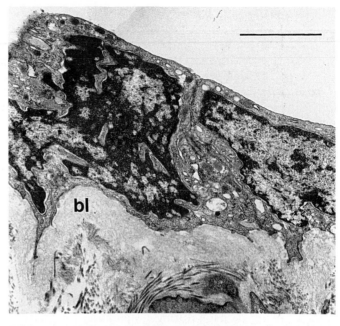

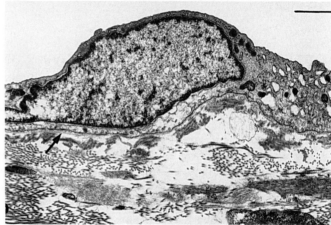

Figure 2-5 Transmission electron micrographs of saphenous vein. Electron micrographs to show the marked thickening of the endothelial basal lamina (bl) of a saphenous vein from a smoker (**A**), compared with normal basal lamina (arrow) in a nonsmoker (**B**) (bar in the upper right corner is equal to 2μm).

abstinence from smoking is sufficient to lower carboxyhemoglobin levels into the accepted nonsmoking range. Whereas we might admonish the 25% of patients who deceive the medical care team about their smoking habits, we should also congratulate the 50% of patients who have appeared to stop smoking. The ability of vascular surgeons to dissuade their patients from smoking is clearly far superior to that of medical specialities, who only persuade 10 to 20% of their patients to quit smoking.[11,12]

All those patients presenting with peripheral arterial disease, claudication, rest pain, or critical ischemia are told very firmly that they must stop smoking. In those patients in whom arterial reconstruction procedures are subsequently performed, only 39% continued to smoke 1 year following reconstruction.[13] This result is in marked contrast with those in whom claudication is not sufficiently severe to consider immediate reconstruction or other intervention, where over 60% of the patients continued to smoke 1 year after the initial presentation. Either the enforced period in

3

Restenosis:

Pathogenesis and Management

Nobuya Zempo, MD, and Alexander W. Clowes, MD

Blood flow in diseased arteries supplying ischemic organs is readily improved by angioplasty, endarterectomy, or bypass grafting. Unfortunately these reconstructions often develop thrombosis. Early postoperative thrombosis is usually related to an error in surgical technique, and later thrombosis occurs because of progression of disease in the inflow and outflow vessels. In the period 1 month to 1 year, luminal narrowing is often the result of intimal hyperplasia and is a significant cause of thrombosis, particularly in reconstructions with low blood flow.[1,2] For example, the incidence of hemodynamically significant restenosis after carotid endarterectomy is between 13 and 25%.[3,4] The patency rate of femoropopliteal percutaneous transluminal angioplasty declines from 73 to 66% during the first 6 to 12 months.[5] Femoropopliteal vein bypass grafts have approximately 60 to 70% 5-year patency,[6,7] and prosthetic bypass grafts show a lower patency rate.[8]

The pathogenesis and management of restenosis as a result of intimal hyperplasia have not been well defined. In this chapter, we will review recent information on the development of restenosis after arterial injury, intimal hyperplasia after vascular grafting, recent molecular mechanisms for regulation of intimal hyperplasia, and experimental and clinical pharmacologic control of restenosis.

DEVELOPMENT OF RESTENOSIS AFTER ARTERIAL INJURY

On gross examination, stenosing intimal lesions are white, firm, and fibrous and are not associated with thrombus. They can accumulate thrombus later on and resemble primary atherosclerotic plaque.[9] All types of vascular reconstruction cause injury to the operated on blood vessels and induce a healing response leading to wall thickening.[10]

In an experimental animal model of arterial injury (balloon-injured rat carotid artery), the endothelium is completely denuded and a part of the media is damaged. The first wave of smooth muscle cell proliferation in the media starts between 24 and 27 hours after arterial injury. Smooth muscle cells begin to migrate from the media to the intima at 4 days and continue to proliferate in the intima.[11,12] In the re-endothelialized region, intimal thickening reaches a maximum at 4 weeks and does not change thereafter. The smooth muscle cell proliferation in this region returns to baseline by 8 weeks. In the de-endothelialized region, intimal thickening progressively increases with time and is maximal between 4 and 12 weeks. Although the smooth muscle cells in the region lacking endothelium continue to proliferate at a slow rate even at 12 weeks, total arterial smooth muscle cell numbers are the same at 2 and at 12 weeks.[13] The intima is further thickened by the accumulation of extracellular matrix synthesized by the smooth muscle cells. At 12 weeks, the intima is approximately 80% matrix and 20% cells. The lumen is narrowed not only by the intimal thickening but also by vessel contraction.[14]

Endothelial proliferation, like smooth muscle cell proliferation, begins immediately after injury. The regrowth of endothelium progresses from either end of the denuded vessel but stops after 6 weeks. Total outgrowth along the vessel is approximately 10 mm. The endothelial layer fails to cover the central third of the artery.[13,15] Modified smooth muscle cells form a luminal surface in the de-endothelialized region. Although this surface is not thrombogenic, the cells lack morphologic characteristics and a permeability barrier to large molecules of normal endothelium.[16]

INTIMAL HYPERPLASIA IN VEIN GRAFTS

Autogenous vein grafts have the advantage of an antithrombogenic luminal surface made of endothelium and are therefore not as susceptible to thrombosis as synthetic grafts. However, vein grafts may develop intimal hyperplasia within 2 years of surgery and atherosclerosis thereafter. Intimal hyperplasia in the vein grafts occurs as long regions of narrowing or as focal stenoses at anastomoses, valve cusps, and sites of clamp injury.[6,7,17,18]

In rabbit vein grafts, many of the endothelial cells are lost, and the subendothelium is exposed to platelets and leukocytes within 1 hour after implantation. Endothelial cells gradually reappear and fully cover over the subendothelium by 2 weeks. They continue to proliferate up to 12 weeks. Smooth muscle cells start proliferating during the first week and form an intimal thickening. Smooth muscle cell mass does not increase after 4 weeks, and the accumulation of extracellular matrix accounts for the subsequent increase in wall thickness. Graft wall thickness reachs a maximum at 12 weeks.[19]

The vein graft adapts to the arterial circulation by becoming thicker, and the calculated wall stress decreases to a level equal to that of a normal artery. This result is consistent with the hypothesis that an increase in wall stress stimulates smooth muscle cell proliferation, matrix deposition, or both, resulting in increased wall mass.[19] Reduction of wall mass and wall stress by narrowing and the addition of an external support decrease vein graft intimal hyperplasia.[20]

Atherosclerosis commonly develops in vein grafts and appears to progress more rapidly than in native arteries. A study of patients over a 10-year period following aortocoronary bypass at the Montreal Heart Institute demonstrated a significant correlation between elevated plasma low-density lipoprotein, and apoprotein B levels and graft atherosclerosis.[21] Cholesterol feeding of rabbits causes increased vein graft intimal thickness because of an accumulation of lipid-laden macrophages, but does not produce an increase in endothelial and smooth muscle cell hyperplasia.[22]

SYNTHETIC GRAFT HEALING AND INTIMAL HYPERPLASIA

Synthetic grafts function well in high-flow situations. They are, nevertheless, prone to thrombosis since they do not develop an endothelial surface except in regions adjacent to anastomoses. The thrombotic tendency is made worse by the formation of flow-reducing neointimal lesions. Although these lesions can form throughout vein grafts, they are confined to the perianastomotic zone in synthetic grafts.[1]

The healing process has been modeled in a number of different animals. Our studies have used nonhuman primates. In standard polytetrafluorethylene (PTFE) grafts (30 μm internodal distance) implanted in the aortoiliac circulation of baboons, neointimal thickening occurrs at the anastomoses and comprises both endothelium and smooth muscle cells. Both endothelial cells and smooth muscle cells are derived from the cut ends of adjacent artery. They migrate along the luminal surface of the graft approximately 1 cm by 1 month and 2.5 cm by 3 months, and by 12 months after surgery 60% of grafts (7 to 9 cm in length) are fully covered.[23,24] Endothelial cells proliferate in association with the growing edge. Smooth muscle cells proliferate in the underlying intima at the growing edge and at anastomoses despite complete endothelial coverage, but not in advance of the endothelial growing edge. Intimal cross-sectional area is greatest at anastomoses and at later stages is due to an accumulation of cells and extracellular matrix. Total smooth muscle cells mass does not increase after 3 months.

More porous PTFE grafts (60 μm internodal distance) exhibit a different pattern of healing. They are fully covered within 2 weeks. The endothelial layer develops from multiple transmural capillaries arising from the granulation tissue surrounding the graft. Despite complete endothelial coverage of the graft, endothelial cells continue to proliferate. Intimal thickening due to smooth muscle cell proliferation develops after endothelialization. Smooth muscle cells in the intima appear to be derived from pericytes accompanying the microvascular endothelium through the wall. Intimal thickening is uniformly distributed throughout the graft and not confined to the anastomosis as the case in 30-μm PTFE grafts.[25]

More than three decades ago, Wesolowski and associates[26] concluded that porous synthetic grafts were incorporated better into the surrounding tissue than impervious grafts. We have suggested that for PTFE grafts the 60-μm internodal distance may be an optimal porosity since 10- and 30-μm grafts fail to achieve luminal endothelial coverage, and 90-μm grafts exhibit instability of the intima with focal endothelial cell loss.[27] However, high-porosity Dacron grafts (porosity 2,000 mL H_2O/cm^2 at 100 mm Hg) implanted in men failed to complete an endothelial lining. This failure might be attributable in part to the graft material itself.[28] Dacron might inhibit endothelialization perhaps by inducing macrophages to secrete substances that inhibit endothelial growth.[29] Alternatively, when compared with other animals, men may simply have a diminished capacity to mount an angiogenic response.

Synthetic grafts implanted in men showed that the intima, even at later stages after surgery, was mainly composed of fibrin and platelets since an endothelial coverage did not occur completely throughout the grafts. This finding was also supported by a platelet study using indium 111 as a label, in which the uptake of Indium 111 was still observed as late as 9 years after graft implantation.[30] Recently, we measured the uptake of indium 111-labeled platelets in the composite 30-μm and 60-μm PTFE grafts implanted into the above-knee femoropopliteal position in men. However, this study did not show a difference between the two graft segments.[31] These results support the conclusion that endothelial coverage of synthetic grafts in men is limited.

The development of intimal thickening may be regulated by a number of factors. In injured arteries proteins from platelets and damaged smooth muscle cells may be important (see Molecular Mechanisms for the Regulation of Intimal Hyperplasia). However, in our PTFE graft model smooth muscle cells proliferate in the absence of thrombus and where endothelium is present. In this situation, growth factors released from regenerating endothelium may stimulate neointimal hyperplasia. Endothelial cells over the grafts do not stop proliferating even though they have reached a confluent state. Chronic endothelial proliferation implies chronic endothelial injury and possibly the release of intracellular mitogens.[32] Since the smooth muscle cell proliferation in healing grafts is found only underneath the endothelium,[23–25] we propose that injured endothelial cells may be regulating smooth muscle cell growth by releasing intracellular mitogens.

The compliance mismatch at vascular anastomoses has been generally implicated in graft failure due to anastomotic neointimal hyperplasia.[33] However, compliance mismatch alone is probably not sufficient for the development of intimal hyperplasia, and other potential causes need to be examined.[34]

Another mechanical force that may affect neointimal hyperplasia in vascular grafts is shear stress. In normal arteries, shear stress is tightly regulated by changes in vascular diameter. Since synthetic vascular grafts are relatively rigid, luminal diameter can only be adjusted by a change in neointimal thickness. To explore the hypothesis that shear regulates neointimal mass, we implanted bilateral aortoiliac 60-µm PTFE grafts 4 mm in diameter distal to an aortoaortic 4-mm 60-µm PTFE graft. The proximal graft supplied two distal iliac grafts and thus carried twice as much blood flow and had twice the average shear stress, although the stress was still within the physiologic range. Proximal grafts showed significantly less neointimal hyperplasia than the distal grafts.[35] These findings were confirmed in another study in which blood flow was increased by means of a distal arteriovenous fistula.[36] From these two studies, we have concluded that the absolute value of the shear stress rather than the magnitude of its oscillation over time is the important determinant of neointimal growth. We also suggest that the mature neointima remains sensitive to change in flow at some time considerably after surgery.

MOLECULAR MECHANISMS FOR THE REGULATION OF INTIMAL HYPERPLASIA

The original "reaction to injury hypothesis" of Ross and Glomset[37] proposed that smooth muscle cell proliferation and intimal thickening after arterial injury is regulated by the release of growth factors from platelets adherent to de-endothelialized artery. This hypothesis was based on the following two observations. First, platelet granules contain potent mitogens for cultured smooth muscle cells.[38] Second, intimal thickening after arterial injury is inhibited in rabbits made thrombocytopenic by treatment with antiplatelet antibody.[39] We have re-examined the effect of thrombocytopenia on smooth muscle cell proliferation and subsequent intimal thickening in the balloon-injured rat carotid artery. We concluded that platelets do not play a role in the initial wave of smooth muscle cell proliferation in the media but do regulate migration from the media to the intima.[40] Recently, we reported that the infusion of platelet-derived growth factor BB (PDGF-BB), the predominant PDGF isoform in rat platelets, stimulates smooth muscle cell migration but has little effect on proliferation.[41] Furthermore, Ferns and colleagues[42] demonstrated that the administration of an antibody to PDGF produces a 40% reduction in intimal thickening. Since smooth muscle cell proliferation was not changed by antibody treatment, they concluded that endogenous PDGF induces intimal thickening principally by stimulating smooth muscle cell migration. These experiments support the conclusion that in injured rat carotid artery PDGF is mainly a migratory factor (Fig. 3–1).

Although platelets are an obvious source of PDGF, vascular wall cells also synthesize and secrete PDGF. Majesky and colleagues[43] documented that within 6

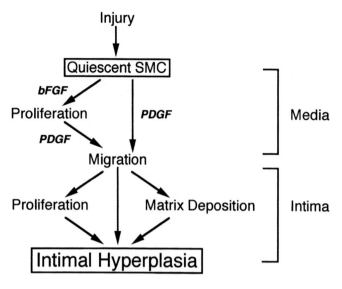

Injury

Quiescent SMC

bFGF

Proliferation   PDGF   Media

PDGF

Migration

Proliferation   Matrix Deposition   Intima

Intimal Hyperplasia

Figure 3–1. Diagram illustrates how arterial injury might cause intimal hyperplasia by stimulating smooth muscle cell (SMC) proliferation and migration. Basic fibroblast growth factor (bFGF) released from injured cells stimulates medial smooth muscle cell proliferation. Platelet-derived growth factor (PDGF) from platelets regulates smooth muscle cell migration from the media to the intima.

hours after balloon injury, rat carotid arteries exhibit a transient increase in gene expression of PDGF A-chain and a rapid loss of PDGF receptor-β mRNA. Platelet-derived growth factor receptor-β mRNA increases later on. A lesser form of injury with a loop of nylon monofilament suture also induces an increase in the mRNA for PDGF A-chain and decreases the PDGF receptor-β mRNA by 6 hours.[44] A comparison of the two methods of experimental arterial injury shows that balloon catheter denudation induces a substantial proliferative rate of smooth muscle cells in the media at 48 hours (13.6% thymidine-labeling index), whereas denudation with the loop of nylon suture has little effect (1.4%). Thus, despite significantly different proliferation rates, the two methods of arterial injury induce similar changes in mRNA. These results suggest that endogenous PDGF synthesis does not play an important role in injury-induced smooth muscle cell proliferation.[44]

Balloon denudation damages medial smooth muscle cells, but nylon loop denudation does not, and smooth muscle cell replication appears to correlate with medial damage rather than endothelial loss or adherence of platelets. Therefore, damaged smooth muscle cells themselves might release endogenous mitogens that could stimulate subsequent proliferation.

A possible candidate for this endogenous mitogen is basic fibroblast growth factor. Basic fibroblast growth factor (bFGF) is synthesized by both endothelial cells and smooth muscle cells *in vitro* and when released is stored in the subendothelial matrix. Recently, bFGF has been shown to be a potent mitogen for smooth muscle cells *in vivo*, and the infusion of bFGF can increase smooth muscle cell proliferation not only in the media 2 days after injury but also in the intima thereafter.[45] Furthermore, the injection of an antibody against bFGF prior to arterial injury reduces smooth muscle cells proliferation by 80%[46] (see Fig. 3–1).

The mRNA for other growth factors, such as transforming growth factor beta (TGF-β)[47] and insulin-like growth factor,[48] are expressed by medial smooth muscle cells in balloon-injured arteries. The role of these factors has not been defined.

The endogenous factors responsible for stimulating endothelial regeneration are not known. Basic fibroblast growth factor is a mitogen for endothelial cells in culture, and when infused intravenously, it accelerates endothelial migration and proliferation. Endothelial cells can express the message for bFGF.[49,50] TGF-β is known to inhibit endothelial cell growth *in vitro*,[51] its effect on endothelial regeneration *in vivo* is not known.

In the healing of vascular grafts, smooth muscle cells proliferate underneath the endothelial layer but not in areas lacking endothelium.[23–25] Thus, platelets probably do not play an important role in intimal thickening in grafts. We have suggested that the vascular wall cells themselves are the source of growth-promoting activity.[52] Porous PTFE grafts implanted in baboon aortoiliac circulation, when perfused *ex vivo*, released more mitogenic activity than normal arteries. Approximately 50% of the mitogenic activity in graft perfusates was inhibited by a polyclonal anti-PDGF antibody.[53] The graft intima expressed a large amount of PDGF A-chain mRNA but a very low level of PDGF B-chain mRNA and exhibited variable levels of mRNA expression for TGF-β. *In situ* hybridization studies indicate that endothelial cells and adjacent intimal smooth muscle cells contain PDGF A-chain mRNA and few endothelial cells, but no smooth muscle cells contain PDGF B-chain mRNA.[54] These results support the hypothesis that intimal PDGF A-chain mRNA may regulate intimal smooth muscle cell proliferation in vascular grafts.

PHARMACOLOGIC CONTROL OF INTIMAL HYPERPLASIA

At present stenosis of vascular reconstructions cannot be prevented. Once formed, the lesion needs to be treated surgically if thrombosis is to be avoided. The challenge for the next decade is to develop pharmacologic strategies to prevent intimal hyperplastic lesions. Progress in this endeavor is summarized in this section.

Antiplatelet Drugs

Many vascular reconstructions fail because of intimal hyperplasia, luminal stenosis, low flow, or thrombosis. Antithrombotic drugs have been used not only to prevent the final thrombotic event but also to inhibit intimal hyperplasia since there may be a link between early platelet accumulation and subsequent smooth muscle migration and proliferation.[10] Antiplatelet drugs, such as aspirin and dipyridamole, appear to reduce platelet consumption after placement of Dacron grafts and reduce to some extent intimal thickening in vein and PTFE grafts in nonhuman primates.[55] However, antiplatelet drugs do not inhibit intimal thickening in the injury-induced intima.[56] They also may retard endothelial healing.[57]

The lack of a response to antiplatelet drugs may have several explanations. First, most antiplatelet drugs inhibit platelet aggregation but have little or no effect on platelet adherence. Second, in injured arteries platelets do not play a role in the initial wave of smooth muscle cell proliferation but do regulate migration.[40,41] Third, in healing PTFE and vein grafts, smooth muscle cells proliferate only underneath the endothelium where platelets do not adhere and aggregate.[23–25]

A number of clinical trials evaluating the effect of antiplatelet drugs on arterial graft failure have been reported.[55] Antiplatelet treatments improve aortocoronary vein graft patency only if they are started preoperatively or within 2 days of surgery.[58] Antiplatelet therapy has little or no effect on femoropopliteal vein bypass patency.[59,60] Prosthetic grafts benefit more from the antiplatelet therapy than do vein grafts.[61] These results support the conclusion that antiplatelet drugs reduce early graft thrombosis but do not prevent late stenosis resulting from intimal thickening.[55]

Heparin

Heparin inhibits intimal hyperplasia by suppressing smooth muscle cell proliferation and migration.[62–67.] The inhibitory activity of heparin is dependent on the amount of heparin administered but is independent of its anticoagulant activity since heparin fragments that do not bind antithrombin III have the same effect as commercial heparin.[67] Castellot and colleagues[68] have demonstrated that low-molecular-weight fractions of heparin possess inhibitory activity for smooth muscle cells *in vitro*. Heparin inhibits smooth muscle cell proliferation most effectively if the administration is started within 18 hours after arterial injury and if it is continued for the period of maximal proliferation.[65] Heparin given for a period of 1 week is as effective as heparin given for 4 weeks.[64] Heparin alters the composition of the extracellular matrix by decreasing elastin and interstitial collagen and increasing proteoglycans, particularly heparan sulfate.[69]

Heparin-like molecules synthesized by endothelial cells and smooth muscle cells inhibit smooth muscle cell growth *in vitro*.[70,71] Heparan sulfate must be liberated from the native proteoglycan by heparanase before it can show inhibitory activity. Hence, heparin and the related heparan sulfates may have a physiologic as well as pharmacologic role in the regulation of smooth muscle cell growth *in vivo*. Smooth muscle cell proliferation might be stimulated by factors such as bFGF and inhibited by endogenous heparan sulfate in the vascular wall.

How heparin inhibits smooth muscle cell proliferation and migration has not been clearly defined. One possibility is that heparin binds bFGF released from the injured smooth muscle cells or endothelial cells and prevents local increase of bFGF in the extracellular matrix.[72,73] Heparin could simply displace bFGF from the matrix into the circulation and inhibit the initial wave of smooth muscle cell proliferation. Other alternatives are that heparin may produce its antiproliferative activity by altering the smooth muscle cell response to epidermal growth factor,[74] or that heparin stimulates TGF-β activity, a potent inhibitor of smooth muscle cell growth, by releasing it from a carrier protein.[75] Heparin might also suppress the expression of c-*fos* and c-*myc* proto-oncogenes in stimulated smooth muscle cells.[76]

Yet another possibility is that heparin interferes with the ability of the smooth muscle cells to degrade the extracellular matrix. Recently, we have shown that smooth muscle cells express a number of proteases. For example, they express urokinase-type plasminogen activator during mitogenesis and tissue-type plasminogen activator (tPA) during migration *in vivo*.[77] Plasminogen, when converted to plasmin by plasminogen activator, degrades a broad range of matrix molecules. Smooth muscle cells also express collagenase and stromelysin. Collagenase specifically degrades connective tissue collagens. Stromelysin specifically degrades extracellular matrix proteoglycans, laminin, fibronectin, and gelatins. Activated stromelysin can activate collagenase. Heparin inhibits the expression of tPA. It also inhibits the expression of interstitial collagenase and stromelysin and displaces urokinase-type plasminogen activator from the cell layer into the medium *in vitro*. Regulation of heparin on tPA and collagenase is at the level of transcription[78] (Fig. 3–2).

Clinical studies using heparin are now in progress.[79] Heparin administered only during the first day after coronary angioplasty fails to prevent restenosis.[80]

Angiotensin-Converting Enzyme Inhibitor

The angiotensin-converting enzyme (ACE) inhibitor, cilazapril, blocks intimal thickening in balloon-injured rat carotid arteries, and the specific angiotensin II receptor antagonist, Dup 753, has the same effect.[10,81] Angiotensin-converting enzyme inhibitor interferes with the conversion of angiotensin I to angiotensin II. Angiotensin II may modulate smooth muscle cell proliferation and matrix protein synthesis.[82] Recently, we have reported that a 1-week treatment of heparin in combination with continu-

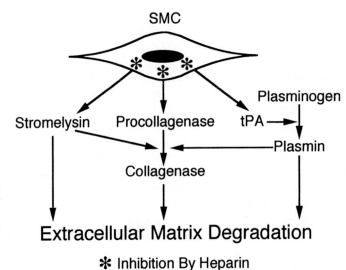

Figure 3–2. Diagram illustrates how heparin might inhibit smooth muscle cell (SMC) function. Smooth muscle cells express tissue-type plasminogen activator (tPA), collagenase, and stromelysin; and plasmin and stromelysin can activate collagenase. Heparin inhibits the expression of tPA, collagenase, and stromelysin.

ously administered cilazapril produces a substantial inhibition of intimal thickening.[83] Clinical trials are in progress to test whether ACE inhibitors can prevent restenosis after coronary angioplasty.[84]

Fish Oil

Fish oil, rich in eicosapentaenoic acid and docosahexaenoic acid, inhibits intimal thickening in animal models.[85,86] Fish oil produces diverse biologic effects, including alterations in lipoprotein levels, inhibition of platelet aggregation, and changes in eicosanoid metabolism. Fish oil appears to inhibit the release of mitogens from platelets, macrophages, and endothelial cells *in vitro*.[87,88] However, clinical studies of fish oil report inconsistent effects on restenosis in patients undergoing coronary angioplasty.[89,90]

Calcium Channel Blockers

Calcium channel blockers appear to inhibit intimal thickening by suppressing the initial wave of smooth muscle cell proliferation. They also inhibit smooth muscle cell migration *in vitro*.[91] On the other hand, they have little effect on preventing restenosis after coronary angioplasty in humans.[92,93]

Cyclosporin A

Cyclosporin A has been reported to decrease smooth muscle cell proliferation and intimal thickening in balloon-injured rat carotid arteries.[94] However, in another study cyclosporin A appeared to have no effect on the inhibition of smooth muscle cell proliferation. Cyclosporin A treatment was associated with increased intimal thickening because of increased number of foaming macrophages.[95]

Steroids

Corticosteroids are effective in suppressing intimal thickening in animal models.[96,97] Steroids may produce this effect by preventing leukocyte adhesion and aggregation both *in vitro* and *in vivo*.[98] Another possibility is that steroids directly inhibit smooth muscle cell proliferation.[99] However, one clinical trial did not find an effect of the drug on restenosis after coronary angioplasty.[100]

Gene Therapy

Gene therapy has been proposed as an innovative approach for controlling restenosis after vascular reconstructions. This technique could be used to introduce inhibitory genes into vascular wall cells in culture and these cells could then be seeded into the vessel. Gene transfer into vascular wall cells *in vivo* might also be accomplished by direct retroviral injection or liposome-mediated DNA transfection.[101–103] For example, endothelial cells genetically modified with human tPA have been seeded onto stents and the stents introduced into sheep arteries. The transfected cells have been shown to express substantial amounts of plasminogen activator.[103] Another potential target for gene therapy is smooth muscle cells. Although endothelial cells exist only as a monolayer, smooth muscle cells can form multiple layers, which may be important where relatively large numbers of genetically modified cells are necessary for gene therapy. Recently we have documented that gene transfer by infection of smooth muscle cells in culture and seeding of the transfected cell onto denuded arteries leads to long-term expression of human adenosine deaminase gene for at least 6 months.[104] Genetically modified smooth muscle cells may be useful for local pharmacologic control of intimal hyperplasia in the near future.

REFERENCES

1. Clowes AW. Pathologic intimal hyperplasia as a response to vascular injury and reconstruction. In: Rutherford RB., ed. *Vascular Surgery.* Philadelphia PA. W B Saunders Co.; 1989:266–275.
2. Bandyk DF, Kaebnick HW, Stewart GW, et al. Durability of the in situ saphenous vein arterial bypass: a comparison of primary and secondary patency. *J. Vasc Surg.* 1987;5:256–268.
3. Healy DA, Zierler RE, Nicholls SC, et al. Long-term follow-up and clinical outcome of carotid restenosis. *J Vasc Surg.* 1989;10:662–669.
4. Cook JM, Thompson BW, Barnes RW. Is routine duplex examination after carotid endarterectomy justified? *J Vasc Surg.* 1990;12:334–340.
5. Adar R, Critchfield GC, Eddy DM. A confidence profile analysis of the results of femoropopliteal percutaneous transluminal angioplasty in the treatment of lower-extremity ischemia. *J Vasc Surg.* 1989;10:57–67.
6. Whittemore AD, Clowes AW, Couch NP, et al. Secondary femoropopliteal reconstruction. *Ann Surg* 1981;193:35–42.
7. Wengerter KR, Veith FJ, Gupta SK, et al. Prospective randomized multicenter comparison of in situ and reversed vein infrapopliteal bypasses. *J Vasc Surg.* 1991;13:189–199.
8. Veith FJ, Gupta SK, Ascer E, et al. Six-year prospective multicenter randomized comparison of autologous saphenous vein and expanded polytetrafluoroethylene grafts in infrainguinal arterial reconstructions. *J Vasc Surg.* 1986;3:104–114.
9. Clagett GP, Robinowitz M, Youkey JR, et al. Morphogenesis and clinicopathologic characteristics of recurrent carotid disease. *J Vasc Surg.* 1986;3:10–23.
10. Clowes AW, Reidy MA. Prevention of stenosis after vascular reconstruction: pharmacological control of intimal hyperplasia—a review. *J Vasc Surg.* 1991;13:885–891.
11. Clowes AW, Reidy MA, Clowes MM. Kinetics of cellular proliferation after arterial injury. I. Smooth muscle growth in the absence of endothelium. *Lab Invest.* 1983;49:327–333.
12. Clowes AW, Schwartz SM. Significance of quiescent smooth muscle migration in the injured rat carotid artery. *Circ Res.* 1985;56:139–145.

13. Clowes AW, Clowes MM, Reidy MA. Kinetics of cellular proliferation after arterial injury. III. Endothelial and smooth muscle growth in chronically denuded vessels. *Lab Invest.* 1986;54:295–303.

14. Clowes AW, Reidy MA, Clowes MM. Mechanisms of stenosis after arterial injury. *Lab Invest.* 1983;49:208–215.

15. Reidy MA, Clowes AW, Schwartz SM. Endothelial regeneration. V. Inhibition of endothelial regrowth in arteries of rat and rabbit. *Lab Invest.* 1983;49:569–575.

16. Clowes AW, Collazzo RE, Karnovsky MJ. A morphologic and permeability study of luminal smooth muscle cells after arterial injury in the rat. *Lab Invest.* 1978;39:141–150.

17. Szilagyi DE, Elliott JP, Hageman JH, et al. Biologic fate of autogenous vein implants as arterial substitutes. *Ann Surg.* 1973;178:232–245.

18. Donaldson MC, Mannick JA, Whittemore AD. Causes of primary graft failure after in situ saphenous vein bypass grafting. *J Vasc Surg.* 1992;15:113–120.

19. Zwolak RM, Adams MC, Clowes AW. Kinetics of vein graft hyperplasia: association with tangential stress. *J Vasc Surg.* 1987;5:126–136.

20. Kohler TR, Kirkman TR, Clowes AW. The effect of rigid external support on vein graft adaptation to the arterial circulation. *J Vasc Surg.* 1989;9:277–285.

21. Campeau L, Enjalbert M, Lesperance J, et al. The relation of risk factors to the development of atherosclerosis in saphenous-vein bypass grafts and the progression of disease in the native circulation. *N Engl J Med.* 1984;311:1329–1332.

22. Zwolak RM, Kirkman TR, Clowes AW. Atherosclerosis in rabbit vein grafts. *Arteriosclerosis.* 1989;9:374–379.

23. Clowes AW, Gown AM, Hanson SR, et al. Mechanisms of arterial graft failure. I. Role of cellular proliferation in early healing of PTFE prostheses. *Am J Pathol.* 1985;118:43–54.

24. Clowes AW, Kirkman TR, Clowes MM. Mechanisms of arterial graft failure. II. Chronic endothelial and smooth muscle cell proliferation in healing polytetrafluoroethylene prostheses. *J Vasc Surg.* 1986;3:877–884.

25. Clowes AW, Kirkman TR, Reidy MA. Mechanisms of arterial graft healing. Rapid transmural capillary ingrowth provides a source of intimal endothelium and smooth muscle in porous PTFE prostheses. *Am J Pathol.* 1986;123:220–230.

26. Wesolowski SA, Fries CC, Karlson KE, et al. Porosity: primary determinant of ultimate fate of synthetic vascular grafts. *Surgery.* 1961;50:91–96.

27. Golden MA, Hanson SR, Kirkman TR, et al. Healing of polytetrafluoroethylene arterial grafts is influenced by graft porosity. *J Vasc Surg.* 1990;11:838–845.

28. Zacharias RK, Kirman TR, Clowes AW. Mechanisms of healing in synthetic grafts. *J Vasc Surg.* 1987;6:429–436.

29. Greisler HP, Lam TM, Henderson S, et al. Vascular graft healing—kinetics of cell proliferation. *FASEB J.* 1990;4:1149. Abstract

30. McCollum CN, Kester RC, Rajah SM, et al. Arterial graft maturation: the duration of thrombotic activity in Dacron aortobifemoral grafts measured by platelet and fibrinogen kinetics. *Br J Surg.* 1981;68:61–64.

31. Clowes AW, Kohler T. Graft endothelialization: the role of angiogenic mechanisms. *J Vasc Surg.* 1991;13:734–736.

32. Reidy MA, Chao SS, Kirkman TR, et al. Endothelial regeneration. VI. Chronic nondenuding injury in baboon vascular grafts. *Am J Pathol.* 1986;123:432–439.

33. Abbott WM, Megerman J, Hasson JE, et al. Effect of compliance mismatch on vascular graft patency. *J Vasc Surg.* 1987;5:376–382.

34. Okuhn SP, Connelly DP, Calakos N, et al. Does compliance mismatch alone cause neointimal hyperplasia? *J Vasc Surg.* 1989;9:35–45.

35. Kraiss LW, Kirkman TR, Kohler TR, et al. Shear stress regulates smooth muscle proliferation and neointimal thickening in porous polytetrafluoroethylene grafts. *Arterioscler Thromb.* 1991;11:1844–1852.

36. Kohler TR, Kirkman TR, Kraiss LW, et al. Increased blood flow inhibits neointimal hyperplasia in endothelialized vascular grafts. *Circ Res.* 1991;69:1557–1565.

37. Ross R, Glomset JA. The pathogenesis of atherosclerosis. *N Engl J Med.* 1976;295:369–377, 420–425.

38. Ross R, Glomset J, Kariya B, et al. A platelet-dependent serum factor that stimulates the proliferation of arterial smooth muscle cells in vitro. *Proc Natl Acad Sci USA.* 1974;71:1207–1210.

39. Friedman RJ, Stemerman MB, Wenz B, et al. The effect of thrombocytopenia on experimental atherosclerotic lesion formation in rabbits. Smooth muscle cell proliferation and re-endothelialization. *J Clin Invest.* 1977;60:1191–1201.

40. Fingerle J, Johnson R, Clowes AW, et al. Role of platelets in smooth muscle cell proliferation and migration after vascular injury in rat carotid artery. *Proc Natl Acad Sci USA.* 1989;86:8412–8416.

41. Jawien A, Bowen-Pope DF, Lindner V, et al. Platelet-derived growth factor promotes smooth muscle migration and intimal thickening in a rat model of balloon angioplasty. *J Clin Invest.* 1992;89:507–511.

42. Ferns GAA, Raines EW, Sprugel KH, et al. Inhibition of neointimal smooth muscle accumulation after angioplasty by an antibody to PDGF. *Science.* 1991;253:1129–1132.

43. Majesky MW, Reidy MA, Bowen-Pope DF, et al. PDGF ligand and receptor gene expression during repair of arterial injury. *J Cell Biol.* 1990;111:2149–2158.

44. Fingerle J, Au YPT, Clowes AW, et al. Intimal lesion formation in rat carotid arteries after endothelial denudation in the absence of medial injury. *Arteriosclerosis.* 1990;10:1082–1087.

45. Lindner V, Lappi DA, Baird A, et al. Role of basic fibroblast growth factor in vascular lesion formation. *Circ Res.* 1991;68:106–113.

46. Lindner V, Reidy MA. Proliferation of smooth muscle cells after vascular injury is inhibited by an antibody against basic fibroblast growth factor. *Proc Natl Acad Sci USA.* 1991;88:3739–3743.

47. Majesky MW, Lindner V, Twardzik DR, et al. Production of transforming growth factor β_1 during repair of arterial injury. *J Clin Invest.* 1991;88:904–910.

48. Cercek B, Fishbein MC, Forrester JS, et al. Induction of insulin-like growth factor I messenger RNA in rat aorta after balloon denudation. *Circ Res.* 1990;66:1755–1760.

49. Lindner V, Reidy MA, Fingerle J. Regrowth of arterial endothelium. Denudation with minimal trauma leads to complete endothelial cell regrowth. *Lab Invest.* 1989;61:556–563.

50. Lindner V, Majack RA, Reidy MA. Basic fibroblast growth factor stimulates endothelial regrowth and proliferation in denuded arteries. *J Clin Invest.* 1990;85:2004–2008.

51. Heimark RL, Twardzik DR, Schwartz SM. Inhibition of endothelial regeneration by type-beta transforming growth factor from platelets. *Science.* 1986;233:1078–1080.

52. Zacharias RK, Kirkman TR, Kenagy RD, et al. Growth factor production by polytetrafluoroethylene vascular grafts. *J Vasc Surg.* 1988;7:606–610.

53. Golden MA, Au YPT, Kirkman TR, et al. Platelet-derived growth factor activity and mRNA expression in healing vascular grafts in baboons. Association in vivo of platelet-derived growth factor mRNA and protein with cellular proliferation. *J Clin Invest.* 1991;87:406–414.

54. Golden MA, Au YPT, Kenagy RD, et al. Growth factor gene expression by intimal cells in healing polytetrafluoroethylene grafts. *J Vasc Surg.* 1990;11:580–585.

55. Clowes AW. The role of aspirin in enhancing arterial graft patency. *J Vasc Surg.* 1986;3:381–385.

56. Clowes AW, Karnovsky MJ. Failure of certain antiplatelet drugs to affect myointimal thickening following arterial injury. *Lab Invest.* 1977;36:452–458.

57. Bomberger RA, DePalma RG, Ambrose TA, et al. Aspirin and dipyridamole inhibit endothelial healing. *Arch Surg.* 1982;117:1459–1464.

58. Fuster V, Chesebro JH. Role of platelets and platelet inhibitors in aortocoronary artery vein-graft disease. *Circulation.* 1986;73:227–232.

59. Kohler TR, Kaufman JL, Kacoyanis G, et al. Effect of aspirin and dipyridamole on the patency of lower extremity bypass grafts. *Surgery.* 1984;96:462–466.

60. McCollum C, Alexander C, Dip N, et al. Antiplatelet drugs in femoropopliteal vein bypasses: a multicenter trial. *J Vasc Surg.* 1991;13:150–162.

61. Clyne CAC, Archer TJ, Atuhaire LK, et al. Random control trial of a short course of aspirin and dipyridamole (Persantin) for femorodistal grafts. *Br J Surg.* 1987;74:246–248.

62. Clowes AW, Karnovsky MJ. Suppression by heparin of smooth muscle cell proliferation in injured arteries. *Nature.* 1977;265:625–626.

63. Clowes AW, Clowes MM. Kinetics of cellular proliferation after arterial injury. II. Inhibition of smooth muscle growth by heparin. *Lab Invest.* 1985;52:611–616.

64. Clowes AW, Clowes MM. Kinetics of cellular proliferation after arterial injury. IV. Heparin inhibits rat smooth muscle mitogenesis and migration. *Circ Res.* 1986;58:839–845.

65. Majesky MW, Schwartz SM, Clowes MM, et al. Heparin regulates smooth muscle S phase entry in the injured rat carotid artery. *Circ Res.* 1987;61:296–300.

66. Majack RA, Clowes AW. Inhibition of vascular smooth muscle cell migration by heparin-like glycosaminoglycans. *J Cell Physiol.* 1984;118:253–256.

67. Guyton JR, Rosenberg RD, Clowes AW, et al. Inhibition of rat arterial smooth muscle cell proliferation by heparin. I. In vivo studies with anticoagulant and non-anticoagulant heparin. *Circ Res.* 1980;46:625–634.

68. Castellot JJ Jr, Choay J, Lormeau JC, et al. Structural determinants of the capacity of heparin to inhibit the proliferation of vascular smooth muscle cells. II. Evidence for a pentasaccharide sequence that contains a 3-*O*-sulfate group. *J Cell Biol.* 1986;102:1979–1984.

69. Snow AD, Bolender RP, Wight TN, et al. Heparin modulates the composition of the extracellular matrix domain surrounding arterial smooth muscle cells. *Am J Pathol.* 1990;137:313–330.

70. Castellot JJ Jr, Addonizio ML, Rosenberg R, et al. Cultured endothelial cells produce a heparin-like inhibitor of smooth muscle growth. *J Cell Biol.* 1981;90:372–379.

71. Fritze LMS, Reilly CF, Rosenberg RD. An antiproliferative heparan sulfate species produced by postconfluent smooth muscle cells. *J Cell Biol.* 1985;100:1041–1049.

72. Saksela O, Moscatelli D, Somner A, et al. Endothelial cell-derived heparan sulfate binds basic fibroblast growth factor and protects it from proteolytic degradation. *J Cell Biol.* 1988;107:743–751.

73. Flaumenhaft R, Moscatelli D, Rifkin DB. Heparin and heparan sulfate increase the radius of diffusion and action of basic fibroblast growth factor. *J Cell Biol.* 1990;111:1651–1659.

74. Reilly CF, Fritze LMS, Rosenberg RD. Antiproliferative effects of heparin on vascular smooth muscle cells are reversed by epidermal growth factor. *J Cell Physiol.* 1987;131:149–157.

75. McCaffrey TA, Falcone DJ, Brayton CF, et al. Transforming growth factor beta activity is potentiated by heparin via dissociation of the transforming growth factor-beta/alpha 2-macroglobulin inactive complex. *J Cell Biol.* 1989;109:441–448.

76. Pukac LA, Castellot JJ Jr, Wright TC, et al. Heparin inhibits c-*fos* and c-*myc* mRNA expression in vascular smooth muscle cells. *Cell Reg.* 1990;1:435–443.

77. Clowes AW, Clowes MM, Au YPT, et al. Smooth muscle cells express urokinase during mitogenesis and tissue-type plasminogen activator during migration in injured rat carotid artery. *Circ Res.* 1990;67:61–67.

78. Au YPT, Kenagy RD, Clowes AW. Heparin selectively inhibits the transcription of tissue-type plasminogen activator in primate arterial smooth muscle cells during mitogenesis. *J Biol Chem.* 1992;267:3438–3444.

79. Muller DWM, Ellis SG, Topol EJ. Experimental models of coronary artery restenosis. *J Am Coll Cardiol.* 1992;19:418–432.

80. Ellis SG, Roubin GS, Wilentz J, et al. Effect of 18- to 24-hour heparin administration for prevention of restenosis after uncomplicated coronary angioplasty. *Am Heart J.* 1989;117:777–782.

81. Powell JS, Clozel JP, Muller RKM, et al. Inhibitors of angiotensin-converting enzyme prevent myointimal proliferation after vascular injury. *Science.* 1989;245:186–188.

82. Daemen MJAP, Lombardi DM, Bosman FT, et al. Angiotensin II induces smooth muscle cell proliferation in the normal and injured rat arterial wall. *Circ Res.* 1991;68:450–456.

83. Clowes AW, Clowes MM, Vergel SC, et al. Heparin and cilazapril together inhibit injury-induced intimal hyperplasia. *Hypertension.* 1991;18 (suppl): II65–II69.
84. Popma JJ, Califf RM, Topol EJ. Clinical trials of restenosis after coronary angioplasty. *Circulation.* 1991;84:1426–1436.
85. Landymore RW, Kinley CE, Cooper JH, et al. Cod-liver oil in the prevention of intimal hyperplasia in autogenous vein grafts used for arterial bypass. *J Thorac Cardiovasc Surg.* 1985;89:351–357.
86. Sarris GE, Fann JI, Sokoloff MH, et al. Mechanisms responsible for inhibition of vein-graft arteriosclerosis by fish oil. *Circulation.* 1989;80(suppl):I109–I123.
87. Smith DL, Willis AL, Nguyen N, et al. Eskimo plasma constituents, dihomo-γ-linolenic acid, eicosapentaenoic acid and docosahexaenoic acid inhibit the release of atherogenic mitogens. *Lipids.* 1989;24:70–75.
88. Fox PL, DiCorleto PE. Fish oils inhibit endothelial cell production of platelet-derived growth factor-like protein. *Science.* 1988;241:453–456.
89. Grigg LE, Kay TWH, Valentine PA, et al. Determinants of restenosis and lack of effect of dietary supplementation with eicosapentaenoic acid on the incidence of coronary artery restenosis after angioplasty. *J Am Coll Cardiol.* 1989;13:665–672.
90. Dehmer GJ, Popma JJ, van den Berg EK, et al. Reduction in the rate of early restenosis after coronary angioplasty by a diet supplemented with *n*-3 fatty acids. *N Engl J Med.* 1988;319:733–740.
91. Jackson CL, Bush RC, Bowyer DE. Mechanism of antiatherogenic action of calcium antagonists. *Atherosclerosis.* 1989;80:17–26.
92. Whitworth HB, Roubin GS, Hollman J, et al. Effect of nifedipine on recurrent stenosis after percutaneous transluminal coronary angioplasty. *J Am Coll Cardiol.* 1986;8:1271–1276.
93. Corcos T, David PR, Val PG, et al. Failure of diltiazem to prevent restenosis after percutaneous transluminal coronary angioplasty. *Am Heart J.* 1985;109:926–931.
94. Jonasson L, Holm J, Hansson GK. Cyclosporin A inhibits smooth muscle proliferation in the vascular response to injury. *Proc Natl Acad Sci USA.* 1988;85:2303–2306.
95. Ferns G, Reidy M, Ross R. Vascular effects of cyclosporine A in vivo and in vitro. *Am J Pathol.* 1990;137:403–413.
96. Makheja AN, Bloom S, Muesing R, et al. Anti-inflammatory drugs in experimental atherosclerosis. 7. Spontaneous atherosclerosis in WHHL rabbits and inhibition by cortisone acetate. *Arteriosclerosis.* 1989;7:155–161.
97. Colburn MD, Moore WS, Gelabert HA, et al. Dose responsive suppression of myointimal hyperplasia by dexamethasone. *J Vasc Surg.* 1992;15:510–518.
98. Prescott MF, McBride CK, Venturini CM, et al. Leukocyte stimulation of intimal lesion formation is inhibited by treatment with diclofenac sodium and dexamethasone. *J Cardiovasc Pharmacol.* 1989;14(suppl.6):S76–S81.
99. Longenecker JP, Kilty LA, Johnson LK. Glucocorticoid inhibition of vascular smooth muscle cell proliferation: influence of homologous extracellular matrix and serum mitogens. *J Cell Biol.* 1984;98:534–540.
100. Pepine CJ, Hirshfeld JW, Macdonald RG, et al. A controlled trial of corticosteroids to prevent restenosis after coronary angioplasty. *Circulation.* 1990;81:1753–1761.
101. Nabel EG, Plautz G, Nabel GJ. Site specific gene expression in vivo by direct gene transfer into the arterial wall. *Science.* 1990;249:1285–1288.
102. Wilson JM, Birinyi LK, Salomon RN, et al. Implantation of vascular grafts lined with genetically modified endothelial cells. *Science.* 1989;244:1344–1346.
103. Dichek D, Neville RF, Zwiebel JA, et al. Seeding of intravascular stents with genetically engineered endothelial cells. *Circ Res.* 1989;80:1347–1353.
104. Lynch CM, Clowes MM, Osborne WRA, et al. Long-term expression of human adenosine deaminase in vascular smooth muscle cells of rats: a model for gene therapy. *Proc Natl Acad Sci USA.* 1992;89:1138–1142.

4

Surveillance Program for Vascular Reconstructive Procedures

David S. Sumner, MD, Mark A. Mattos, MD, and Kim J. Hodgson, MD

Despite gains made in surgical technology over the past several decades, a number of vascular reconstructions continue to fail. Although some failures can be ascribed to lapses in technique and are preventable, others are the result of biologic factors currently beyond the control of the surgeon. Whatever the cause, failure can have devastating consequences. The result may be limb loss in patients operated on for peripheral ischemia, or the outcome may be stroke in patients who have undergone a carotid endarterectomy. Secondary interventions are often ineffective. It seems logical, therefore, to institute surveillance programs designed to detect restenoses or other causes of impending failure and to correct the defects before failure occurs.

In the past, routine surveillance of vascular reconstructions was hampered by the lack of sensitive methods for detecting stenoses in the formative stage. Arteriography, although adequately sensitive and specific, is invasive, inherently risky, and too expensive to be employed on a routine basis. Noninvasive physiologic tests are safe and inexpensive but are insensitive to the presence of low-grade stenoses, seldom identify the site of the problem, and often become positive only after the reconstruction occludes or the patient becomes symptomatic. With the development of duplex scanning, routine surveillance became practical. By combining the imaging capabilities of B-mode ultrasonography and the ability of Doppler ultrasonography to measure flow velocity, duplex scanning not only permits the examiner to identify and locate stenoses but also provides information concerning the severity of the stenotic process. Adding a color-flow map greatly facilitates the scanning process, reducing the time and effort required for a thorough examination.

As experience with these sophisticated instruments accumulates, new questions have arisen. Which lesions should be repaired? What criteria should be used to determine the reconstructions that are likely to thrombose or the patients that are in danger of suffering a stroke? Is it safe to follow some stenoses? Do revisions prolong graft patency or avoid the development of symptoms? How frequently should patients be examined? And finally, is routine surveillance cost-effective? The jury is still out on most of these questions. Definitive answers await the results of further clinical research.

This chapter discusses and compares various methods for surveying peripheral vascular reconstructions and carotid endarterectomies. In so far as possible, the questions posed above are addressed.

SURVEILLANCE OF PERIPHERAL ARTERIAL BYPASS GRAFTS

Although some aortoiliac and aortofemoral reconstructions fail, long-term patency rates are quite good and secondary operations are usually successful. On the other hand, thrombosis of infrainguinal grafts, especially those terminating in the tibial or pedal arteries, may be a catastrophic event. Occlusion of a bypass graft in this area returns the limb to its previous state of circulatory compromise; or, if disease progression or thrombosis has occurred in the native inflow or outflow arteries, perfusion will be further impaired.[1-3] Occasionally, when collaterals have developed during the process of failure, the circulation will be better than it was prior to operation; but it is never as good as it was while the graft functioned. Because the majority of infrainguinal bypasses are performed for critical ischemia, the limb with a failed graft again suffers from rest pain or develops tissue loss, both of which may require amputation if a secondary procedure cannot be performed. The results of thrombectomy or thrombolysis with or without subsequent graft revision are dismal. Sladen and Gilmour noted that 6 of 13 thrombosed grafts reoccluded within 1 month of thrombectomy and revision, and by 1 year 10 had failed.[4] Five-year cumulative patency rates following revision of occluded grafts range from 5% to 32%.[5-8] When graft patency cannot be restored, an entirely new graft may be required; but the potential for successful regrafting is often limited by the lack of a suitable autogenous vein—especially when revascularization has been performed multiple times, both legs have been operated on, and the supply of greater and lesser saphenous veins and arm veins has been exhausted. Although secondary bypasses with autogenous veins have a reasonable (60–70%) 5-year patency rate, the results with prosthetic materials are generally disappointing (18%–37%).[3,9-11] Furthermore, with each graft failure, the surgeon may be forced to move progressively down the leg in the quest for a suitable recipient artery.

For these reasons, every effort should be made to prevent graft failure. These efforts begin in the operating room, where it behooves the surgeon to ensure the technical adequacy of the procedure. This is the time to detect suture line stenoses, residual disease in inflow or outflow arteries, narrowed segments or twists in the venous conduit, retained valves, or large arteriovenous fistulas. Pharmacologic measures, such as low-dose heparin, aspirin or other antiplatelet agents, and long-term anticoagulation with warfarin, may decrease the risk of developing fibromuscular dysplasia or thrombosis in patients in a hypercoagulable state. Attention to these details reduces the incidence of failure occurring within the first postoperative month.

Early failures, those developing from 1 month to 1 year, are usually due to strictures developing at the site of valves, retained valves, or stenoses at the anastomotic sites. Failures occurring after 1 year (late failure) are often attributable to progression of atherosclerosis in the inflow or outflow arteries and sometimes within the vein graft itself. If these lesions can be detected and repaired prior to graft failure, the long-term cumulative patency of the graft will be far superior to the secondary patency achieved by revising thrombosed grafts and will approach that of grafts that have never developed lesions or undergone repair.[7,12,13] Moreover, many of these early lesions (especially those in *in-situ* grafts) are readily assessable and easily repaired. These considerations constitute the rationale for routine surveillance.

History and Physical Examination

Return of symptoms in a patient who has been rendered asymptomatic by the bypass graft is, of course, an important warning sign.[14] Progression of disease in the inflow or outflow arteries remote from the graft itself may be responsible for the return of symptoms.[15] Unfortunately, symptoms often appear only after the graft has failed.[2,16] About two-thirds of patients with localized graft-threatening lesions remain asymptomatic, since these lesions typically do not seriously impair blood flow.[2,17–21] Bandyk and colleagues noted that 51 (91%) of 56 patients with stenotic grafts were asymptomatic.[22]

Similarly, the loss of or diminution of palpable pedal pulses that were present after reconstruction implies the development of a lesion somewhere in the vascular supply to the distal limb. Pulse palpation, however, is highly subjective, especially when different observers are involved. Moreover, a patient in whom the distal anastomosis was made to a "blind" popliteal segment or to the peroneal artery may never have palpable pedal pulses despite a successful reconstruction. Because a graft may continue to exhibit strong pulses even in the face of a severe distal stenosis, graft pulses are unreliable.[8,17]

Bruits auscultated along the graft are strongly suggestive of an intrinsic stenosis but may also be heard distal to an anastomosis between the native artery and graft when the diameters are widely disparate.[4] A bruit emanating from the graft disappears when the graft is compressed. Bruits are very helpful for identifying and locating an arteriovenous fistula developing following an *in situ* bypass graft.

Noninvasive Hemodynamic Tests

The first methods employed to detect impending graft failure were the simple noninvasive tests familiar to those working in the vascular laboratory.[17,23,24] These tests become positive only when a lesion becomes hemodynamically significant, which usually implies a diameter stenosis of greater than 50% somewhere along the vascular circuit, either in the graft itself or in the inflow or outflow arteries. Lesions of lesser degree, some of which may eventuate in graft thrombosis, escape detection. An additional drawback of these tests is their limited ability to localize the offending lesion. The results of these tests reflect the hemodynamic proficiency of the graft and thus are very valuable in assessing the functional results of the revascularization procedure.[15,23]

Ankle–Brachial Indices

Measurement of systolic blood pressure at the ankle has long been a recognized part of the vascular evaluation. The ankle–brachial index (ABI) (calculated by dividing the ankle pressure obtained from Doppler assessment of flow in the dorsalis pedis or posterior tibial arteries by the higher of the two brachial systolic pressures) correlates well with the functional status of the limb. Early work by Strandness showed that patency of a bypass graft determined by pulse palpation or the lack of recurring symptoms did not necessarily reflect the functional status of the limb.[25] When the circulation was stressed, the physiologic limitations of the graft became more apparent. Ankle pressures in asymptomatic patients were found to decrease markedly after treadmill exercise. It was but a small step to apply this method to a graft surveillance protocol.

There are several problems that decrease the reliability of the ABI when used for surveillance purposes. First, the ABI has been shown to vary considerably from time to time and from one observer to the next in the same patient, even under optimum laboratory conditions and in the absence of disease progression. The 95% confidence limits of this variation have been established at ±0.15.[26] For this reason, most investigators require a drop of 0.15 or more in the ABI before a change is considered significant, and some require a drop of 0.20.[27] Clearly, insisting on a change of this magnitude allows many early lesions to escape detection even though they are on the borderline of hemodynamic significance. Second, pressures usually drop precipitously rather than gradually, both because of hemodynamic principles and because the final event is often sudden thrombosis. A significant drop in ankle pressure occurring in the interval between the last measurement and graft thrombosis would be missed.[2] Third, the ankle pressure may not be reliable in patients with calcified arteries—a common problem in diabetics. Fourth, measurement of ankle pressures in limbs with bypasses to the ankle or pedal arteries is not reliable, since the pneumatic cuff is placed above the distal anastomosis and completely compresses the graft when it is inflated.[21,28] Because there is no blood flow in the graft, the pressure measured at the ankle reflects that in the inflow artery and not that existing in the graft when blood is flowing. Even if a significant stenosis were present, it would not be detected. The situation, therefore, is analogous to the measurement of stump pressures during operations on the carotid bifurcation. Although toe pressures can be substituted for ankle pressure, they are even more variable and may be decreased by pedal or digital artery disease.[29] Fifth, a decreased ankle pressure may reflect disease progression in inflow or outflow arteries remote from the graft.[15] Although such lesions are by definition hemodynamically significant, they do not necessarily portend immediate graft failure.

Although a number of investigators have found the ABI to be valuable for detecting lesions that threaten graft survival,[7,17,24] others report less favorable results.[22,30–34] Barnes and colleagues, in a retrospective study of 232 infrainguinal bypass grafts, found that a significant drop in ABI (>0.20) did not correlate with cumulative 5-year graft patency.[27] The primary patency in limbs with stable ABIs was 60%, which was almost identical to the 62% patency rate in limbs with interval drops in ABI. Our results are similar. We followed 38 grafts with stenoses demonstrated by color duplex scans and found that the ABI dropped by 0.20, or more in 20% of limbs, within 2 months of graft occlusion.[13] A similar drop, however, occurred in 25% of limbs whose graft remained patent (Table 4–1). The mean ABI in 103 legs with negative graft scans (0.94 ± 0.17) was only slightly higher than that in 59 limbs with positive scans (0.91 ± 0.22). Although the mean preocclusive ABI of 62 limbs with failed grafts (0.80 ± 0.20) was significantly less ($P = 0.002$) than the lowest ABI measured in 162 grafts that remained patent (0.95 ± 0.18), an abnormal ABI (<0.92 in our laboratory) had a positive predictive value of only 22%. Results from other investigators are listed in Table 4–1.

A progressive decline in the ABI or persistently decreased ABIs are unfavorable prognostic signs. In the series by Blackshear and colleagues, 9 of 20 grafts with decreasing ABIs eventually occluded.[2] Green and associates reported 68 patients with infrainguinal grafts in whom the ABI decreased by more than 10% during the follow-up period.[20] Although thrombosis occurred in none of 42 patients with transient ABI drops, grafts occluded in 11 of 26 patients with persistent drops, and another 8 required graft revision because of symptoms. Thus, ankle pressure measurements, although not highly sensitive or specific for impending graft failure, have the virtue of simplicity and, if properly interpreted, can be a valuable adjunct to other noninvasive modalities. A decrease in the ABI is always a matter of concern and should prompt further investigation.[21] No surveillance protocol is complete without measurement of ankle blood pressures.

TABLE 4–1. PREDICTIVE VALUE OF ANKLE-BRACHIAL INDICES FOR IDENTIFYING THE FAILING INFRAINGUINAL BYPASS GRAFT

Author	ABI Criterion	Sensitivity (%)	Specificity (%)	Positive Predictive Value (%)	Negative Predictive Value (%)	Endpoint
Green et al 1990[20]	↓ >10%	66	80	12	98	About to occlude within next follow-up interval
Zwolak et al 1991[47]	↓ >0.15	37	89	34	90	Thrombosis or stenosis requiring revision
Laborde et al 1991[39]	↓ >0.15	60	50	—	—	Preocclusive lesion
Wyatt et al 1991[35]	<0.80	29	100	100	48	Graft at risk for thrombosis
Stierli et al 1992[21]	↓ >0.10	100	73	—	—	Significant stenosis
Mattos et al 1992[13]	<0.92	67	52	32	82	Thrombosis of stenotic grafts
	↓ >0.20	20	75	22	72	Thrombosis of stenotic grafts

Plethysmography

A few authors have used the *pulse volume recorder,* which is an air plethysmograph, for following grafts.[8] The cuff is placed around the calf or ankle, and a 5-mm drop in pulse volume is considered positive. This method has the advantage of not being affected by the presence of arterial calcification, which renders ankle pressures meaningless. Measurements, however, are even more variable with this instrument than with Doppler-derived ankle pressures. Berkowitz and associates found that the pulse volume recorder was positive in 79% of stenotic grafts, but there is little information in the literature to substantiate its value as a method for surveillance.[8]

Impedance Analysis

By the process of Fourier analysis, pressure and flow velocity waveforms can be broken down into a series of sine waves, or harmonics, each with a modulus defining the maximum excursion of the wave on either side of the mean value and a phase angle defining the shift of the harmonic wave in relation to the beginning of the pulse cycle. Impedance is the ratio of the pressure and flow moduli at each harmonic. Wyatt and associates have devised an ingenious method of computer-assisted analysis that calculates an *impedance score* from pulse volume recorder tracing obtained at the thigh and calf and Doppler waveforms recorded from the upper and lower ends of the bypass graft.[35] In a prospective study of infrainguinal bypass grafts, impedance scores greater than 0.45 detected 33 (97%) of 34 diameter stenoses greater than 50%. Unlike duplex scanning, impedance analysis detects runoff stenoses as well as those in the graft itself. A disadvantage to this method is its inability to localize the stenosis. The eventual role of impedance analysis in graft surveillance remains to be determined.

Duplex Scanning

Because duplex scanning provides both anatomic and hemodynamic information, it has become the preferred method of graft surveillance. The entire graft, the proximal and distal anastomoses, and the adjacent inflow and outflow arteries are routinely examined (Figs. 4–1 to 4–3). (In our experience and in that of others, proximal

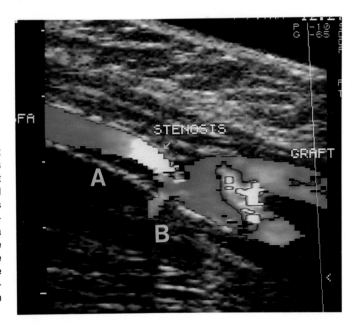

Figure 4–1. Color-flow duplex scan of the proximal anastomosis of an *in situ* saphenous vein graft originating from the superficial femoral artery. The arterial wall is clearly defined on the B-mode image. A 40% stenosis caused by a plaque on the posterior wall of the native artery is indicated by the color change from red to white and by the width of the color image (A). A small branch is seen emerging from the artery (B).

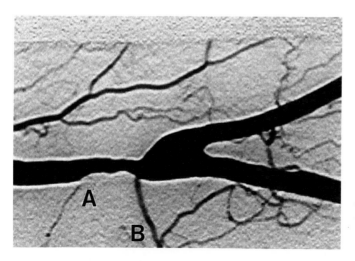

Figure 4–2. Arteriogram of the same area shown in Figure 4–1, showing a close correlation between the color duplex scan and the contrast study. The posterior plaque (A) and the arterial branch (B) are clearly evident.

anastomoses are always seen and distal anastomoses are visualized in about 90% of the limbs.[36] Ordinarily, studies begin with the inflow artery and then progress down the leg terminating in the native artery below the distal anastomosis. Cross-sectional views may be obtained to help locate the graft and arteries, but, for the most part, scanning is done with the probe oriented along the long axis of the graft. Higher frequency probes are used for examining the more superficial conduits, such as *in situ* grafts or vessels at the level of the foot or ankle, and lower frequency probes are used to visualize deeper structures. The examination of the graft and all vessels except the popliteal artery is performed with the patient supine and with the leg externally rotated at the hip. Although it may be necessary to have the patient assume a prone position for optimum visualization of the popliteal artery, we find that turning the patient to the side usually provides adequate access to this difficult area.

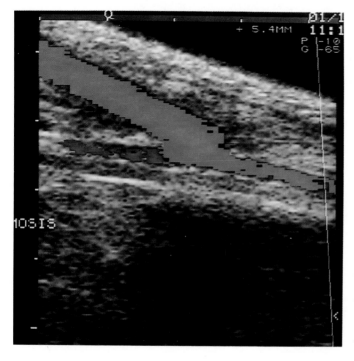

Figure 4–3. Color duplex scan of a distal anastomosis of an *in situ* vein graft to a tibial artery. The native vessel shows both antero-grade (red) and retrograde (blue) flow.

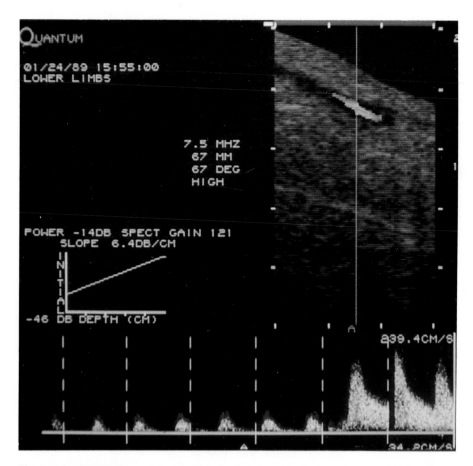

Figure 4–4. Doppler frequency spectrum showing low-velocity flow above and high-velocity flow within a stenosis. There is marked spectral broadening. (*Reproduced with permission from Londrey GL, Hodgson KJ, Spadone DP, et al. Initial experience with color-flow duplex scanning of infrainguinal bypass grafts.* J Vasc Surg. *1990;12:284–290.*)

Blood flow velocity is measured in the inflow and outflow arteries, at the proximal and distal end of the graft, and at any point along the graft where the image suggests narrowing or velocities appear elevated. The B-mode image is used to ensure that the pulsed-Doppler sample volume is placed in the center of the flow stream. Comparisons are made between the velocity at the site of a presumed stenosis and that in the adjacent [apparently] normal vessel several centimeters above or below (Fig. 4–4). Although it is possible to estimate total blood flow from velocity measurements and the cross-sectional diameter of the vessel or by using built-in features of the duplex instrument, blood flow has proved to be too variable and the measurements too inconsistent to be of value in graft surveillance.[37]

The diameter of the graft or host arteries can be measured at selected sites from the B-mode image. Atherosclerotic plaques may also be visualized.

Owing to the length of many infrainguinal bypass grafts, a complete examination may be a time-consuming and tedious exercise.[19] It may be especially difficult to study grafts and anastomotic sites that are located deep in the leg.

Color-Flow Duplex Scanning

These instruments combine a color-coded Doppler flow map and a conventional B-mode image. A red color is assigned to flow in the normal antegrade direction down the leg to identify predominately arterial flow and a blue color to flow up the leg, corresponding to the usual direction of venous flow. Color saturation is proportional to the velocity of flow, deeper colors corresponding to slow velocities and lighter colors, approaching white, to higher velocities. Some instruments employ other colors to label specific velocities, such as a *green tag* that can be set to appear when velocities exceed a defined limit (Fig. 4–5). A black image (absence of color) is indicative of no flow or of velocity vectors at right angles to the direction of the sound beam.

Color greatly simplifies the imaging process, making it easy to locate the graft and to follow it longitudinally.[30,38,39] This method immediately identifies underlying vessels and discriminates between arteries and veins. It is particularly useful for locating grafts that are placed deep in the leg in the "anatomic" position within the subsartorial (Hunter's) canal and for identifying deeply situated anastomoses, such as those to the above-knee popliteal and peroneal artery. A shift in color from red to white identifies stenotic areas where the vascular diameter is decreased and flow velocities are increased (Fig. 4–5).[19,30] The appearance of blue pixels may correspond to aliasing (associated with very high velocities exceeding the Nyquist limit) or to a localized area of reversed flow, both suggesting a disturbed or turbulent flow pattern. Color clearly defines the interface between the flow stream and the graft wall (Fig.

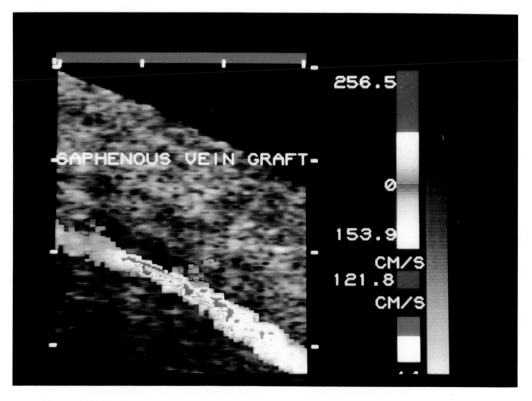

Figure 4–5. Stenosis in a saphenous vein graft indicated by a shift in color from red to white. A green tag indicates velocities over 120 cm/s. Aliasing produces a few light blue pixels within the stenosis.

4–1).[19] The width of the apparent flow stream can be estimated from the color image, though the image tends to exaggerate the diameter of stenotic areas due to the size of the color pixels.

By identifying sites of apparent narrowing, color guides the placement of the pulsed-Doppler sample volume for measurement of stenotic flow velocities. Likewise, it ensures that relatively normal segments of graft are examined to obtain comparative velocities. Color also facilitates the identification of aneurysms, seromas, hematomas, and arteriovenous fistulas (Fig. 4–6).

With the assistance of color, the entire leg can be examined in about 20 minutes—or about the time required for a carotid study.[38,40] The only real difficulties we have encountered are in imaging an occasional peroneal and above-knee popliteal anastomosis.[30] Both are deeply located and, in the latter case, the graft may intersect the artery at a 90-degree angle, making it hard to see both structures simultaneously.

Interpretation and Accuracy

Various criteria for interpreting duplex scan results have been advocated. These involve characteristics of the frequency spectrum, velocity measurements, and the appearance of the B-mode image and the color-flow map.

Low-Velocity Criterion. In 1985, Bandyk and associates proposed a "low-velocity" criterion based on measurement of peak systolic velocity in the segment of graft with the smallest diameter, where velocities should be highest.[41] This point is usually at the distal end of *in situ* bypass grafts. Their investigations indicated that peak systolic velocities less than 45 cm/s or a drop of more than 30 cm/s compared with postoperative velocities identified grafts at risk of failure due to intrinsic lesions or progression of atherosclerosis in the inflow or outflow arteries.[28,41] In one of a series of studies conducted by this group, velocities less than 45 cm/s were found in 54 (96%) of 56 femoropopliteal or femorotibial grafts with stenotic lesions.[22] Although

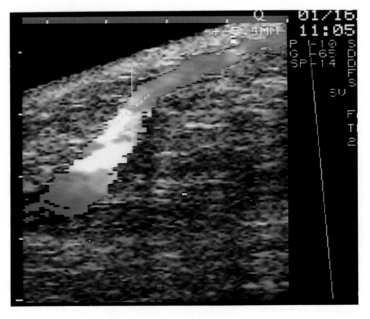

Figure 4–6. Small subcutaneous arteriovenous fistula emerging from an *in situ* vein graft. The white color is due in part to the acute angle that the flow makes with the ultrasonic beam.

included) have found the color-flow map to be the most sensitive indicator of the presence of stenosis (Fig. 4–5).[13,30,44] Not only do changes in color saturation and hue alert the examiner to the presence of a flow disturbance, but also the width of the flow stream has some diagnostic value (Fig. 4–1). In the study by Buth and associates, measurement of graft diameter based on color and B-mode images proved to be the best method for detecting low-grade stenoses.[44] Diameter stenoses of 30% were identified with a sensitivity of 88% and excluded with a specificity of 99%. Positive and negative predictive values were 97% and 93%, respectively. The color image, however, does not discriminate reliably between various degrees of stenosis.

Arteriovenous Fistulas.   Arteriovenous fistulas are easily detected and accurately located with color duplex scanning (Fig. 4–6).[30] They are reliably differentiated from stenoses by visualizing high-velocity flow in a persistent vein branch rather than in the graft itself. A *visual bruit,* consisting of colored pixels produced by vibrations in the adjacent tissues, is often observed. Velocities in the graft above a fistula exceed those measured below. Chang and colleagues found that the average flow in the proximal end of a series of *in situ* vein grafts studied 5 to 9 days after surgery was 345 ± 37 mL/min, whereas that in the distal end was only 83 ± 8 mL/min.[46] Thus, the flow through persistent fistulas was estimated to be 257 ± 31 mL/min. By 4 to 6 months, fistula flow decreased to 143 ± 54 mL/min; and by 12 to 18 months, it was only 48 ± 11 mL/min.

Combined Criteria.   Most laboratories using duplex or color-flow imaging employ several criteria in evaluating the results of surveillance studies.[20,22,38,40,44,46,47] When there are discrepancies, the final assessment depends on weighing the relative accuracy of the criteria. In our laboratory, we emphasize the velocity ratio and the appearance of the color image and downplay the significance of low-velocity recordings.[13,30] One method is to call the study positive when either the velocity ratio exceeds 2.0 or 3.0 or the peak systolic velocity elsewhere in the graft is less than 45

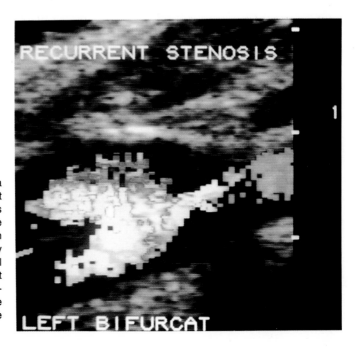

Figure 4–8. Color-flow scan of a high-grade stenosis recurring at the carotid bifurcation 5 years after endarterectomy. A large echolucent plaque is present in the distal common carotid artery and at the origins of the internal and external carotid arteries. At surgery, a hemorrhagic atherosclerotic plague was found. The blue pixels represent aliasing due to the high-velocity jet.

TABLE 4–5. ACCURACY OF COMBINED PEAK SYSTOLIC VELOCITY <45 CM/S AND VELOCITY RATIO FOR PREDICTING GRAFT STENOSIS

Author	Velocity Ratio	Sensitivity (%)	Specificity (%)	Positive Predictive Value (%)	Negative Predictive Value (%)	Endpoint
Sladen et al 1989[38]	≥3.0	98	87	80	99	"High-risk grafts"
Taylor et al 1992[40]	≥2.0	100	99	96	100	>50% Stenosis

cm/s and to call the study negative if both the velocity ratio and the peak systolic velocity are within normal limits. Two reports have shown that this approach increases the overall sensitivity of the study without decreasing the specificity significantly (Table 4–5).[38,40]

Clinical Observations

Routine surveillance of infrainguinal bypass grafts discloses a remarkably high incidence of hemodynamically significant stenoses (>50% diameter reduction), ranging from 10% to 34% in several recent studies (Table 4–6).[13,33,38,40,44,48,49] Most of these develop soon after surgery. In our study, 61% of the lesions in autogenous vein grafts were detected within the first 6 months, 77% within 12 months, and 90% within 18 months.[13] Similar distributions have been reported by other investigators, all of whom note that the majority of graft stenoses become evident in the first year.[4,48,50] Stenoses occurring after 1 year are more likely to be due to progression of arteriosclerosis and occur with increasing frequency in the inflow and outflow arteries.[51] About 50% to 60% of the lesions are detected in the graft itself.[12,13,38,44,48,50] Retained valve leaflets, valve site stenoses, diffuse intimal thickening, fibrotic stenosis, arteriosclerosis, graft entrapment, and torsion are among the multiple causes that have been identified.[12,52] Strictures due to myointimal hyperplasia, atherosclerosis, or suture stenoses account for about 30% of the lesions detected.[12,13,44] The remainder of the stenoses involve the inflow and outflow arteries; and, as mentioned above, are usually due to arteriosclerosis. Residual arteriovenous fistulas may be detected in 22% to 37% of *in situ* vein grafts.[19,30,38] The incidence depends on the surgical technique employed and the care with which they are sought during operation. Fistulas seldom jeopardize the survival of the graft or interfere with its function. Flow through fistulas decreases with time and most small fistulas resolve spontaneously.[30,46,53]

TABLE 4–6. INCIDENCE OF STENOSIS IN INFRAINGUINAL BYPASS GRAFTS

Author	Grafts at Risk (*n*)	Stenosis (*n*)	Incidence (%)
Sladen et al 1989[38]	173	33	19
Mills et al 1990[33]	379	48	13
Taylor et al 1990[48]	412	42	10
Bandyk et al 1991[49]	372	83	22
Buth et al 1991[44]	116	37	32
Taylor et al 1992[40]	74	19	26
Mattos et al 1992[13]	170	57	34
Total	1696	319	19

Natural History of Graft-Related Stenoses

Although intuition and clinical observation tell us that graft lesions portend a poor prognosis, there is little hard data concerning the natural history of stenoses developing in infrainguinal bypass grafts or in the inflow and outflow vessels.[20] For the most part, stenoses detected by surveillance protocols have been subjected to revision.

It is known, however, that the incidence of graft occlusion parallels that of the appearance of stenosis.[3,13,50] In a series of femoropopliteal grafts, Brewster and associates found that 63% of occlusions occurred within the first year and that 79% occurred within 2 years of surgery.[3] This temporal relationship supports the concept that graft stenoses are related to occlusion. Other data associate graft failure with the presence of stenoses. Donaldson and colleagues, in a careful review of 70 occluded *in situ* vein grafts and 20 with preocclusive lesions, found that only 7 "failures" (7.6%) were unexplained.[54] Most of the failures (63%) could be attributed to lesions in the graft itself and another 20% to stenoses in the inflow and outflow arteries. Szilagyi and associates found structural defects in 85 (33%) of 260 autogenous vein grafts followed with serial arteriograms for 1 to 10 years.[52] During the period of observation, 77% of the lesions progressed and 38% of the grafts with lesions thrombosed.

Perhaps the only truly prospective study of the natural history of graft stenoses is that of Moody and colleagues, who used intravenous digital subtraction angiography to follow saphenous vein grafts and adopted a "deliberate policy of nonintervention" when an asymptomatic lesion was discovered.[16] After a median interval of 13 months, 5 (23%) of 22 strictured grafts occluded. In contrast, only 4 (7%) of 58 angiographically normal grafts suffered the same fate. New stenoses developed in 6 grafts, 2 of which had previously been normal. Five (14%) of 36 stenoses progressed, but 65% of the strictures remained stable and asymptomatic.

For various reasons (physician or patient reluctance, stenosis location), 33 stenotic grafts in our most recent series with velocity ratios greater than 2.0 were not subjected to revision.[13] Ten (30%) of these grafts occluded during the time of the study. Subsequently, an additional graft has occluded and another has been revised. The 2-year cumulative patency rate of the nonrevised grafts, (measured from the time of the initial operation) was 57%. Following detection of the stenoses, the 2-year cumulative patency was only 33%. These figures stand in marked contrast to a 2-year cumulative patency of 83% in grafts with no detectable stenosis.

Results of Revision

Interpreting the voluminous data in the literature concerning the benefits conferred by revising patent but stenotic grafts is somewhat difficult owing to vagaries in terminology. For example, the term *failed graft* has been applied to patent grafts with severe (preocclusive) lesions and to hemodynamically compromised but patent grafts as well as to those grafts that have actually thrombosed. As originally suggested by the Ad Hoc Committee on Reporting Standards of the Society for Vascular Surgery and the North American Chapter of the International Society for Cardiovascular Society, any intervention, however minor, performed on a patent graft counts against "primary patency."[55] By this definition *primary patency* is reduced any time a patent graft is revised (even if the revision consists of ligation of a arteriovenous fistula). *Secondary patency* encompasses the patency of all revised grafts, whether the revision was performed on a patent or on an occluded graft.[55] Since the outcome of revision of patent, never thrombosed, grafts is far more favorable than that of revision of thrombectomized grafts, Rutherford has suggested that the former be designated, "assisted primary patency."[56]

Autogenous vein grafts revised while they remain patent have cumulative 5-year assisted primary patency rates ranging from 76% to 95%—rates approaching those of nonstenotic, never revised, grafts.[4,5,8,49,53,54,57,58] To determine the benefits of revision, these patency rates have been compared with 5-year primary patency rates of 59% to 70%, rates that are 17 to 25 percentage points lower than those achieved by revision.[53,54,58] Green and associates have pointed out the fallacy of this comparison.[20] Even if none of the revised grafts were destined to fail, the primary patency rate would have to be lower than the secondary or assisted primary patency rate, since the former is arbitrarily reduced with each revision. Thus, this type of comparison would indicate the true benefits of revision only if it were assumed that all nonrevised stenotic grafts would ultimately fail.[20] To circumvent this problem, we compared the assisted primary patency rate of 24 stenotic but never occluded grafts that had undergone revision with the primary patency rate of 33 stenotic nonrevised grafts.[13] The cumulative 2-year patency rate of the revised grafts (88%) was significantly higher ($P = 0.05$) than that of the nonrevised stenotic grafts (57%), suggesting that revision preserved patency in 31 of 100 stenotic grafts. When 2-year patency rates were calculated from the time of detection of the lesion, the difference was even more striking (90% for the revised grafts versus 33% for the nonrevised grafts).

Clinical Application

Because knowledge of the natural history of graft stenoses and the benefits of graft revision remains imperfect, it is difficult to establish precise guidelines for the clinical application of surveillance methods. Some general recommendations can be made, however.

Since at least half of the graft-threatening lesions develop within the first 6 months and about three-quarters within the first year, surveillance should be frequent in the early months and less frequent later. Most authors recommend surveillance within a few weeks of the primary procedure and then every 3 months for the first year.[21,33,36,44,48,50] Although Taylor and colleagues suggest that surveillance be discontinued after 1 year,[48] others advocate repeating the studies every 6 to 12 months for an indefinite period in order to detect late atherosclerotic progression in the inflow and outflow arteries.[14]

In addition to an interval history and physical examination, all patients should have ankle pressures measured and a duplex scan performed, preferably with a color-flow instrument. A pulse volume recorder or impedance measurement can also be obtained if the equipment is available, but these tests are less specific than duplex scanning. In our experience, the most reliable criteria for detecting and grading stenoses have been the appearance of the color image and the velocity ratio, although we continue to respect low-velocity recordings. A major advantage of duplex scanning is its ability to accurately locate lesions, thus, obviating the need for prerevision arteriography in many patients. Even if the graft fails prior to revision, knowledge of the precise location of the causative lesion simplifies the approach to thrombectomy.

Once a lesion is detected, one must decide whether it should be revised or whether it can be followed safely.[20] Clearly, not all stenoses require revision. Minor stenoses (<50% diameter reduction) can be followed.[13] Although many of these do progress,[45] a few seem to disappear on repeat studies. Some apparent stenoses (pseudostenoses) reflect diameter changes in normal grafts where large branches emerge from the harvested vein. Others are due to disparities in the calibre of two veins joined to form a composite conduit. Still others are the result of the rapidly changing diameter of the flow conduit that may occur at the proximal anastomosis where the host artery is much larger than the graft and at the distal anastomosis where the graft is much larger than the recipient native vessel. These size disparities are more often seen with reversed saphenous veins than with *in situ* or nonreversed vein grafts. It is well known that inflow and outflow stenoses and even occlusions may develop without loss of the graft.

Since no firm guidelines are available, it is probably wisest to revise those lesions that are hemodynamically significant in terms of a decrease in ankle pressure or those lesions that cause symptoms. Green and associates found that 66% of grafts with a decreased ABI and an abnormal duplex scan thrombosed or caused symptoms before the next follow-up visit.[20] Only 4% of grafts with an abnormal duplex scan and normal ABIs suffered a similar fate. In our experience, lesions with clearly high-grade stenoses responsible for turbulence or high velocities (velocity ratios exceeding 2.0 or 3.0) have a very poor prognosis, regardless of the ABI or the presence or absence of symptoms, and should be revised.[13] Lower grade lesions, such as those with velocity ratios less than 2.0 and those occurring in inflow and outflow vessels, can be followed, but the interval between examinations should be decreased.

Cost Effectiveness

Based on their experience with ankle–brachial pressure indices, Barnes and associates concluded that routine noninvasive surveillance and prophylactic intervention on asymptomatic lesions detected in leg bypass grafts may not be justified.[27] Lack of specific information concerning the natural history of graft stenoses makes it difficult to determine what price is paid for detection and revision of grafts. Since the reported revision rate of autogenous vein grafts ranges from 7% to 26%, this is a matter of concern.[13,20,33,48,54,58] From the difference in the secondary patency rates and assisted primary patency rates of the grafts in our series, it can be estimated that revision of 100 stenotic grafts prevents 30 graft occlusions within 2 years of the initial operation and almost 60 occlusions from the time the stenoses was first detected.[13] The cost of revision is relatively low, most operations are minor, the hospital stay is brief, and the patient suffers little discomfort. On the other hand, the cost of thrombectomy followed by a complicated revision or a redo graft is high, hospitalization may be prolonged, and the patient is subjected to considerable pain, anxiety, and possible limb loss. Despite the high cost of routine testing, surveillance seems justified based on these considerations.

Prospective Trials

A prospective randomized trial, perhaps involving multiple centers, is required to provide definitive answers to the questions posed above. Such a trial would define the natural history of graft-related stenoses and would indicate which lesions are safe to follow and which portend immediate graft failure. It would also verify the accuracy of various diagnostic methods, determine the optimum frequency of surveillance, and establish the benefits of graft revision. There are, however, ethical considerations that militate against such trials.[59] Although one might feel comfortable following a 50% diameter reducing lesion; it is harder to avoid reoperating on a 90% stenosis, since all retrospective studies and clinical observations suggest that lesions of this magnitude have a poor prognosis.

SURVEILLANCE AFTER CAROTID ENDARTERECTOMY

Restenosis at the site of a carotid endarterectomy may be a benign event or may lead to total occlusion or result in a stroke. Disobliteration of a total carotid occlusion is seldom possible and revision of a stenosis after a stroke has occurred does nothing to improve the patient's neurologic impairment. The ability to follow the endarterectomized site noninvasively enables the surgeon to detect and treat these lesions before they become irretrievable. Most recurrent lesions, however, remain asymptomatic. This has led a number of investigators to question the indications for routine surveillance.[60–62]

Methods and Interpretation

Duplex scanning is the only noninvasive method suitable for follow-up studies of the carotid endarterectomy site.[63] Other methods, such as oculoplethysmography and B-mode scanning alone, are less specific and too insensitive to be of value. Color-flow mapping facilitates the examination and is perhaps even more accurate than conventional duplex scanning, especially for identifying total occlusions.[64,65] Care should be taken to scan the internal carotid artery for several centimeters above the bifurcation to ensure that the distal end of the endarterectomy site is included in the study. Narrowing of the color-flow map and a shift in color from red to white alerts the examiner to the presence of a stenosis (Fig. 4–8, p. 47). The criteria used for surveillance studies are similar to those employed for routine carotid examinations. In our laboratory, a peak systolic velocity greater than 120 cm/s measured at the site of stenosis (indicated by color change) corresponds to a greater than 50% diameter stenosis; and an end-diastolic velocity exceeding 120 cm/s identifies 80% to 99% stenosis. These velocity changes are typically associated with marked spectral broadening. Absence of a Doppler signal or a color image in a carotid artery visualized on the B-mode scan is indicative of total occlusion. The external carotid artery may be distinguished from the internal by its more pulsatile flow pattern and by the presence of visible branches. Since minor flow disturbances and mild increases in velocity are common in postoperative carotid arteries (especially in patched arteries), no attempt is made to classify lower degrees of stenosis.[63] Before a definite diagnosis of greater than 50% diameter reduction is made, changes appropriate to this degree of stenosis should be present on two sequential examinations.[66] It is also possible to evaluate plaque morphology with the B-mode image.[67,68]

An initial study is recommended within the first few weeks after carotid endarterectomy to detect residual disease. During the first year, when the incidence of restenosis is highest, scans are repeated every 6 months. Thereafter, a yearly study is adequate. If a significant stenosis is detected, the interval between scans may be reduced to 3 months until the stability of the lesion established.

Incidence of Recurrent Stenosis

The reported incidence of hemodynamically significant recurrent carotid artery stenosis (>50% diameter reduction) varies widely from 6% to 37% (mean = 21%).[61] Much of this variation is probably attributable to study design, length of follow-up, and the accuracy of the methods used to detect stenoses. Inclusion of residual lesions left at the time of the initial endarterectomy artificially increases the incidence.[69,70] Studies in which random sampling of postoperative carotid arteries have been used generally report a lower incidence of recurrent stenosis than those in which the carotid arteries have been examined by serial scans. Cook and associates found recurrent stenoses (>50% diameter reduction) in 14 (18.4%) of 76 carotid arteries followed with duplex scanning.[61] Using color duplex scanning, we detected 44 recurrent lesions (>50% diameter stenosis) in 353 endarterectomized carotid arteries followed from 1 to 8 years, a crude incidence of 12.5%.[71]

Minor lesions with diameter reduction less than 50% account for a large portion (59% to 72%) of the recurrent stenoses but are seldom included in statistical analyses.[63,68,72–74] Although stenoses greater than 50% are found in approximately 14% of postoperative carotid arteries (Table 4–7), stenoses exceeding 70% to 80% are less common (1.4% to 6%).[62,68,71,72] In our series, only six (1.7%) of the carotid endarterectomies developed recurrences of this magnitude.[71] Total occlusions have been reported in 0 to 6% of cases.[62,68,72,73] Surveillance revealed six total occlusions in our study, an incidence of 1.7%.[71] Although most lesions remain stable, progression may occur in 8% to 14%, and regression has been observed in 26% to 30% of recurrent stenoses.[60,61,66,73] Regression may represent remodeling of the arterial wall at the proximal shelf where plaque remains in the common carotid artery, lysis of clots formed on the endarterectomized surface, or disappearance of neointimal hyperplasia.[66,70]

Life Table analyses provide the best information.[66,75,76] In the study by DeGroote and colleagues, the 7-year cumulative incidence of hemodynamically significant restenosis was 32%.[76] Healy and associates arrived at a remarkably similar figure of 31% for the same time span.[66] Since the comparable incidence of regression was 10%, the cumulative prevalence of restenosis (21%) was somewhat lower.

About 50% to 70% of the restenoses are detected in the first year.[60,66,71] These figures may be spuriously high owing to the possible inclusion of residual disease and to the relatively limited number of patients available for follow-up after 1 or 2 years. Green and colleagues found no "true" recurrent lesions in patients without residual disease earlier than 8 months after surgery; and by Life Table analysis, the incidence of recurrence appeared to be linear with time,[70] an observation supported by the work of other investigators.[75,76] Stenoses forming before 2 years are largely due to neointimal hyperplasia and have a benign prognosis.[67,68,77,78] Those developing after 2 years more likely represent atherosclerotic degeneration of neointimal disease or new atheroma.[77,79] These lesions have a more ominous prognosis.[78] Pseudostenoses, characterized by increased velocities and spectral broadening but no visible plaque, have been attributed to kinks or to the disparity in the calibre of the lumen at the terminal end of the endarterectomy site, where tacking sutures may have been used to secure residual atheroma in the internal carotid artery.[63,70]

Symptoms

That recurrent stenoses can cause neurologic symptoms in the hemisphere ipsilateral to the carotid endarterectomy is widely accepted. In a recent report, Washburn and associates carefully analyzed the cause of late postoperative strokes and found that 15% of those occurring within 3 years were attributable to recurrent stenoses or occlusions. In contrast, recurrent stenoses were responsible for 53% of the strokes appearing after 3 years.[78] Yet, the incidence of neurologic symptoms associated with recurrent stenosis is relatively low. Nine (20%) of 44 recurrent stenoses in our series were symptomatic.[71] Thus, the incidence of recurrent symptomatic lesions was only 2.5% (9/353). Only one of the nine (a patient with total carotid occlusion) presented with a stroke, an incidence of 0.3%. In the study by Cook and colleagues, one transient ischemic attack (TIA) and one stroke occurred in 14 patients with recurrent stenoses, an incidence of 14.3%.[61] The crude incidence of symptoms (one TIA and three strokes) was somewhat less (6.5%) in the 62 patients in whom no stenoses were detected.

Similarly, Ricotta and associates reported no strokes in 26 patients with severe residual or recurrent stenoses (>80% diameter reduction), but 5 (19%) experienced transient neurologic deficits.[62] This represented only 1.1% of 452 carotid endarterectomies. Of 9 total occlusions, 6 were asymptomatic, 2 had minor symptoms, and 1 suffered a stroke. The overall incidence of stroke related to recurrent disease was therefore only 0.2%. A partial summary of the recent literature (Table 4–7) shows that 243 recurrent stenoses were associated with 36 TIAs (14.8%) and 6 strokes (2.5%). The incidence of TIAs ipsilateral to the total number of endarterectomies (1775) was 2.0%, and the incidence of stroke was 0.3%.

Washburn and colleagues estimated that the probability of stroke related to recurrent stenoses or occlusion is about 0.45%/year in the first 3 years and 2.1%/year after 3 years.[78] By Life Table analysis, the cumulative 5-year stroke-free rate of patients in our [unpublished] series with recurrent stenosis (94.4%) was almost exactly the same as that of patients in whom no stenosis had been detected (94.2%). These results are practically identical to those reported by Cook and associates, who also found that the presence or absence of recurrent stenosis had no effect on the 5-year symptom-free rate.[61] Although Healy and colleagues found a higher 7-year cumulative incidence of TIAs in patients with recurrent stenoses (17%) than in patients with no recurrent stenosis (7%), the difference was not statistically significant.[66] Interestingly, the 7-year stroke incidence was lower (3%) in patients with restenosis than it was in the postoperatively normal group (16%), but again the difference was not statistically significant. This paradoxical finding has recently been substantiated by Bernstein and associates, who theorized that recurrent neointimal hyperplasia was in some way protective.[74]

In the series by Green and colleagues, none of the patients with flow abnormalities but no visible plaque experienced symptoms during follow-up.[70] Sterpetti and colleagues reported that the incidence of symptoms was higher in patients with heterogeneous plaques.[68]

Reoperation

Only about 1% to 3% of carotid endarterectomies and 5% to 22% of those with recurrent stenoses undergo reoperation.[60–62,66,71,76] Secondary operations on the carotid bifurcation are more difficult and may be associated with a higher morbidity than primary endarterectomies.[80,81] Although some surgeons advocate reoperations on asymptomatic critically stenotic (>80% diameter reduction) lesions, others prefer to wait until symptoms occur.[61,62,66,81] Washburn and associates recommend a conservative approach to early uncomplicated hyperplastic lesions and a more aggressive approach to those occurring later.[78] In our series, 6 (1.7%) of 353 patients underwent reoperation, 3 for symptoms and 3 for severe asymptomatic stenosis.[71]

Role of Carotid Surveillance

Routine surveillance during the early postoperative period reveals residual defects and serves as a quality control for the surgical procedure. Disclosure of a high incidence of residual stenoses should prompt the surgeon to re-examine his or her operative technique and suggests the need for intraoperative monitoring. Periodic follow-up of asymptomatic lesions in the contralateral carotid artery is also important for detecting advancing disease, which, if it exceeds 80% diameter reduction, may lead to stroke or carotid occlusion.[75,82] Because of the low incidence of stroke associated with recurrent carotid disease, the similar incidence of stroke in patients with and without restenosis, and the observation that strokes in patients with recurrent stenosis are usually preceded by symptoms, it is difficult to justify routine surveillance of the endarterectomized artery.[60–62]

69. Barnes RW, Nix ML, Wingo JP, et al. Recurrent versus residual carotid stenosis: incidence detected by Doppler ultrasound. *Ann Surg*. 1986;203:652–660.
70. Green RM, McNamara J, Ouriel K, et al. The clinical course of residual carotid arterial disease. *J Vasc Surg*. 1991;13:112–120.
71. Mattos MA, Hodgson KJ, Londrey GL, et al. Carotid endarterectomy: operative risks, recurrent stenosis, and long-term stroke rates in a modern series. *J Cardiovasc Surg*. (in press).
72. Glover JL, Bendick PJ, Dilley RS, et al. Restenosis following carotid endarterectomy: evaluation by duplex ultrasonography. *Arch Surg*. 1985;120:678–684.
73. Bertin VJ, Plecha FB, Rogers GJ, et al. Recurrent stenosis by duplex scan following carotid endarterectomy. *Arch Surg*. 1989;124:866–869.
74. Bernstein EF, Torem S, Dilley RB. Does carotid restenosis predict an increased risk of late symptoms, stroke, or death? *Ann Surg*. 1990;212:629–636.
75. Ackroyd N, Lane R, Appelberg M. Carotid endarterectomy: long-term follow-up with specific reference to recurrent stenosis, contralateral progression, mortality, and recurrent neurologic episodes. *J Cardiovasc Surg*. 1986;27:418–425.
76. DeGroote RD, Lynch TG, Jamil Z, et al. Carotid restenosis: long-term noninvasive follow-up after carotid endarterectomy. *Stroke*. 1987;18:1031–1036.
77. Stoney RJ, String ST. Recurrent carotid stenosis. *Surgery*. 1976;80:705–710.
78. Washburn WK, Mackey WC, Belkin M, et al. Late stroke after carotid endarterectomy: the role of recurrent stenosis. *J Vasc Surg*. 1992;15:1032–1037.
79. Clagett GP, Robinowitz M, Youkey JR, et al. Morphogenesis and clinicopathologic characteristics of recurrent carotid disease. *J Vasc Surg*. 1986;3:10–23.
80. Piepgras DG, Sundt TM, Marsh WR, et al. Recurrent carotid stenosis. Results and complications of 57 operations. *Ann Surg*. 1986;203:205–213.
81. Bartlett FF, Rapp JH, Goldstone J, et al. Recurrent carotid stenosis: operative strategy and late results. *J Vasc Surg*. 1987;5:452–456.
82. Roederer GO, Langlois YE, Lusiani L, et al. Natural history of carotid artery disease on the side contralateral to endarterectomy. *J Vasc Surg*. 1984;1:62–72.

II

Durability of Cerebral Revascularization Procedures

5

Carotid Endarterectomy:

Ten-Year Follow-Up

Allan D. Callow, MD, PhD

The usefulness of carotid endarterectomy in prevention of stroke has been a subject of intense discussion since its separate and nearly simultaneous introduction by Molins,[1] DeBakey,[2] and Rob.[3] Anecdotal reports of low perioperative mortality and morbidity achieved in some centers[4–6] have been controverted by other series detailing unacceptably high death and complication rates.[7–9]

Surgical enthusiasts with a wide spectrum of skill and judgment brought the number of carotid endarterectomies performed in the United States close to 100,000 in 1987, and worldwide experience amounted to an estimated 1 million operations since its introduction.[10]

Several reports not only questioned the value of carotid endarterectomy in preventing stroke, but suggested it might even be harmful.[11] Despite a number of individual but anecdotal reports documenting satisfactory results, criticism of the operation continued. Long-term benefits were challenged on the basis that recurrent stroke was not prevented and the quality of patient life after operation was low. Long-term survival was unlikely. Patients did not live long enough to obtain long-term benefit.

We reviewed our carotid registry to determine our own long-term experience. Particular attention was directed to the incidence of recurrent stroke, length of survival following operation, and the influence of coronary artery occlusive disease upon late morbidity and mortality. We wished to challenge the validity of the opinion that although short-term benefits might accrue to the postendarterectomy patient, poor quality of life and limited survival counterbalanced real or apparent benefit. Our study is retrospective and nonrandomized. It utilizes historic controls and provides raw data on the long-term experience of patients who have been operated on.

Using a literature review, we also compared the short- and long-term results of carotid endarterectomy in symptomatic and asymptomatic patients with results obtained by solely medical treatment of similar patients.

MATERIALS

Beginning in 1970, 619 patients underwent 993 operations with complete or determinant follow-up evaluations. Patients were placed into a symptomatic or asymptomatic group based on clinical findings at presentation. Details of management, assessment, and outcome were obtained from retrospective review of records and follow-up data from office records, where possible, or from detailed questionnaires sent to the patient or surviving spouse and to the referring physician. Detailed information was requested regarding stroke or neurologic deficit of any kind, cardiac disease, particularly myocardial infarction, and death since operation, together with the dates of these events or of hospitalizations following operation. A clerical research assistant was employed whose responsibility was to identify some source of information concerning the patient via telephone calls to the patient's last known phone number, to the referring physician, to the local hospital, and where indicated, to government offices for death certificate data. Patients in whom such follow-up data could not be obtained were excluded from further investigation, leaving us with 619 patients with adequate documentation. Surgery was offered to virtually all symptomatic and to some selected asymptomatic patients: those with substantial bifurcation atherosclerosis. Staged bilateral carotid endarterectomy was offered to patients with contralateral carotid disease with more than 75% stenosis or those with lesser degrees of stenosis with unequivocal surface irregularity or ulceration and who were an acceptable cardiac risk. Patients with carotid and vertebrobasilar transient ischemic events and patients with a remote carotid territorial infarction but with little or no clinical residual, who therefore had substantial carotid territory still at risk from an appropriate carotid lesion, were also evaluated for surgery. Nine patients were operated on during an acute carotid territorial stroke. Retrograde transfemoral arteriography via the Seldinger technique was used to visualize the aortic arch, the four brachiocephalic vessels, and selected intracranial branches. Neurologists examined all patients. Operative risk was assessed by cardiologists and anesthesiologists. Routine thallium-dipyridamole (Persantine IV) stress testing was added in 1985.

Our methods of clinical assessment and surgical management had gradually evolved beginning with our first carotid endarterectomy in 1957. By 1970, we had developed a standardized protocol, including cerebral protection and cerebral blood flow monitoring during surgery. We abandoned, except in very rare instances, induced hypertension, hypercapnia, hypothermia, and measurement of carotid back pressure after cross-clamping. Virtually all patients were operated on under normocapnic, normotensive general anesthesia. Shunting was selectively performed based on electroencephalographic monitoring criteria as described in earlier publications.[12–15] Systemic heparin was used and was not reversed on completion of the operation.

We believe that one of the causes of recurrent stenosis is residual plaque left at the time of endarterectomy. We were also reluctant to use tacking sutures at the distal end of the plaque because their need suggests incomplete plaque removal. Thus, we have emphasized a long arteriotomy from well above the distal end point of the plaque to well down into the common carotid artery. Primary closure without a patch was standard. Vein was preferred to synthetic patch, and its use was reserved for the small artery, after reopening the incision to inspect the endarterectomy site, and for the recurrent stenosis operation. Low-molecular-weight dextran was used in every case during surgery and for 24 hours afterward. The endarterectomy surface was copiously irrigated with several hundred milliliters of heparinized saline followed by low-molecular-weight dextran before arteriotomy closure. Completion angiography was used only in recent years of the study. Preoperative aspirin, if used, was resumed on the first postoperative day and continued indefinitely. Follow-up questionnaires were distributed in 1984 and again in 1987. All data, both perioperative and follow-up, were computer filed using DataBase III. Life table analysis conformed to the guidelines published by the Joint Committee of the Society for Vascular Surgery and the North American Chapter of the International Society of Cardiovascular Surgery.[16]

Abstat software was used for analysis and log rank testing of life table comparisons. Statistical significance was inferred from a P value of less than 0.05. The two essential points were (1) the date of entry into the study group (the patient's initial operation), and (2) the occurrence of any neurologic deficit with residua that was referable to *any* cerebral territory and that was included regardless of cause, alleged or established. This second piece of information was the stroke end point. From the patients' standpoint, strokes of any type or location and whether related to the initial operation or not, may impair their quality of life. Thus, strokes in the contralateral hemisphere, that is, opposite that of the operated on artery, or in the vertebrobasilar territory, or the result of embolus of actual or suspected cardiac origin, were included as stroke end points. The significant item in describing quality of life following carotid endarterectomy is total stroke incidence. By analyzing life table data in this manner, we wished to show the effect of our carotid disease management protocol. The time from operation to stroke end point was calculated to the nearest month. The study group consisted of 619 patients who underwent 993 operations.

RESULTS

The mean length of follow-up was 56.4 ± 1.6 months with a maximum of 206 months. Operations for symptomatic lesions were performed 404 times, and 179 operations were for asymptomatic lesions. Thirty-six operations were for clinical states not typically or exclusively one or the other. There were no substantial differences in age, sex, and risk factor prevalence between the groups. Four hundred and four patients (65.2%) were symptomatic at their initial presentation. A large number of patients had second operations, this time for asymptomatic disease, indicating our aggressive attitude toward disease in the contralateral artery. Twenty-five of the 619 patients (4%) required reoperation for recurrent stenosis. The stroke rate, at 30 days from operation, for the entire group was 2.3%. Stroke and death rates within 30 days after surgery were not different between the asymptomatic and symptomatic group ($P>0.2$). Similarly, late stroke-free (Table 5–1) and stroke-free survival (Table 5–2) rateswere also not different ($P>0.1$). When the symptomatic and asymptomatic

TABLE 5–1. LIFE TABLE STROKE-FREE RATES

Interval	Number at Risk	Number Lost	Stroke-Free (%)	
			Interval	*Cumulative*
Total Group				
30 days	619	2	97.7	97.7
1 y	559	19	99.8	96.7
3 y	461	90	98.1	93.6
5 y	302	53	93.5	90.1
10 y	110	52	98.8	84.8
Symptomatic Group				
1 y	359	12	99.7	96.0
3 y	291	58	97.3	92.3
5 y	195	29	97.2	89.3
10 y	42	31	98.3	84.0
Asymptomatic Group				
1 y	166	7	100.0	98.3
3 y	139	26	99.2	96.2
5 y	89	20	98.7	93.1
10 y	11	18	100.0	87.1

TABLE 5–2. THE LIFE TABLE STROKE-FREE SURVIVAL RATES

Interval	Number at Risk	Number of Deaths from Strokes	Number Lost	Alive + Stroke-Free (%) Interval	Alive + Stroke-Free (%) Cumulative
Total Group					
30 days	619	16	0	97.4	97.4
1 y	559	14	12	99.1	92.9
3 y	461	26	72	93.9	83.8
5 y	302	22	38	92.2	73.0
10 y	110	9	44	89.8	53.5
Symptomatic Group					
1 y	359	3	10	99.2	92.4
5 y	195	11	23	94.0	73.0
10 y	74	5	27	91.7	55.8
Asymptomatic Group					
1 y	166	2	5	98.8	93.8
5 y	89	7	14	91.5	75.6
10 y	29	4	148	81.8	46.7

groups were compared, and operation-specific stroke rate (30 days perioperative) was 1.6%, or 16, of 993 operations and the operation-specific death rate (30 days perioperative) was 0.62%, or 6, of 993 operations (Figs. 5–1 and 5–2).

DISCUSSION

Clearly the objective of all surgeons concerned with the treatment of carotid artery occlusive disease and the goal for all patients is stroke prevention. In this series, this goal was achieved at the 5-year interval in 93.1% of asymptomatic patients and 89.3% of patients with symptoms. At the 10-year interval, stroke prevention was achieved in 87.1 and 84% of asymptomatic and symptomatic patients, respectively. The crude annual stroke incidence for the entire group, including perioperative strokes (2.3%), was 1.9%. This crude annual stroke rate for the symptomatic subgroup was 2.1%. For the asymptomatic group, it was 1.4%.

Although our patients experienced a gratifying freedom from stroke occurrence, their stroke-free survival is less impressive. Only 73% of surgical patients were alive *and* stroke-free at 5 years. At 10 years stroke-free survivors had dwindled to 53.5%.

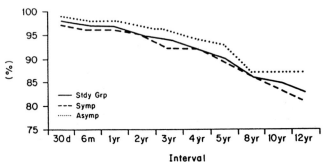

Figure 5–1. Life table stroke-free rates for the entire group (solid line), the symptomatic subgroup (dashed line), and the asymptomatic subgroup (dotted line). Log rank analysis yields *P* > 0.1 for comparison of symptomatic and asymptomatic subgroups. (*Reproduced with permission: Callow AD, Mackey WC. Long-term follow-up of surgically managed carotid bifurcation atherosclerosis: justification for an aggressive approach. Ann Surg. 1989; 210:308–316.*)

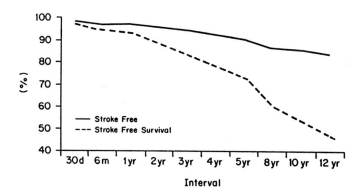

Figure 5–2. Comparison of life table stroke-free (solid line) and stroke-free survival (dashed line) curves. Difference in curves suggests that late death in endarterectomy patients is not stroke-related. (*Reproduced with permission: Callow AD, Mackey WC. Long term follow-up of surgically managed carotid bifurcation atherosclerosis: justification for an aggressive approach.* Ann Surg. *1989;219:308–316.*)

This experience is illustrated in Figure 5–2 and illustrates the comparison of our life table stroke-free results with our life table stroke-free survival results. Analysis revealed that the mortality among these patients was not stroke related. The cause of death was known in 120 of the 144 recorded deaths (83.3%). Fifty of the deaths of known cause (41.7%) were due to myocardial infarction and 14 (11.75%) to congestive heart failure. Only 16 (13.3%) could be attributed to stroke of any cause or any cerebral territory.

LITERATURE COMPARISONS

Carotid Endarterectomy Results

Cleveland Clinic[17]

Of the asymptomatic patients, 91.8% were stroke-free at 5 years. At 10 years 74.4% were stroke-free. In symptomatic patients (those who had experienced transient ischemic attacks: TIAs) the 5-year stroke-free rate was 89.3%, and the 10-year rate was 76.1%. For patients with a history of prior stroke, the 5-year and 10-year stroke-free rates were 76.7 and 69.4%, respectively. The postoperative annual stroke incidence was 3%. Long-term survival was reduced as in our series, with a 5-year mortality rate of 28.4% and a 10-year rate of 57.5%.

Scripps-La Jolla

In a series reported by Bernstein[18] a postoperative neurologic event occurred in 7.8% of 370 patients and consisted of 21 nonfatal and 8 fatal strokes during a mean follow-up of 43 months. The crude annual stroke incidence was 2.2%. At the 5-year period, the life table stroke-free rate was 91.3% for patients with carotid territorial TIAs and 93.7% for the asymptomatic group.

St. Thomas Hospital–London

Browse and associates[19] reported a crude annual stroke incidence of 2% among 100 patients operated on because of TIAs and followed for a mean of 5.5 years. Four of these were fatal and seven were nonfatal. The 5-year life table stroke-free rate was approximately 90%.

Admittedly, differences in criteria for patient selection for operation and for techniques of operation exist within these series. In addition, the experience reported is not randomized or prospective. Nevertheless, a crude annual postoperative stroke incidence of approximately 2% reported in all these series is impressive. So too, are the 5-year and 10-year life table stroke-free rates of approximately 90 and 80%, respectively for symptomatic patients, and of 93% and 75 to 85% at 5 and 10 years, respectively, among asymptomatic patients. We report a similar experience: a crude annual stroke incidence of 1.9%, a 5-year stroke-free rate by life table analysis of 89.3%, and of 84% at 10 years among the symptomatic. In the asymptomatic patients these rates were 93.1 and 87.1% among 5- and 10-year survivors, respectively.[20]

It is apparent from these series that stroke prevention can be achieved by carotid endarterectomy in symptomatic patients and in asymptomatic patients with a substantial carotid lesion. Long-term survival, however, is limited, largely due to death from cardiac causes. Thus, only 73% of our patients were alive and stroke-free at 5 years. By 10 years, the stroke-free survival was only 53.5%. Among the 144 deaths recorded, the cause of death was known in 120, or 83.3%, of the patients. Of these known causes, 50, or 41.7%, were related to myocardial infarction and 14, or nearly 12%, to congestive heart failure. Conversely, only 16 (13.3%) could be attributed to stroke.

CLEVELAND CLINIC[17]

	5 years (%)	10 years (%)
Stroke-free[a]		
asymptomatic	91.8	74.4
symptomatic (TIA)	89.3	76.1
prior stroke	76.7	69.4
Long-term mortality	28.4	57.5

[a] *Crude annual postoperative stroke rate: 3%*

SCRIPPS–LAJOLLA[18]

	5 years (%)
Stroke-free[a]	
symptomatic (TIA)	91.3
asymptomatic	93.7

[a] *Crude annual postoperative stroke rate: 2.2%*

ST. THOMAS HOSPITAL–LONDON[19]

	5 years (%)
Stroke-free[a]	90

[a] *Crude annual postoperative stroke rate: 2%*

To obtain some perspective of the effectiveness of medical therapy in the prevention of stroke, and because at the time no randomized trial had been completed, we reviewed the literature and selected four randomized trials of medical therapy for symptomatic patients. The relevant factor in medical therapy appears to be administration of antiplatelet agents.[21]

1. The Canadian Cooperative Study revealed the beneficial effect of aspirin or aspirin plus sulfinpyrazone, but the effect occurred only in men. The crude annual stroke incidence at 26 months was 4.6%, whereas in woman it was 8.2%.[22]

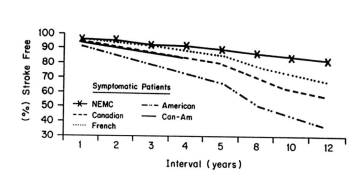

Figure 5–3. Comparison of surgical results in this series of five trials and results of "optimal" medical therapy as defined by the Canadian Cooperative Trial, the AICLA Trial, the American Multicenter Trial, and the Canadian–American Cooperative Trial for symptomatic patients. Late results in medical trials are extrapolated from annual incidence data. (*Reproduced with permission: Callow AD, Mackey WC. Long-term follow-up of surgically managed carotid bifurcation atherosclerosis: justification for an aggressive approach. Ann Surg. 1989;210:308–316.*)

2. The French trial by Bousser and colleagues administered aspirin or aspirin plus dipyridamole to 400 patients suffering transient ischemic attacks. The test revealed an annual crude incidence of stroke of 3.2% but was not carried out beyond 3 years. At that time, life table stroke-free rates were approximately 90.5% for men and 88.0% for women.[23]

3. An early American trial of aspirin reported a life table stroke-free rate of 91.2% at 1 year and 84.1% at 2 years. These rates yielded an annual crude stroke incidence of 8%.[24]

4. The American–Canadian Cooperative Trial of aspirin plus dipyridamole yielded life table stroke-free rates of 93.1, 87.7, 84.5, and 79.4%, respectively, at 1, 2, 3, and 4 years after surgery.[25] By comparison, our surgical patients had life table stroke-free rates of 96.0, 94.8, 92.3, and 91.8%, respectively, at 1, 2, 3, and 4 years after surgery.

The data from all four studies are reproduced graphically in Figure 5–3. Clearly, although these are nonrandomized, nonperspective studies, surgical therapy appears superior to medical therapy in stroke prevention among symptomatic patients.

CONCLUSION

Carotid endarterectomy provides substantial and long-lasting protection against stroke due to carotid artery occlusive disease in symptomatic carotid artery patients and in individuals with substantial (albeit asymptomatic) carotid occlusive disease. This protective effect based on this and other retrospective studies lasts for at least 10 years. In nearly 50% of patients, late death after carotid endarterectomy is due to the consequences of coexisting coronary artery and other cardiac disease. In symptomatic patients, postendarterectomy freedom from stroke reaches 89 and 84% at the 5- and 10-year levels, respectively. Improvement in long-term survival may depend upon improvement in the management of coexisting cardiac disease.

REFERENCES

1. Carrerra R, Molins M, Murphy G. Surgical treatment of spontaneous thrombosis of the internal carotid artery of the neck. *Acta Neurol Latinoam.* 1955;1:71–78.

2. DeBakey ME. Successful carotid endarterectomy for cerebrovascular insufficiency. Nineteen year follow-up. *JAMA*. 1975;223:1083–1085.

3. Eastcott HHG, Pickering GW, Rob C. Reconstruction of internal carotid artery in patient with intermittent attacks of hemiplegia. *Lancet*. 1954;2:994–996.

4. Thompson JE, Talkington CM. Carotid endarterectomy. *Ann Surg*. 1976;184:1–15.

5. Thompson JE, Putman RD, Talkington CM. Asymptomatic carotid bruit: long-term outcome of patients having endarterectomy compared with unoperated controls. *Ann Surg*. 1978;188: 308–316.

6. Callow AD. An overview of the stroke problem in the carotid territory. *Am J Surg*. 1980; 140:181–191.

7. Dyken ML, Pokras R. The performance of endarterectomy of the extracranial arteries of the head. *Stroke*. 1984;15:948–950.

8. Brott T, Thalinger K. The practice of carotid endarterectomy in a large metropolitan area. *Stroke*. 1984;15:950–955.

9. Easton JD, Sherman DG. Stroke and mortality rate in carotid endarterectomy: 228 consecutive operations. *Stroke*. 1977;8:565–568.

10. North American Symptomatic Carotid Endarterectomy Trial Collaborators. Beneficial effect of carotid endarterectomy in symptomatic patients with high-grade carotid stenosis. *N Engl J Med*. 1991;325:445–453.

11. AbuRahma AF, Robinson P. Indications and complications of carotid endarterectomy as performed by four different surgical specialty groups. *J Cardiovasc Surg*. 1988;29:277–282.

12. Matsumoto GH, Cossman D, Callow AD. Hazards and safeguards during carotid endarterectomy. *Am J Surg*. 1977;133:458–462.

13. Callow AD. Risk factors and current status of carotid endarterectomy. *Int Angio*. 1982;1:95–108.

14. Kelly JJ, Callow AD, O'Donnell TF, et al. Failure of carotid stump pressures. Its incidence as a predictor for a temporary shunt during carotid endarterectomy. *Arch Surg*. 1979;114:1361–1366.

15. Matsumoto G, Baker J, Watson C, et al. EEG surveillance as a means of extending operability in high risk carotid endarterectomies. *Stroke*. 1976;7:554.

16. Rutherford RB, et al. Suggested standards for reports dealing with lower extremity ischemia. *J Vasc Surg*. 1986;4:80–94.

17. Hertzer NR, Aronson R. Cumulative stroke and survival 10 years after carotid endarterectomy. *J Vasc Surg*. 1986;2:661–668.

18. Bernstein EF, Humber PB, Collins GM, et al. Life expectancy and late stroke following carotid endarterectomy. *Ann Surg*. 1983;198:80–86.

19. Stewart G, Ross-Russell RW, Browse NL. The long-term results of carotid endarterectomy for transient ischemic attacks. *J Vasc Surg*. 1986;4:600–605.

20. Callow AD, Mackey WC. Long-term follow-up of surgically managed carotid bifurcation atherosclerosis: justification for an aggressive approach. *Ann Surg*. 1989;210:308–316.

21. Fields WS. Aspirin for prevention of stroke: a review. *Am J Med*. 1983;74:61–65.

22. Canadian Cooperative Study Group. A randomized trial of aspirin and sulfinpyrozone in threatened stroke. *N Engl J Med*. 1978;229:53–59.

23. Bousser MD, Eschwege R, Haguenau M, et al. "AICLA" controlled trial of aspirin and dipyridamole in the secondary prevention of atherothrombotic cerebral ischemia. *Stroke*. 1983;14:5–14.

24. Fields WS, Lemak NA, Fernkowski RF, et al. Controlled trial of aspirin in cerebral ischemia. *Stroke*. 1977;8:301–315.

25. The American–Canadian Cooperative Study Group. Persantine aspirin trial in cerebral ischemia. *Stroke*. 1985;16:406–415.

6

Long-Term Results of Reconstructions of the Vertebral Artery

Ramon Berguer, MD, PhD

Reconstructions of the vertebral artery (VA) are generally carried out at either the first (proximal) or third (distal) extracranial segment of this artery. Proximal reconstructions are usually done to relieve symptomatic stenoses at the ostium of the VA. Distal reconstructions are indicated for the purpose of bypassing a symptomatic obstruction, whether temporary or fixed, of the intraspinal course of the VA. Some of these operations are done in conjunction with endarterectomy of the carotid, and rarely, of the subclavian arteries. The subgroup of patients undergoing concomitant carotid and VA reconstruction should be considered separately. Their surgical risk is higher and, in some of them, the reconstruction of the internal carotid artery (ICA) or VA is done for prophylactic reasons.

Our long-term results will be analyzed for both proximal and distal reconstructions. The subgroup of combined carotid–vertebral reconstructions will be discussed within each of these two groups.

Our experience encompasses 233 vertebral artery reconstructions, starting in 1975 but accumulated mostly in the last 10 years. There were 176 proximal VA operations and 57 distal ones. Forty-three of the 233 VA reconstructions were done simultaneously with a carotid operation. The ratio of males to females was 1.1 for proximal and 1.5 for distal operations. The mean age was 62 ± 12 years. Preoperative evaluation showed hypertension or coronary artery disease in 58% of the patients.

PROXIMAL RECONSTRUCTIONS

We have done and followed 176 proximal VA reconstructions. Of these, 140 operations were done to revascularize the VA alone; the remaining 36 patients had concomitant ICA reconstructions.

With 1 exception, all 140 patients undergoing single VA reconstruction were operated upon for symptoms of vertebrobasilar ischemia (VBI). The exception was a

38-year-old woman who had developed preocclusive lesions of both vertebral arteries seen in arteriograms done to elicit the cause of bilateral neck bruits. She had no demonstrable posterior communicating artery and, although asymptomatic, was advised to undergo transposition of the dominant left VA into the common carotid artery (CCA).

The remaining 139 patients had a syndrome of VBI, the most common symptoms of which were dizziness, vertigo, blurring of vision, and diplopia. Two or more of these symptoms were present in 72% of patients. Less common findings were drop attacks, lateral medullary syndrome, alternating paresthesia, or cerebellar infarction.

Table 6–1 lists the operations done in 176 proximal VA reconstructions. At the beginning of our experience we favored subclavian to VA vein bypass,[1] an operation that does not require clamping of the CCA. From 1980, the subclavian to VA bypass was used only in patients whose opposite ICA was occluded and in whom clamping the remaining carotid artery without some means of cerebral protection would be risky. Since 1980, and with the exception just mentioned, our standard operation to reconstruct the proximal VA has been a transposition of the proximal VA to the CCA.

In one patient with ipsilateral occlusion of the ICA and severe disease of the subclavian artery, the opposite subclavian was used as a source and the graft was routed behind the pharynx. In another patient with bilateral ICA occlusion and severe and bilateral subclavian artery disease the graft to revascularize the proximal VA was brought from the ascending aorta.

The anatomic indications for reconstruction of the proximal VA were stenosis of 75% of diameter in the dominant VA, with the opposite VA being absent, hypoplastic, or ending in a posterior–inferior cerebellar artery, or a similar degree of stenosis in both vertebral arteries if they were of equivalent size.

Mortality

The mortality for all proximal VA operations has been 2 of 176 (1.1%). One death was secondary to a myocardial infarction 4 days after surgery, in a patient who underwent combined carotid and VA repair. The other death occurred in a patient who also underwent a combined operation. Because of contralateral ICA disease, an intraluminal shunt was used. An atheromatous embolus seen through the shunt at the time of its insertion caused a middle cerebral artery occlusion and a massive stroke, which eventually resulted in the patient's death. Both of these deaths occurred in patients undergoing combined carotid–vertebral operations. If we consider patients undergo-

TABLE 6–1. TECHNIQUES USED IN THE PROXIMAL VERTEBRAL ARTERY

Endarterectomy and patch	1
Eversion endarterectomy	4[a]
Subclavian VA bypass graft	17
Transposition of VA into another subclavian site	9
Subclavian to contralateral VA retropharyngeal bypass	1
Ascending aorta to VA vein bypass	1
Common carotid to VA bypass	3
Transposition of VA into common carotid artery	140[b]

[a] In combination with revascularization of proximal subclavian artery.
[b] 36 of 140 transpositions had a simultaneous ipsilateral internal carotid operation.

ing VA reconstructions alone (140 patients), the mortality and central neurologic morbidity in this group has been nil.

Morbidity

There was 1 central neurologic deficit among the 174 survivors (0.5%). It occurred in a patient who underwent combined myocardial, ICA, and VA revascularization. During surgery and through the postoperative period, the patient had recurrent atrial fibrillation and flutter and developed a right upper extremity monoparesis. We noted 3 inferior laryngeal nerve palsies (2%) and 26 instances of Horner's syndrome (15%), which was temporary in 20 cases and permanent in 6. There were 7 lymphoceles (4%) and 1 chylothorax; the latter patient required a secondary operation to stop the accumulation of lymph in the chest, which was drained at the rate of 2 L/day.

Four patients underwent successful thrombectomy of the proximal VA reconstruction within 2 days of the operation. All four patients had had a vein graft. The vertebral artery in its intraspinal segment had remained opened through muscular and intercostovertebral branches. A successful thrombectomy was accomplished in all four cases. In three of the four cases, thrombus had developed in a kink of the graft. The remaining patient had had a small (and, in retrospect, inadequate) saphenous vein anastomosed to a large (6-mm) VA. Lack of a suitably sized vein required replacing the first graft with a 6-mm polytetrafluoroethylene prosthesis, which remained open.

Three patients required revision of the proximal reconstructions when recurrence of symptoms prompted an arteriogram that disclosed narrowing of the vein graft (two cases) or of the VA at the site of transposition into the subclavian (one case). These seven reoperations (four thrombectomies and three revisions) remained patent during follow-up.

Figure 6–1 shows the life expectancy of 176 patients undergoing proximal VA reconstruction. The survival of this group is 90% at 5 years and 79% at 10 years.

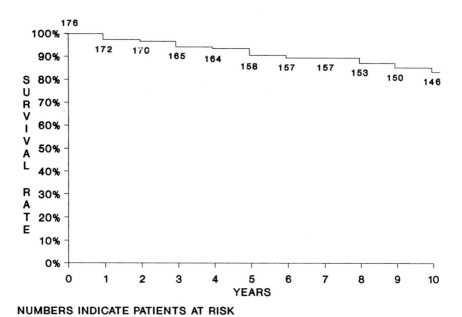

Figure 6–1. Life table analysis of patients after proximal VA reconstruction.

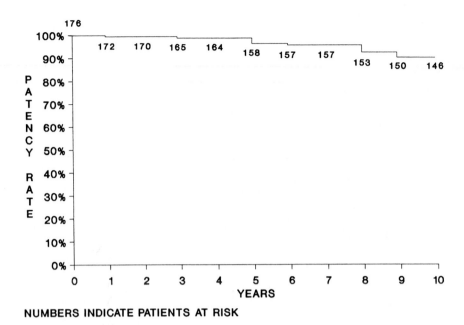

NUMBERS INDICATE PATIENTS AT RISK

Figure 6–2. Cumulative (secondary) patency rates of proximal VA reconstructions.

Patency was assessed in all patients during the postoperative period by arteriography. During follow-up a minority of patients underwent repeat arteriography (usually to evaluate new carotid lesions or neurologic symptoms) and all had periodic ultrasound exams. The latter procedure can image well a subclavian to VA bypass and a transposition of the VA into the CCA.

Figure 6–2 shows the secondary cumulative patency rate of proximal VA operations.

For the purpose of discussing the clinical results only the 140 patients who had a single proximal VA reconstruction are considered (the 36 patients who underwent combined ICA and proximal VA reconstruction will be discussed separately). There was cure or substantial improvement of symptoms in 93 of 112 (83%), whereas 19 of 112 (17%) were neurologically the same.

The causes of death in the 20 patients that died during the follow-up period were coronary artery disease in 11 (55%), stroke in 5 (35%), and other diseases in 4 patients (20%).

COMBINED CAROTID–PROXIMAL VERTEBRAL RECONSTRUCTION

Among the 36 patients undergoing combined carotid and proximal VA reconstructions there were two deaths (the only deaths in the proximal VA series). If this subgroup of patients is considered separately[2] the mortality is 2 of 36 (5%). All of these patients had severe carotid disease. Among the 24 cases who had had hemispheric symptoms or previous strokes, the majority also had VBI. In 12 patients that had severe VA lesions and VBI, the carotid endarterectomy was done for a severe stenosis without hemispheric symptoms or computed tomography findings of a previous infarction. Relief of symptoms in this combined group after 10 years was 86%.

DISTAL VERTEBRAL ARTERY RECONSTRUCTION

There were 57 patients undergoing distal VA reconstruction, and all of these patients had symptoms of VBI. In 8 patients the mechanism was thromboembolic, and in 49 patients it was hemodynamic or a combination of both.

Preoperative arteriography consisted of a four-vessel study. In patients with symptoms related to head position, the selective subclavian injection (to outline the VA) was done with the head in the same position that caused the symptoms, generally a combination of rotation and extension of the neck. In the last 4 years we have added some Trendelenburg's positioning to this arrangement of the arteriographic table, with the head supported by a block. This simulates the axial compression of the cervical spine due to the weight of the head, which occurs when the subject is standing or sitting up—the position in which hemodynamically induced VBI generally appears.

The anatomic indication for distal VA reconstruction in symptomatic patients has been severe stenosis of the intraspinal segment of the VA either fixed (plaque, thrombus) or transient (external compression) (Fig. 6–3). In patients with hemodynamic symptoms, the dominant VA must be involved, and the other VA should be absent or hypoplastic. In patients with thromboembolic symptoms and a demonstrated embolic source in one VA (Fig. 6–4), the status of the opposite VA is irrelevant to the surgical decision.

The distal VA was exposed and revascularized in 55 instances between C-2 and

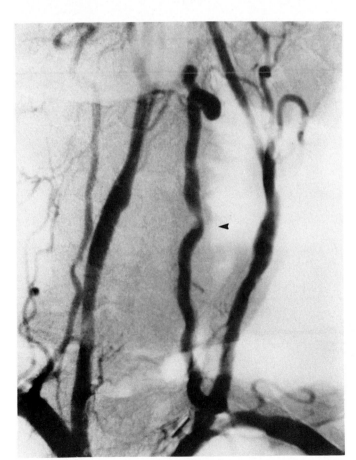

Figure 6–3. This patient had recurrent VBI 3 years after transposition of the dominant left VA to the left CCA. The arteriogram with the neck rotated to the left shows the impingement caused by an osteophyte on the second segment of the VA (arrow). The metal clip adjacent to the left subclavian is on the stump of the VA.

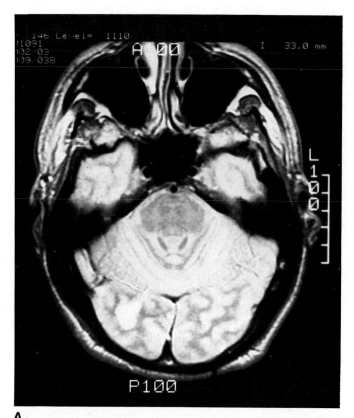

Figure 6–4. (**A**) Patient presenting with a right cerebellar infarction shown in this magnetic resonance image. (**B**) Emboligenous mural thrombus in the VA at an abnormally high level into the spine. (**C**) The right posterior–inferior cerebellar artery (arrow) is severely attenuated from an embolus. (**D**) An intraoperative arteriogram after common-to-distal VA bypass and ligation of the proximal VA at the C-2 level.

A

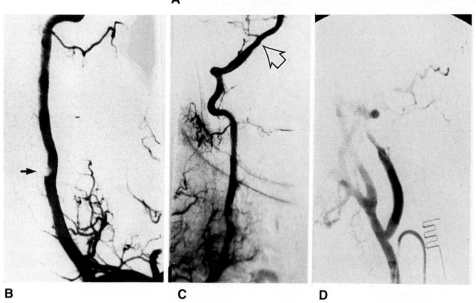

B   **C**   **D**

C-1 and in two instances above C-1.[3] Table 6–2 lists the techniques used for distal revascularization. All of the distal vertebral arteries in our study but one were revascularized from the ipsilateral carotid vessels. In this one patient the only available source was the contralateral CCA. The graft was tunneled from the CCA, behind the pharynx, to the contralateral distal VA (Fig. 6–5).

TABLE 6–2. TECHNIQUES USED IN THE DISTAL VERTEBRAL ARTERY

Common carotid to distal VA vein bypass	41
Internal carotid to distal VA vein bypass	1
Transposition of external carotid to distal VA	10
Transposition of occipital artery to distal VA	2
Transposition of distal VA to ICA	2
Carotid to contralateral distal VA retroesophageal bypass	1
Total	57

Mortality

There were 3 deaths following these 57 operations, for an operative mortality of 5%. One patient died of a hemispheric infarction secondary to the occlusion of a severely stenotic middle cerebral artery known to exist on the preoperative arteriogram. Another patient who underwent a CCA to distal VA bypass had a massive hemispheric brainstem stroke 6 hours after surgery. At exploration an intraoperative arteriogram showed severe spasm of the distal VA and also of the ICA, which had not been manipulated during the previous operation. Papaverine-mediated dilation, thrombectomy of the graft, and reestablishment of a normal arteriographic appearance did not improve the severe clinical picture, and the patient died decerebrated 3 days later. The reason for the spasm seen in two unrelated arteries was never found. The third death occurred in a patient who was found to have a thrombosed graft on the arteriogram obtained on the second postoperative day while he was neurologically normal. The operation had been done for VBI secondary to compression of a

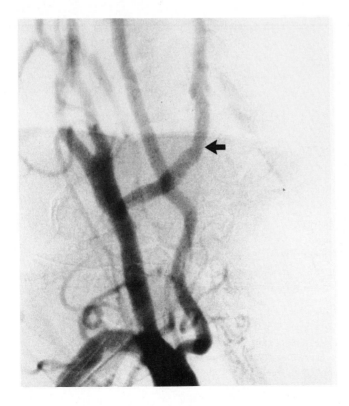

Figure 6–5. A retropharyngeal bypass across the neck in a patient with an emboligenous source (arrow) in the left intraspinal VA. His left common and internal carotid arteries were occluded and the left subclavian artery was severely diseased. This determined the choice of the right common carotid artery as a source vessel.

single but small VA by an osteophyte at the level of C-3. Following clearing of the graft, no spontaneous backflow was obtained from the distal VA. A 5-cm length of a No. 2 embolectomy catheter was passed distally, and the thrombus plug was removed with brisk backflow. Flow was reestablished. Immediately after this there were dramatic changes in blood pressure. The patient was comatose after anesthesia and died 4 days after surgery. The postmortem showed subarachnoid hemorrhage, which was most likely the result of perforation of the intradural segment of the VA with the thrombectomy catheter.

Morbidity

There were five early occlusions (8.5%) after distal VA reconstruction. Two occlusions occurred in the two patients that died, described in the paragraph above. The other three occlusions were secondary to competitive flow between the VA bypass and the collaterals from the occipital artery. One of these patients had an ipsilateral ICA occlusion and a stenosis at the origin of the external carotid artery (Fig. 6–6). The occipital branch of the external carotid artery supplied the distal VA at the level of C-2, but the VA proximal to this level was occluded. The patient underwent a distal VA bypass and a concomitant external carotid angioplasty. The arteriogram obtained 2 days after the operation showed the external carotid artery angioplasty to be open and supplying the distal VA through the previously seen occipital collateral. The

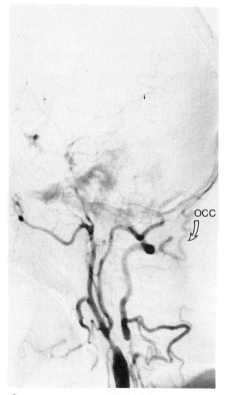
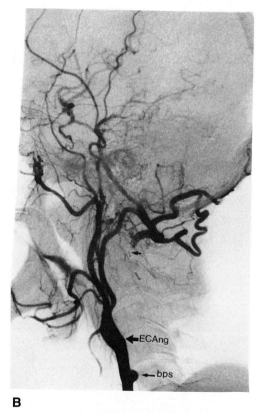

A   **B**

Figure 6–6. (A) Preoperative arteriogram showing an intraspinal VA occlusion, an ICA occlusion and a stenosis of the origin of the external carotid artery. The occluded VA is fed by muscular collaterals in the middle of the neck and by branches of the occipital artery (OCC) at the level of C-1. **(B)** Postoperative arteriogram showing the external carotid angioplasty (ECAng) and the stump of the occluded distal VA bypass (bps).

distal VA bypass was occluded. Electromagnetic flow measurements obtained after thrombectomy showed that the flow through the VA bypass graft rose from 26 to 78 mL/min when the external carotid or its occipital branch were clamped; clearly a matter of competitive flow. We documented this competitive flow situation during the operation, using an electromagnetic flowmeter in another patient who also had an external carotid angioplasty and a distal VA bypass. After thrombectomy the flow measured through the bypass increased fourfold when the occipital artery was clamped. In this patient the occipital artery was ligated, and the bypass graft to the distal VA remained patent.

One patient had recurrence of symptoms 2 years after a successful distal VA bypass. The arteriogram showed extensive intimal hyperplasia causing a preocclusive condition (Fig. 6–7). The vein graft was replaced by one of optimal caliber, and the reconstruction has remained open for a total of 7 years.

Other than dysesthesia or anesthesia in the territory of the external auricular nerve, which was present in approximately 30% of patients, there were no other peripheral nerve deficits found.

Follow-up

All patients had an arteriogram within a week of the operation. Follow-up with ultrasound has been done in all patients. In 18 patients late arteriograms were done to investigate new neurologic symptoms in the carotid or vertebral territories.

Figure 6–8 shows the life-expectancy curve of this group of patients. Figure 6–9

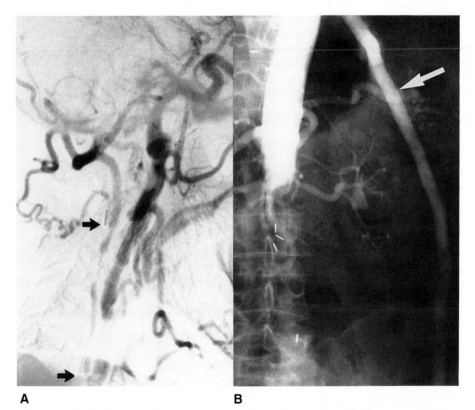

A   **B**

Figure 6–7. (A) Severe intimal hyperplasia in a vein bypass graft (between arrows) to the distal VA. **(B)** The bypass was replaced with a segment of saphenous vein.

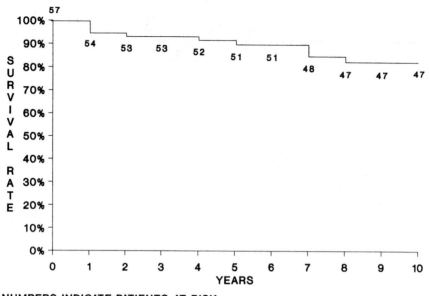

NUMBERS INDICATE PATIENTS AT RISK

Figure 6–8. Life table analysis of patients after distal VA reconstruction.

shows the cumulative secondary patency rate of the 57 patients undergoing distal VA revascularization. This graph includes one vein graft that was revised for intimal hyperplasia that caused a recurrence of symptoms 2 years after reimplantation.

Clinical results showed that 58% of the patients were cured and 20% had substantial improvement to the point of being able to carry on with their work and daily activities. A total of 78% of patients were therefore cured or had substantially improved after 10 years.

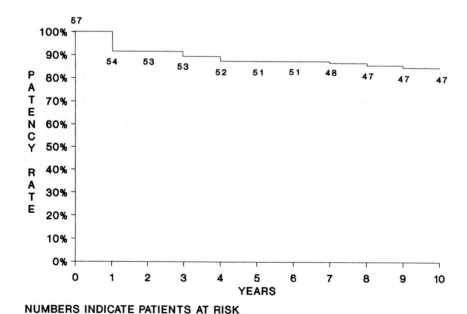

NUMBERS INDICATE PATIENTS AT RISK

Figure 6–9. Cumulative (secondary) patency rate of distal VA reconstructions.

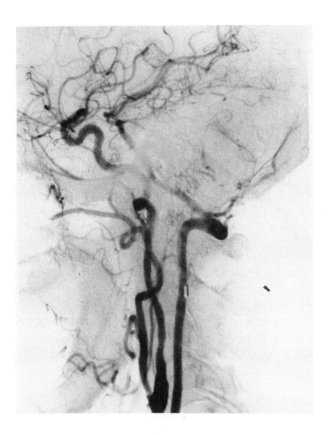

Figure 6–10. Postoperative arteriogram after combined carotid endarterectomy and distal vertebral bypass.

COMBINED CAROTID AND DISTAL VERTEBRAL ARTERY REVASCULARIZATION

Only seven patients underwent combined carotid and VA reconstruction (Fig. 6–10). Three of them were patients undergoing concomitant operations on the external carotid artery in whom the phenomenon of competitive flow was noted (see the Morbidity section under Distal Vertebral Artery Reconstruction). The other four patients underwent a concomitant ICA reconstruction. There were no operative deaths in these seven patients, but these numbers are too small to draw any conclusions.

COMMENTARY

Reconstruction of the proximal VA in patients is a safe procedure with a good outcome. The life expectancy of these patients and the good functional and clinical results of VA reconstruction validates its use in patients who satisfy the clinical and anatomic indications for surgery.

If a VA operation is to be combined with an ICA operation, one must be aware of the increased mortality and morbidity seen in this subgroup. Our death-to-stroke rate was 6.9%. Bahnini and colleagues[4] reported a death-to-stroke rate of 7.2% in a larger group of similar patients and referred to similar rates reported in patients undergoing ICA endarterectomy for VBI.[5] Patients in whom a combined carotid and VA reconstruction is indicated represent a substantially higher risk than those undergoing treatment for isolated carotid or vertebral disease. In addition, the multiplicity of their extracranial lesions and the ensuing loss of autoregulation makes this subgroup of patients more susceptible to a hyperperfusion syndrome following double revascularization of their ICA and VA. We nevertheless advised a combined operation in patients with the appropriate anatomic indications and symptoms of hemispheric, vertebrobasilar, or mixed location.

Distal VA reconstructions are more demanding technically than proximal reconstructions. Our early occlusion rate of 8% is disappointing and similar to the 7.5% reported by Kieffer and associates.[6] With one exception, these early occlusions can be traced to then unrecognized contraindications, such as a small VA or a concomitant external carotid revascularization creating competitive flow.

The one disastrous experience with gentle thrombectomy of the fourth segment of the VA would suggest that this is not a safe maneuver. If the thrombus distal to a failed reconstruction at the C-1 level cannot be removed by picking it up with forceps and with the help of back pressure, it is probably better to leave it alone.

Distal reconstructions are high-flow-rate bypasses, and their patency rates indicate that late occlusions are rare. The finding of intimal hyperplasia in these grafts used in both proximal and distal locations, however, calls for routine ultrasound follow-up.

In summary, reconstructions of the proximal VA have low risk and good patency rates and clinical results. The experience acquired with distal VA reconstruction has helped us to redefine indications and to avoid the technical problems observed in the early part of our series.

REFERENCES

1. Berguer R, Bauer RB. Vertebral artery reconstruction. *Ann Surg.* 1981;193:441–447.
2. McNamara MF, Berguer R. Simultaneous carotid-vertebral reconstruction. *J Cardiovasc Surg.* 1989;30:161–164.
3. Berguer R. Distal vertebral artery bypass: Technique, the "occipital connection" and potential uses. *J Vasc Surg.* 1985;2:621–626.
4. Bahnini A, Koskas F, Kieffer E. Combined carotid and vertebral surgery. In: Berguer R, and Caplan L, eds. *Vertebrobasilar Arterial Disease.* St. Louis, Mo: Quality Medical Publishing; 1982.
5. Brancherau A, Rudondy PH, Bartoli JM, et al. Chirurgie carotidienne daus l'insuffisance vertebro-basilaire. In: Kieffer E, ed. *Indications et resultats de la chirurgie carotidienne.* Paris: AERCU; 1988.
6. Kieffer E, Koskas F, Ranchurel G, et al. Reconstruction of distal vertebral artery. In: Berguer R, Caplan L, eds. *Vertebrobasilar Arterial Disease.* St. Louis, Mo: Quality Medical Publishing; 1982.

reason it seems appropriate to establish similar guidelines for surgical intervention. Unfortunately, controlled prospective randomized trials are currently not available to confirm these impressions. Therefore, surgical indications must be individualized based on the severity of symptoms, experience of the surgeon, and overall medical condition of each patient. At the University of California at Los Angeles, proximal carotid artery lesions are managed as follows. Asymptomatic stenoses or occlusions represent a stable clinical situation and require only careful follow-up for treatment. These patients are given complete information regarding the signs and symptoms of cerebrovascular and upper extremity ischemic syndromes and are re-examined frequently. Appropriate lesions that manifest typical symptoms are considered an indication for surgical repair.

Although the pathophysiology of the development of symptoms due to stenoses or occlusions of the proximal subclavian arteries is well understood, the natural history of these lesions remains poorly characterized. Again, this is probably due to the infrequency with which this problem is encountered in clinical practice. In the Joint Study of Extracranial Arterial Occlusion, only 17% of 6,534 patients were found to have a stenosis of 30% or greater in either the innominate or subclavian origins.[12] In a radiographic study, Ackermann and associates found that only 17% of 67 patients being followed for subclavian stenoses showed any degree of progression after a follow-up interval of approximately 2 years.[13] The long-term clinical outcome of these lesions also appears to be quite benign. One recent report noted 64% of 324 patients with documented reversal of flow in or both vertebral arteries, remained asymptomatic.[14] Bornstein and Norris reported that only 11% of 45 patients with asymptomatic subclavian steal became symptomatic during 2 years of observation, and none suffered a stroke.[15] In a related study, only 4 of 55 patients with a documented subclavian steal developed vertebrobasilar symptoms after a mean follow-up of over 4 years.[16] Also, none of these patients ever developed a posterior circulation infarct. Thus, unlike carotid bifurcation occlusive disease, one cannot make a convincing argument for prophylactic surgical intervention in asymptomatic patients with proximal subclavian artery disease. Furthermore, due to the very low risk of suffering an infarct, most surgeons agree that operation is only indicated for those patients experiencing frequent and disabling symptoms.[17,18]

HISTORIC PERSPECTIVES: THE EVOLUTION OF TREATMENT FOR BRACHIOCEPHALIC OCCLUSIVE DISEASE

Upper extremity and cerebral vascular insufficiency due to atherosclerotic occlusive disease of the proximal great vessels was first described in detail by Martorell and Fabre in 1944.[19] Soon after this report, a variety of syndromes related to occlusive disease in the major branches of the aortic arch became reorganized. Also, in addition to atherosclerosis, other pathologic processes, such as Takayasu's disease, were noted to be capable of producing similar symptoms.[20]

Arterial reconstructive surgery of proximal arch vessel lesions was introduced in the early 1950s. The first report on this topic was published by Shimizu and Sano in 1951.[20] In that paper the authors described their experience treating two proximal carotid occlusions. One patient underwent a retrograde thrombectomy through the external carotid artery, and the second was treated by replacing the occluded segment with a venous homograft. Intrathoracic repair of an arch lesion was probably first performed by Davis and associates in 1956.[21] That paper described the case of a patient with an innominate artery occlusion who was treated by thromboendarterectomy through a right anterior thoracotomy. Two years later, DeBakey and colleagues reported the first transthoracic repair of a great vessel lesion utilizing a prosthetic graft.[22] In that paper the authors described a patient who was treated for significant disease of both the innominate and right carotid arteries. At operation, an ascending aortic bifurcated Dacron graft was placed with the distal anastomoses to both the right carotid and subclavian arteries. The patient survived the operation and enjoyed long-term function of the reconstruction. Following that report, the approach was utilized with increasing frequency. In 1962, that same group reported on their results in 67 patients with occlusive arch lesions who were treated by either anterograde bypass or thromboendarterectomy.[23] All of these procedures were performed through a transthoracic approach. Although the functional results were acceptable, with most surviving patients reporting relief of preoperative symptoms, the surgical mortality was alarmingly high. This high mortality rate was probably due to the high incidence of concomitant coronary artery disease in this selected group of patients.

The high mortality of transthoracic procedures caused great concern during the early experience in the surgical management of these lesions. This concern grew stronger as information regarding the natural history of arch vessel lesions became available. Although a selected number of symptomatic proximal lesions involving the origin of the innominate and carotid vessels were well known to pose a significant risk of subsequent neurologic events, disease in other locations was clearly much less worrisome. In particular, proximal lesions of the subclavian arteries, even when symptomatic, possess little or no potential for resulting in a significant cerebrovascular deficit. Thus, in this setting, the high mortality associated with transthoracic repair of subclavian stenoses or occlusions was difficult to justify.

In 1967, Diethrich and associates introduced the carotid–subclavian bypass.[24] Because of the good results and very low mortality described in that report, the technique was recommended as the procedure of choice in patients with appropriate lesions. Specifically, proximal lesions of either the carotid or subclavian vessels are amenable to this method. The first large series reported by Crawford and colleagues in 1969 confirmed the initial impressions regarding the mortality of this procedure.[25] In that paper, the authors reported a reduction in operative mortality from 22% to 5.6% when comparing transthoracic and extrathoracic approaches, respectively.

CURRENT SURGICAL MANAGEMENT

Currently, a variety of treatment options are available for the patient with symptomatic occlusive lesions of the great vessels, including anterograde anatomic reconstructions, endarterectomy, and autologous transpositions, as well as a variety of extraanatomical bypass procedures. In general, the transthoracic approach is reserved for low-risk patients with proximal disease involving the innominate artery. Also, patients with concomitant coronary artery disease who require coronary artery bypass grafting are often treated with a simultaneous repair. Endarterectomy of arch vessel lesions has proven to be a durable procedure and is still advocated by some surgeons. At UCLA we use this technique most often for short, isolated lesions of the innominate artery that do not extend into the aortic arch. Limited lesions of the other vessels can also be easily managed in this way, particularly when the patient is undergoing a simultaneous intrathoracic procedure. For patients with disease limited to either the carotid or subclavian vessels, the transthoracic approach is generally avoided. Although improvements in preoperative cardiac evaluation, intraoperative techniques, and postoperative management have led to a decrease in mortality from this approach, modern studies continue to report mortality rates as high as 14.7%.[26] Two additional contemporary series reported surgical deaths of 6.7%[27] and 18.7%,[5] respectively, for transthoracic procedures compared with no deaths in patients undergoing an extrathoracic reconstruction.

The management of occlusive disease of the common carotid artery depends on the location of the lesion. Occlusions secondary to a carotid bifurcation lesion that result in retrograde thrombosis are best approached by exposing the bifurcation in the usual fashion. After performing a standard bifurcation endarterectomy, restoration of blood flow can usually be accomplished by retrograde thrombectomy. Even though the internal carotid is often found to be occluded in this setting, the external carotid beginning just beyond the superior thyroid branch is almost always patent. If the retrograde thrombectomy fails to restore normal anterograde flow, a subclavian-to-carotid bifurcation bypass graft can easily be constructed. Alternatively, some surgeons prefer to perform a carotid-to-subclavian transposition in this situation. In either case, it is important to completely exclude the occluded carotid segment from the circulation to prevent further embolization. For lesions at the origin of the common carotid artery, surgical options include performing either a subclavian-to-carotid bypass or a carotid-to-subclavian transposition. The latter procedure has the advantage of excluding the occluded segment from the cerebral circulation and is therefore preferred if it is suspected that the patient's lesion is a source of emboli.

Proximal lesions of the subclavian artery requiring treatment are best managed with an extrathoracic repair. Options include a carotid-to-subclavian bypass, subclavian-to-carotid transposition, or a variety of crossover extraanatomic bypass procedures. When selecting the ipsilateral carotid as a donor vessel for subclavian reconstruction, several principles should be followed. First, care must be taken to ensure that the donor carotid is free of significant disease. A proximal stenosis can compromise the function of the subclavian reconstruction and may lead to the development of a significant "carotid steal." Likewise, a significant occlusive lesion at the level of the bifurcation may lead to preferential flow through the subclavian reconstruction and also siphon blood away from the internal carotid. The development of symptoms of ischemia in the ipsilateral anterior circulation from a carotid steal, following extrathoracic reconstruction of the subclavian artery, has long been a theoretical concern. Recently this phenomenon was described clinically in a patient who developed a carotid bifurcation lesion 2 years after a carotid–subclavian bypass.[28] However, laboratory and clinical evidence has demonstrated that, in the absence of any significant lesion in the donor carotid, this phenomenon does not occur.[18,29] If disease exists in the donor carotid, it should be corrected before a carotid–subclavian reconstruction is performed.

RESULTS

Early

The early results of carotid–subclavian bypass procedures, reported in nine contemporary studies, are reviewed in Table 7–1. For the purpose of contrast, a comprehensive review of the experience accumulated prior to 1981 is also included in this table.[30] In this latter report, F. J. Criado summarized the results of all extrathoracic procedures performed for arch vessel disease from every English-language study that appeared in the literature between 1962 and 1980. For carotid–subclavian bypasses, he recorded 426 operations, from which there were 8 surgical deaths, for a mortality rate of 1.9%.

TABLE 7–1. EARLY RESULTS OF CAROTID–SUBCLAVIAN BYPASS PROCEDURES[a]

Author	Year	Number of Patients	Deaths	Strokes	Patency	Other Complications
Criado[30]	1962–1980	426	8(1.9%)	8(1.9%)	423(99%)	3 false aneurysms, 2 nerve injuries, 2 thoracic duct injuries
Depalma and Broadbent[38]	1981	14	0(0.0%)	0(0.0%)	14(100%)	1 pleural effusion
Vogt et al[26]	1982	37	0(0.0%)	2(5.4%)	37(100%)	
Crawford et al[39]	1983	95	1(1.1%)	3(3.2%)	93 (98%)	
Ziomek et al[33]	1986	31	1(3.2%)	2(6.4%)	29 (94%)	
Sterpetti et al[32]	1989	30	0(0.0%)	1(3.3%)	30(100%)	2 nerve injuries
Defraigne et al[40]	1990	29	1(3.4%)	1(3.4%)	27 (93%)	
Perler and Williams[18]	1990	28	0(0.0%)	1(3.6%)	27 (96%)	2 nerve injuries
Kretschmer et al[35]	1991	19	0(0.0%)	1(5.3%)	17 (89%)	1 wound hematoma
Fry et al[34]	1992	20	1(5.0%)	0(0.0%)	20(100%)	4 nerve injuries
Total		303	4(1.3%)	11(3.6%)	294 (97%)	8 nerve injuries, 1 wound hematoma, 1 pleural effusion

[a] Series includes all types of grafts (prosthetic and autologous vein) placed for both proximal common carotid and subclavian lesions.

Eight perioperative strokes (4 fatal) were reported, yielding a 30-day stroke rate of 1.9%. Finally, 3 grafts failed in the immediate postoperative period, and, therefore, the early patency rate was calculated at 423 to 426, or 99%. The cumulative early mortality since 1981 has remained relatively unchanged. Of 303 patients reported between 1981 and 1992, there have been 4 perioperative deaths, yielding a mortality rate of 1.3%. Approximately half of all these deaths were due to myocardial infarction. Interestingly, the 30-day stroke rate has increased slightly from 1.9% to 3.6%. There are several possible explanations for this observation. First, early reports maintained the practice of not recording posterior circulation or contralateral operative strokes. Second, a parallel trend towards treatment of higher risk patients has influenced these results. Lastly, advances in technology have increased the sensitivity for detecting subtle neurologic events that previously may have gone unrecorded.

The early results of subclavian-to-carotid transposition procedures are shown in Table 7–2. Again a comparison between the early experience and contemporary series is provided. Although the numbers are considerably smaller, the early 30-day results of this procedure are clearly superior to carotid–subclavian bypass operations. The cumulative surgical mortality rate in recent series is 0.6%, with a 0% incidence of perioperative stroke. Also, an initial patency rate of 100% has been achieved. This operation does seem to be associated with a higher incidence of other complications, but damage to peripheral nerves is more common, as is injury to the main thoracic lymphatic duct. This morbidity is only temporary, however, as nearly all of these injuries resolve spontaneously. Furthermore, the largest reported series of subclavian–carotid transpositions recorded no wound, nerve, or lymphatic injuries, suggesting that increased experience with this procedure may reduce the incidence of these

TABLE 7–2. EARLY RESULTS OF SUBCLAVIAN–CAROTID TRANSPOSITION PROCEDURES

Author	Year	Number of Patients	Deaths	Strokes	Patency	Other Complications
Criado[30]	1962–1980	97	0 (0.0%)	0 (0.0%)	97 (100%)	3 nerve injuries, 1 thoracic duct fistula
Ziomek et al[33]	1986	5	0 (0.0%)	0 (0.0%)	5 (100%)	
Sandmann et al[31]	1987	72	1 (1.4%)	0 (0.0%)	72 (100%)	
Weimann et al[41]	1987	38	0 (0.0%)	0 (0.0%)	38 (100%)	3 nerve injuries, 1 wound hematoma, 1 thoracic duct fistula
Sterpetti et al[32]	1989	16	0 (0.0%)	0 (0.0%)	16 (100%)	3 nerve injuries
Kretschmer et al[35]	1991	32	0 (0.0%)	0 (0.0%)	32 (100%)	6 nerve injuries, 2 thoracic duct fistulas
Total		163	1 (0.6%)	0 (0.0%)	163 (100%)	12 nerve injuries, 1 wound hematoma, 3 thoracic duct fistulas

complications.[31] A likely explanation for the lower surgical risk observed in transposition series is the overall condition of those patients selected for this procedure. Most surgeons prefer the less complicated bypass procedure when faced with an operation in a high-risk patient. This practice no doubt preselects those cases for subclavian–carotid transposition from a group of patients that carries a lower overall risk.

Late

The late results of carotid–subclavian bypass procedures are shown in Table 7–3. Unfortunately, long-term clinical outcomes in earlier studies are not available. However, a patency rate of 96%, with follow-up ranging from 9 to 204 months has been reported.[30] Contemporary studies report long-term patency rates from 74% to 100%, with a combined overall experience of 87%. Furthermore, approximately 82% of patients remained free of all cerebral vascular symptoms at follow-up at 1 to 264 months. Life Table analysis of the long-term patency of carotid–subclavian bypass is only available in two recent series.[18,32] In the paper by Sterpetti and associates, a 7-year actuarial patency rate for 30 carotid–subclavian bypasses was reported to be 86%.[32] The 5- and 8-year patency rates by Life Table methods, reported by Perler and Williams, were 92% and 83%, respectively.[18]

The choice of conduit appears to have a significant effect of the long-term patency of carotid–subclavian bypass procedures (Table 7–4). This difference in the performance of prosthetic versus autologous vein grafts was first noted by Ziomek and colleagues in 1986.[33] In their review of 31 cases (18 prosthetic grafts and 13 vein grafts), these authors reported a 5-year patency rate by Life Table methods of 91% for prosthetic grafts compared with only 57% for venous bypasses. Table 7–4 shows the cumulative results of those series in which results were analyzed according to the choice of conduit. In the experience since 1981, the patency rate for 92 prosthetic grafts is 91%, compared with 85% for vein bypasses, with a follow-up of up to 180 months. Several reasons have been postulated to account for the superiority of prosthetic

TABLE 7–3. LATE RESULTS OF CAROTID–SUBCLAVIAN BYPASS PROCEDURES[a]

Author	Year	Number of Patients	Deaths	Strokes	Patency	Free of Symptoms	Follow-up (months)
Criado[30]	1962–1980	426	NA	NA	409 (96%)	NA	9–204
Depalma and Broadbent[38]	1981	14	3 (21%)	NA	14 (100%)	12 (86%)	3–144
Vogt et al[26]	1982	37	NA	NA	32 (87%)	30 (81%)	2–189
Crawford et al[39]	1983	95	7 (7%)	10 (11%)	NA	80 (84%)	9–264
Ziomek et al[33]	1986	31	3 (10%)	5 (17%)	24 (79%)	22 (70%)	9–156
Sterpetti et al[32]	1989	30	0 (0%)	0 (0%)	26 (87%)	23 (77%)	2–148
Defraigne et al[40]	1990	29	5 (17%)	0 (0%)	26 (90%)	26 (90%)	mean 40
Perler and Williams[18]	1990	28	6 (21%)	1 (4%)	24 (86%)	22 (80%)	1–121
Kretschmer et al[35]	1991	19	3 (16%)	NA	14 (74%)	NA	1–120
Fry et al[34]	1992	20	5 (25%)	1 (5%)	20 (100%)	19 (95%)	1–122
Total		303	32 (12%)	17 (7.3%)	180 (87%)	234 (82%)	

[a] Series includes all types of grafts (prosthetic and autologous vein) placed for both proximal common carotid and subclavian lesions.
NA: Not available

TABLE 7–4. PATENCY RATES OF CAROTID–SUBCLAVIAN BYPASS PROCEDURES ACCORDING TO TYPE OF CONDUIT USED

Author	Year	Number of Patients	Prosthetic		Autologous Vein		Follow-up
			No.	Patency	No.	Patency	(months)
Criado[30]	1962–1980	361	302	298 (99%)	59	48 (81%)	9–204
Depalma et al[38]	1981	14	14	14 (100%)	NA	NA	3–144
Vogt et al[26]	1982	37	1	1 (100%)	36	30 (83%)	2–180
Ziomek et al[33]	1986	36	17	16 (94%)	12	7 (58%)	6–108
Sterpetti et al[32]	1989	30	24	21 (88%)	6	5 (83%)	2–148
Defraigne et al[40]	1990	29	14	12 (86%)	15	14 (93%)	mean 40
Perler and Williams[18]	1990	28	26	23 (88%)	2	2 (100%)	1–121
Fry et al[34]	1992	20	5	5 (100%)	15	15 (100%)	1–122
Total		194	101	92 (91%)	86	73 (85%)	

NA: Not available

conduits in this position, including the small size of the venous conduits and the possibility of graft kinking due to neck motion in several axes. It should be mentioned that, in the most recent series of 15 carotid–subclavian bypass grafts constructed with autologous vein, the long-term patency rate after a follow-up of between 1 and 122 months was 100%.[34] It is interesting to note, however, that all of these grafts were subclavian-to-carotid bypasses performed for proximal lesions in the common carotid. It is possible that the configuration of these grafts, and the relative low resistance of the cerebral circulation compared with that in the upper extremity, contribute to the favorable outcome observed in this setting.

The late mortality and postoperative incidence of stroke are also shown in Table 7–3. Overall, between 7% and 25% of patients had died during the follow-up period. The vast majority of these deaths were related to coronary artery disease, a fact that highlights the importance of an adequate preoperative cardiac evaluation in these patients as well as careful postoperative follow-up. The stroke rates following these procedures are very difficult to interpret for several reasons. First, information regarding the location of the infarct is frequently not available. Second, follow-up is often incomplete, and Life Table methods are rarely used. Finally, adequate knowledge of the natural history of an untreated lesion, as well as randomized prospective trials to accurately predict the long-term stroke risk in operated patients, are both unavailable.

The late results of subclavian-to-carotid transposition procedures are summarized in Table 7–5. Again, due to the preselection of healthier patients, the postoperative mortality rates are lower than those for bypass operations. The low late-stroke rates that have been reported are impressive; however, these have yet to be tested in randomized prospective trials. As expected, the patency rates are higher than those reported for bypass procedures, no doubt due to the absence of a small-diameter bypass conduit, and a somewhat more favorable anatomical configuration.

COMPLICATIONS

Complications following extrathoracic operations for proximal lesions of the common carotid and subclavian arteries include those problems common to all surgical procedures, as well as some specific injuries related to the complex anatomy of the supraclavicular fossa. As always, wound complications, such as bleeding and infec-

TABLE 7–5. SUMMARY OF LATE RESULTS OF SUBCLAVIAN–CAROTID TRANSPOSITION PROCEDURES

Author	Year	Number of Patients	Deaths	Strokes	Patency	Free of Symptoms	Follow-up (months)
Criado[30]	1962–1980	97	0 (0%)	0 (0%)	97 (100%)	NA	6–192
Ziomek et al[33]	1986	5	0 (0%)	0 (0%)	5 (100%)	4 (80%)	9–156
Sandmann et al[31]	1987	72	8 (11%)	2 (3%)	68 (95%)	59 (82%)	mean 46
Weimann et al[41]	1987	38	0 (0%)	0 (0%)	37 (97%)	38 (100%)	mean 13
Sterpetti et al[32]	1989	16	0 (0%)	1 (6%)	16 (100%)	15 (94%)	2–148
Kretschmer et al[35]	1991	32	6 (19%)	0 (0%)	32 (100%)	NA	1–120
Total		163	14 (9%)	3 (2%)	158 (97%)	116 (89%)	

NA: Not available

tion, do occur. However, because of the rich vascularity of this region, their incidence follows an inverse relationship, that is, wound hematomas and reoperations for bleeding are not uncommon, whereas postoperative infections are exceedingly rare. Specific complications unique to these procedures include injury to the adjacent nerve and lymphatic structures. Unfortunately, although it is not possible to accurately assign a precise incidence for each of these complications, surgeons performing these procedures must be aware of the possibility of injury to these structures. It is, therefore, useful to describe each of these special complications separately in the hope of minimizing such injuries in the future.

Phrenic Nerve Palsy

The phrenic nerve passes directly over the anterior scalene muscle along its course from the neck into the mediastinum. Because supraclavicular exposure of the subclavian artery frequently involves division of this muscle, damage to the phrenic nerve at this level is not uncommon. Even though direct injury to the nerve is rare, traction and devascularization may produce temporary or permanent paralysis of the ipsilateral hemidiaphragm. In the papers reviewed in Table 7–1, 6 of the 8 nerve injuries reported in the contemporary studies involved the phrenic nerve for an overall incidence is approximately 2%. Of the 12 nerve complications reported following transposition procedures, 3 represented phrenic nerve injuries yielding an identical incidence of 2% (see Table 7–2). Injury to this nerve can be minimized by careful retraction and incomplete removal of the surrounding scalene musculature to preserve the vascular supply.

Recurrent Nerve Palsy

Injury to the recurrent laryngeal nerve can occur either directly from trauma or indirectly from injury to the vagus nerve. Injury to the recurrent laryngeal nerve leads to vocal cord paralysis, and patients most often manifest this by signs of hoarseness. Direct injury to the recurrent nerve usually occurs where this structure courses around the subclavian artery. Because the medial exposure of the subclavian through the supraclavicular surgical approach comes in close proximity to the carotid sheath, the vagus nerve is at risk of injury in this location. Also, the vagus is obviously in close proximity during dissection of the proximal common carotid. The incidence of recurrent nerve injury in bypass procedures was 1 in 303 patients, or 0.3%. This

8

Innominate Artery Bypass:

A Ten-Year Follow-Up

George J. Reul, MD, Michael J. H. M. Jacobs, MD, PhD, Igor D. Gregoric, MD, and Denton A. Cooley, MD

Symptomatic innominate artery disease is uncommon compared with other types of extracranial disease. Thus, surgical reports involving innominate artery lesions alone are rare.[1,2] At the Texas Heart Institute, surgery for innominate artery lesions has accounted for only 2% of operations on extracranial vessels to manage cerebral vascular occlusive disease.

Most reports of innominate artery occlusive lesions are incorporated in reports of other types of arch vessel constructions.[3-10] In this chapter, which summarizes our experience with innominate artery revascularization procedures at the Texas Heart Institute during a 10-year period, we also include procedures that were done to correct other lesions of the arch vessels. We emphasize, however, the important role of the innominate artery in multiple arch vessel disease and the extra precautions that must be taken during vascular reconstruction in such cases.

INDICATIONS FOR SURGERY

The classic indications for revascularization of the innominate artery remain either hypoperfusion or embolization resulting from the lesion. Grosveld and colleagues[11] reported that ultrasonic duplex scanning, with hemodynamic measurements before and after arm exercise, allowed for differentiation between hemodynamically significant and insignificant innominate artery lesions. At our institution, this technique has been used to determine the presence of steal syndromes and to attempt to reproduce the patient's symptoms. The standard indications established for carotid endarterectomy can be applied as indications for innominate artery surgery. Surgery of the innominate artery is indicated in cases involving severe anatomic lesions (i.e., ≥80% stenosis) or severely ulcerated plaque (≥50%) and should be performed in all patients with symptoms referable to the lesion.

SURGICAL APPROACH

Important considerations in revascularization of the innominate artery are the choice of inflow, type of reconstruction, concomitant procedures, and cerebral protection. Although the transthoracic approach was recommended in early reports of arch vessel revascularization,[12,13] this approach resulted in high morbidity and mortality.[14] Extrathoracic repair improved results,[15–17] and in at least one instance of a patent cervical inflow artery, the extrathoracic approach has been proposed as the treatment of choice for high-risk patients.[18,19] This approach is especially applicable to occlusive lesions of the subclavian and carotid arteries, which have been successfully managed by carotid–subclavian or axillary–carotid bypass.[20,21] The intrathoracic approach to endarterectomy has been advocated by Cherry and coworkers.[2]

SURGICAL TECHNIQUE

Revascularization procedures involving the innominate artery are performed with the use of general anesthesia; high-dose barbiturate support is used during arterial occlusion. Two-lead encephalography is used to determine the depth of anesthesia and barbiturate administration. Proper positioning of the head is stressed, especially in cases involving multiple lesions, to prevent occlusion of the collateral sources. Arterial blood pressure and cardiac rhythm should be constantly maintained, especially during periods of arterial clamping. Heparin (1 mg/kg) is administered prior to occlusion. The distal portion of the artery is occluded first to prevent embolization. We do not use shunts except in selected cases of combined procedures involving internal carotid endarterectomy when the shunt can be easily placed.

PATIENT CHARACTERISTICS

During a 10-year period, 54 patients with innominate artery occlusive lesions underwent revascularization procedures at the Texas Heart Institute at St. Luke's Episcopal Hospital. The patient population consisted of 28 men (52%) and 26 women (48%), ranging in age from 16 to 75 years (mean, 49.8 years). Of the 54 patients, 42 had a history of smoking, and 35 had more than one cardiac risk factor. Fifteen patients had undergone previous coronary artery bypass surgery for severe coronary artery disease. Diabetes mellitus was present in 12 patients.

Three patients had undergone an operation for occluded grafts prior to the 10 years included in the study; one of those had had a third operation because of two failed attempts. Three patients had previous carotid endarterectomy; in all three, the carotid vessels were patent. Four additional patients had previously placed extrathoracic bypasses; one of those had undergone extrathoracic bypass with carotid endarterectomy.

DIAGNOSIS AND CLINICAL FINDINGS

Diagnosis of innominate artery disease includes selective arch aortography, often with digital subtraction techniques. Computed tomography or magnetic resonance imaging is also performed when indicated.

TABLE 8–1. DISTRIBUTION OF DISEASE

	Number of Patients	Percentage
Innominate artery alone	21	39
Innominate artery + right carotid	2	4
Innominate artery + left carotid[a]	17	31
Innominate artery + left carotid[a] + left subclavian	8	15
Innominate artery + left subclavian	6	11
Totals	54	100

[a] Seven patients had occlusion of left carotid artery.

Significant stenosis in our series was calibrated as reported by Baker and associates.[22] Stenosis was believed to be significant if there was 80% or more encroachment on the lumen of the artery. The innominate artery alone was involved in 21 patients (39%); it was occluded in 6 patients and significantly stenosed in 15. In the remaining 33 patients with combined lesions, the innominate artery was occluded in 13, and high-grade stenosis was noted in 20. The left common carotid artery was occluded in 6 patients and the left internal carotid artery in 1 (Table 8–1).

In these patients, 19 vessels (35%) were totally occluded. Because of the severity of these lesions, the collateral circulation would be expected to be well developed. However, all but four patients were symptomatic with respect to the vascular territory. Multiple-vessel involvement did not appear to affect the development of neurologic deficits, although cerebral flow was supported during reconstructive procedures in the four patients who had undergone previous extrathoracic bypass and in the three patients who had had previous carotid endarterectomy.

SURGICAL EXPERIENCE

Revascularization procedures in our series were performed to correct not only the innominate artery stenosis but also other lesions of the arch vessels. The extrathoracic approach was used in 16 patients (30%), and the intrathoracic approach was used in 38 (70%). Endarterectomy of the innominate artery was performed in 8 patients who had innominate artery lesions alone, and it was done in combination with left common (at the origin) or internal carotid endarterectomy in 3 additional patients. Endarterectomy was not done if there was any evidence of distal disease. Three patients had Dacron patch closure of the endarterectomy site, 5 patients had direct closure, and 3 had interposition grafts after endarterectomy in conjunction with resection of an ascending thoracic aneurysm (Table 8–2).

Our preferred procedure, the intrathoracic approach with bypass graft, was undertaken in 27 patients. A variety of bypass grafts were created in these procedures (Fig. 8–1). Twenty-five patients underwent standard median sternotomy with extension or separate incisions in the areas to be bypassed (Fig. 8–2). The other two patients had a limited right anterior parasternal thoracotomy, wherein exposure of the ascending aorta was achieved through the second or third interspace. Appropriate tunneling of the graft and a separate incision at the distal artery were done.

Extrathoracic repair was used in 16 patients considered to be at high risk for intrathoracic repair. Contraindications included severe calcification of the ascending aorta and arch; a previous intrathoracic procedure, such as coronary artery bypass; and poor general condition or advanced age. Carotid-to-carotid bypass was preferred

TABLE 8–2. SURGICAL PROCEDURES CLASSIFIED BY APPROACH

Surgical Procedure[a]	Innominate Artery Alone	Innominate Artery with Other Lesions	Number of Patients	Percentage
Extrathoracic	*7*	*9*	*16*	*30*
Carotid–carotid bypass	3	5	8	
Carotid–carotid–subclavian	1	3	4	
Subclavian–subclavian	3	1	4	
Intrathoracic	*14*	*24*	*38*	*70*
Endarterectomy				
Innominate artery	8	—	8	
Innominate artery + left carotid	—	3	3	
Bypass				
Aorta–right carotid artery	3	4	7	
Aorta–right carotid artery–left carotid artery	—	3	3	
Aorta–right carotid artery–left subclavian artery	—	1	1	
Aorta–right carotid artery–right subclavian artery	1	1	2	
Aorta–right carotid artery–right subclavian artery–left carotid artery	—	1	1	
Aorta–innominate artery	2	1	3	
Aorta–innominate artery–right subclavian artery–left subclavian artery	—	2	2	
Aorta–innominate artery–left carotid artery		2	2	
Aorta–innominate artery–left subclavian artery		2	2	
Aorta–innominate artery–left subclavian artery–left carotid artery		1	1	
Aorta–right subclavian artery	—	1	1	
Aorta–right subclavian artery–left subclavian artery		1	1	
Aorta–right subclavian artery–left subclavian artery–left carotid artery		1	1	
Total	21	33	54	

[a] All bypasses involving the carotid arteries involved the common carotid (except combined procedures).

if the left carotid flow was adequate and there was no distal carotid disease. A carotid–carotid–subclavian bypass was done in 4 patients with double-vessel disease in whom an intrathoracic approach was contraindicated. Four patients had a subclavian-to-subclavian bypass; in 2, the left carotid artery was totally occluded (see Table 8–2).

Our principal goal in each of these procedures was to bypass all significantly occluded arteries while using inflow from the ascending aorta. In cases involving ulcerative lesions or symptoms of distal embolization, the innominate artery was transected and anastomosed end to end to the Dacron graft. In instances with no apparent ulceration noted on the arteriogram and no distal embolization, an end-to-side anastomosis was completed to either the innominate, right carotid, or right subclavian artery, depending on the degree of distal or associated lesions. Bypass grafts to the left carotid and left subclavian arteries were also created when indicated. Simultaneous carotid endarterectomy was accomplished in six patients, using the standard indications for isolated carotid endarterectomy.

All but four patients had Dacron grafts. The remainder had Goretex grafts (W.L.

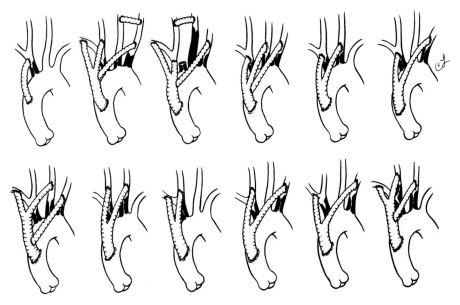

Figure 8–1. Schematic drawings of the various types of vascular reconstruction used in 27 patients who underwent revascularization by an intrathoracic approach and bypass grafting of the innominate artery and accompanying lesions. In patients with innominate artery lesions alone, when the intrathoracic bypass technique was used, a bypass was placed from the ascending aorta to the innominate artery, right carotid, or right subclavian artery depending on the degree of distal vessel involvement and exposure. (*Reprinted with permission: J Vasc Surg. 1991;14:408.*)

Gore & Associates, Elkton, MD). A double-velour Dacron graft was preferred, although in some instances, we used a woven Dacron graft (Meadox Medicals, Oakland, NJ) because of previous heparinization and inability to preclot the graft prior to the decision to use a Dacron graft. Most double-vessel bypasses were carried out with a 12 × 7-mm double velour bifurcation graft (Meadox Medicals, Oakland,

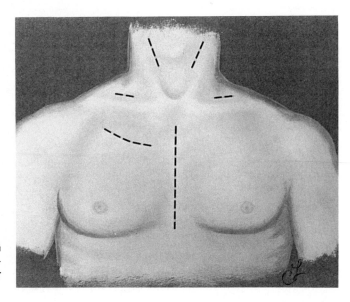

Figure 8–2. Standard median sternotomy approach for operation, with separate incisions for areas to be bypassed.

NJ). If the thoracic outlet and substernal area were compromised in any way by the patient's size or other factors, single 7- or 8-mm Dacron grafts were preferred.

In two patients, a previously placed right-carotid-to-left-carotid bypass provided the only inflow for cerebral circulation. One patient had previously undergone carotid–carotid bypass to supply inflow to the left carotid artery. She developed occlusion of the left subclavian and left common carotid arteries and high-grade ulcerated stenosis of the innominate artery with transient ischemic attacks related to the right hemisphere. The left vertebral artery was also occluded (Fig. 8–3). In order to provide circulation during the innominate artery resection, the right side of a bifurcation graft from the ascending aorta was placed to the right subclavian artery first. This provided for retrograde flow through the right subclavian artery to the right and left common carotid arteries through the previously placed carotid–carotid bypass. Another Dacron graft was placed from the bifurcation graft to the left subclavian artery. The ulcerated and stenotic innominate artery was then resected and anastomosed end to end directly to the other side of the bifurcation graft. This provided for complete revascularization of all three arch vessels and cerebral protection by the right subclavian graft (Fig. 8–4). Both patients with similar occlusive problems recovered well without further evidence of neurologic deficits.

Placement of a bifurcation graft requires an exacting technique, since kinking may easily occur if the graft is not placed at the most proximal portion of the ascending aorta. Also, the graft must be placed on the right side of the ascending aorta rather than the anterior surface to avoid compromise by the sternum. The graft must be beveled appropriately and a large incision made on the aorta to prevent kinking at the bifurcation site. The limbs of the graft must not be too tightly connected to the distal arteries, since movement of the head and neck may be restricted if the graft is too tight and fibrosis fixes it in an inflexible position. Individual grafts must be used if the aorta is calcified and a wide aortotomy cannot be completed.

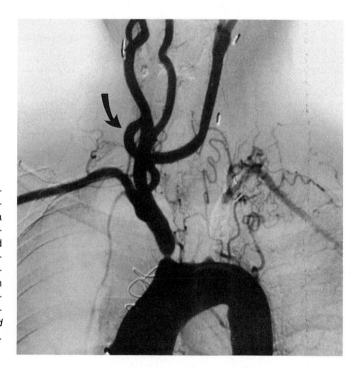

Figure 8–3. Preoperative aortogram in a patient who had a previous carotid bypass (arrow) for a totally occluded left internal carotid artery. The left vertebral and subclavian arteries were also occluded. Severe stenosis developed in the innominate artery with distal embolization. Ocular symptoms and cortical transient ischemia attacks followed. (*Reprinted with permission:* J Vasc Surg. *1991;14:409.*)

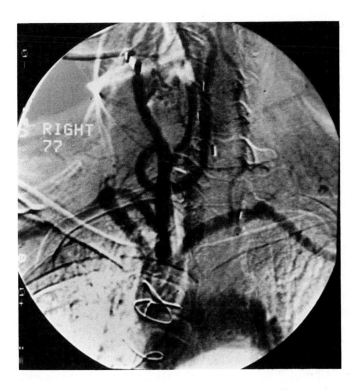

Figure 8–4. Postoperative digital subtraction aortogram shows patency of the right subclavian, innominate, and left subclavian bypass grafts with good distal filling. The patient improved clinically and suffered no neurologic sequelae. (*Reprinted with permission:* J Vasc Surg. *1991;14:410.*)

In most instances of combined occlusive disease of the left internal carotid and innominate arteries, a staged procedure was done. This consisted of a left carotid endarterectomy followed by appropriate surgery on the right side. If all vessels were occluded with no allowance for proper inflow to an internal carotid artery, we then preferred to complete all procedures simultaneously, including the carotid endarterectomy.

COMPLICATIONS OF SURGERY

Neurologic Complications

Despite the importance of the vascular territory supplied by the innominate artery and the frequent involvement of other arch vessels, few neurologic complications have occurred following innominate artery reconstruction. Results are comparable to those of uncomplicated carotid endarterectomy. On the other hand, the innominate artery may be the last supplying blood vessel in cases of multiple arch vessel disease, and extra precautions must be taken during vascular reconstruction.

Neurologic symptoms, which are commonly associated with innominate artery disease, were noted in 25 patients in our series (Table 8–3). Arm ischemia was the underlying mechanism for pain in 8 patients (claudication in 6 patients and microembolization in 2). Combined neurologic symptoms, not related to the innominate vascular territory, were present in 17 patients. Four patients with high-grade stenosis of the innominate artery had no symptoms.

The 25 patients who had neurologic symptoms related to the innominate vascular territory exhibited a wide distribution of vascular involvement. Sixteen of the 25 patients had ocular involvement in the form of amaurosis fugax or permanent

TABLE 8–3. NEUROLOGIC SYMPTOMS AND RELATED VASCULAR TERRITORY

Symptoms (Site)[a]	Number of Patients
A	4
B	4
C	4
A + B	7
A + C	5
B + C	1
Total	25 (46%)

[a] *Legend:* A = carotid ocular, B = carotid cortical, C = vertebrobasilar.

embolic deficits. Ten patients had vertebrobasilar symptoms, and 12 patients had cerebral hemispheric symptoms. By using the CHAT system proposed by Baker and associates,[22] we noted carotid ocular vascular territory involvement in 4 patients, carotid cortical in 4, and vertebrobasilar involvement in 4. Combined carotid ocular–cortical symptoms were present in 7 patients, carotid ocular–vertebrobasilar symptoms in 5, and carotid cortical–vertebrobasilar symptoms in 1.

Preoperative status of neurologic symptoms up to 1 year was recorded according to the CHAT classification.[22] Twenty-two of the 25 patients had a transient ischemic attack, which lasted less than 24 hours. One patient had a stroke, but fully recovered within 3 weeks; 2 other patients had minor strokes, both of which lasted more than 3 weeks.

The neurologic deficits that occurred in the perioperative period stemmed from the contralateral hemisphere and were unrelated to the area supplied by the innominate artery. Despite the multiplicity of disease patterns and severity of the lesions, clinically detectable cerebral ischemia did not result from surgical clamping of the arch vessels.

Graft Occlusion

Early graft occlusion (within 30 days after surgery) occurred in 3 of 43 patients (7%) who underwent bypass revascularization. Failure after endarterectomy occurred early in 1 of the 11 patients (9%) who underwent endarterectomy.

The patient who had innominate artery occlusion also had a simultaneous left common carotid endarterectomy; the carotid artery later reoccluded. Extensive disease had been found in both arteries, and an adequate removal of the plaque was followed by primary closure. Forty-eight hours after surgery, the patient developed a right hemiparesis. A bifurcation graft was then placed from the aorta to the innominate artery and to the left carotid artery. After thrombectomy the patient had a permanent residual deficit of right hemiparesis. This was the only patient with a permanent deficit, and it was not related to the innominate artery vascular territory.

Graft occlusion occurred in one patient who underwent extrathoracic bypass. He had a left subclavian–left carotid–right carotid bypass with Dacron graft to manage innominate and left carotid stenosis. Immediately after surgery, the graft occluded and right hemiparesis developed. The patient then underwent a thrombectomy followed by aorta-to-graft bypass. The neurologic symptoms completely resolved, and he recovered without difficulty. The inflow from the left subclavian artery apparently was not enough to sustain flow, thus causing the thrombosis.

Two patients had early graft occlusion after surgery with the transthoracic approach. The first patient, a 24-year-old woman with severe diffuse arteritis, had innominate–right common carotid and left common carotid artery occlusion. An aorta-to-right subclavian–right carotid–left carotid bypass was done, using a Dacron bifurcation graft and a separate implanted limb. The patient developed extremity claudication and weakness in the immediate postoperative period, and a thrombectomy was undertaken. The right carotid artery was not revascularized at the second procedure because it was extremely stenotic, and we believed it would not remain open. The left carotid bypass eventually occluded 1 year later because of diffuse distal disease.

The last patient with an early revascularization failure had undergone an end-to-side aorta-to-right carotid bypass with a 6-mm polytetrafluoroethylene graft to manage innominate artery occlusion. No neurologic symptoms were evident. However, the right subclavian pulse was absent in the postoperative period, and the patient was immediately returned to surgery for redo aorta-to-right carotid bypass. The original graft was replaced with a 7-mm Dacron graft without further difficulty. Thus, in all cases of early reocclusion, revascularization procedures were successfully completed, with a secondary patency rate of 100%.

In long-term follow-up, only four late occlusions occurred. One left carotid-to-right carotid extrathoracic graft occluded at 1 year due to progressive proximal stenosis of the left carotid artery; this resulted in dizziness and transient ischemic attacks. Repeat aorta-to-right carotid bypass was done successfully, and the patient had no further symptoms. A second graft occluded at 10 years; however, due to a lack of symptoms, no further surgery was done. One patient, who had undergone both an endarterectomy to manage extensive disease of the innominate artery and a simultaneous left carotid endarterectomy, developed a right hemiparesis 6 months after the first carotid–left subclavian bypass was done with a Dacron graft. The right hemiparesis persisted. As previously described, the last patient had occlusion of the right subclavian, right carotid, and left carotid grafts at 1 year due to arteritis.

A patient with a previously placed left subclavian–left carotid–right carotid bypass graft to manage arteritis developed an infected graft 11 months after surgery. She had undergone dental surgery without appropriate antibiotic coverage. The original graft was replaced with a carotid-to-carotid bypass away from the area of infection. Her postoperative course was uneventful.

SURGICAL RESULTS

All 54 patients survived the operative procedures. There were 7 late deaths, from 1 to 10 years following the operation. No late deaths were related to cerebrovascular events. Causes of late death included myocardial infarction (4 patients) and carcinoma (3 patients). Actuarial survival for the 10-year period was 83%.

There was no difference in mortality rates in the intrathoracic or extrathoracic groups. Morbidity did not appear to be decreased by the extrathoracic approach. The early occlusion rates were similar for both groups. In cases of extrathoracic bypass, early and long-term patency rates are dependent on the diffuse nature of the disease, especially in the inflow artery. Surgical risks are not increased by using the intrathoracic approach, and use of the aorta for inflow may prolong long-term patency.

CONCLUSION

Transthoracic innominate artery revascularization by appropriate grafting techniques to all bypassable occluded arch vessels, combined with endarterectomy of the internal carotid artery, either simultaneously or in staged procedures, can be done safely with minimal likelihood of morbidity and mortality. Isolated obstructing lesions of the innominate artery can be considered for endarterectomy. We have concluded that innominate endarterectomy should not be done in conjunction with left common carotid endarterectomy at the origin in the aortic root, since our only major complications occurred in two patients who had this procedure. The intrathoracic approach for bypass can be used safely without increased complications. The extrathoracic approach should be reserved for elderly patients who would be at high risk for thoracotomy or patients who have severely calcified ascending aortas. Results of revascularization procedures for innominate artery lesions, even when combined with procedures for other arch vessel lesions, appear to be similar to those for simple internal carotid artery lesions with regard to both intraoperative cerebral protection and excellent long-term results.

Acknowledgments

Tables 8–1, 8–2, and 8–3 are reproduced with permission from the Journal of Vascular Surgery *(1991;14:406–407). (Copyright © 1991, by the Society for Vascular Surgery and North American Chapter for Cardiovascular Surgery). Reul GJ, Jacobs MJ, Gregoric ID, Calderon M, Duncan JM, Ott DA, Livesay JJ, Cooley DA.*

REFERENCES

1. Brewster DC, Moncure AC, Darling RC, et al. Innominate artery lesions: problems encountered and lessons learned. *J Vasc Surg.* 1985;2:99–112.
2. Cherry KJ, McCullough JL, Hallett JW, et al. Technical principles of direct innominate artery revascularization: a comparison of endarterectomy and bypass grafts. *J Vasc Surg.* 1989;9: 718–724.
3. Criado FJ. Extrathoracic management of aortic arch syndrome. *Br J Surg.* 1982;69(suppl): S45–51.
4. Evans WE, Williams TE, Hayes JP. Aortobrachiocephalic reconstruction. *Am J Surg.* 1988; 156:100–102.
5. Cormier F, Ward A, Cormier JM, et al. Long-term results of aortoinnominate and aortocarotid polytetrafluoroethylene bypass grafting for atherosclerotic lesions. *J Vasc Surg.* 1989;10:135–142.
6. Walker HSJ, Peterson GJ. Considerations in extrathoracic reconstruction for disease of the branches of the aortic arch. *Am J Surg.* 1984;147:299–301.
7. Vogt DP, Hertzer NR, O'Hara PJ, et al. Brachiocephalic arterial reconstruction. *Ann Surg.* 1982;196:541–552.
8. Crawford ES, Stowe CL, Powers RW. Occlusion of the innominate, common carotid, and subclavian arteries: long-term results of surgical treatment. *Surgery.* 1983;94:781–791.
9. Zelenock GB, Cronenwett JL, Graham LM, et al. Brachiocephalic arterial occlusions and stenoses: manifestations and management of complex lesions. *Arch Surg.* 1985;120:370–376.
10. De Sobregrau RC, Lopez-Collado ML, Matas-Docampo MM, et al. Surgery of the innominate artery. *J Cardiovasc Surg.* 1986;27:31–37.
11. Grosveld WJ, Lawson JA, Eikelboom BC, et al. Clinical and hemodynamic significance of innominate artery lesions evaluated by ultrasonography and digital angiography. *Stroke.* 1988;19:958–962.
12. DeBakey ME, Crawford ES, Cooley DA, et al. Surgical considerations of occlusive disease of innominate, carotid, subclavian, and vertebral arteries. *Ann Surg.* 1959;149:690–710.
13. DeBakey ME, Crawford ES, Morris GC, et al. Surgical considerations of occlusive disease of the innominate, carotid, subclavian, and vertebral arteries. *Ann Surg.* 1961;154:698–725.
14. Crawford ES, DeBakey ME, Morris GC, et al. Surgical treatment of occlusion of the

9

Aortic Dissection:

Long-Term Results of Surgical Treatment

George E. Sarris, MD, and D. Craig Miller, MD

Aortic dissection, the most common catastrophe involving the aorta,[1-3] is associated with very high mortality rates (1%–3%/h for the first 24–48 hours) if undiagnosed and untreated.[4] Optimal outcome depends on early diagnosis and identification of the type of dissection, namely type A or B (Stanford classification[4-6]). There is general agreement that essentially all patients presenting with an acute type A dissection should undergo emergency operation, which generally consists of graft replacement of the ascending aorta with repair (or replacement, AVR, of the aortic valve if aortic insufficiency is present; composite AVR and ascending aortic replacement or concomitant arch repair may be warranted in selected patients.[4,6-24] In contrast, controversy persists regarding the optimal treatment of patients presenting with acute type B dissections. Although many hospitals adhere to a universal policy of medical therapy that reserves surgery only for patients who develop life-threatening complications,[8,9,18] some experienced centers have advocated early operation (replacement of the most diseased segment of the descending thoracic aorta) for carefully selected patients with acute type B dissections (e.g., younger, low-risk patients, those with localized aortic false aneurysms (>5 cm), individuals without severe coexisting cardiopulmonary or renal disease, and patients with Marfan's syndrome) in addition to those who develop complications (end-organ ischemia).[4,6,10-17,20-21] Furthermore, many medically treated patients with chronic dissections (>14 days old), eventually require surgery for enlarging or rupturing aortic false aneurysms or to correct progressive aortic valve insufficiency.

The early results of surgical therapy have been extensively reviewed.[7-10,12,15-24] Surgical centers experienced in the treatment of aortic dissection have reported continuous improvement in early operative results (due to a combination of earlier diagnosis, better medical management, and more refined surgical techniques and postoperative care), with recent operative mortality rates in the 7%–11%[12] range and as low as 4%–8%.[17] Several risk factors have been identified as independent predictors of early surgical mortality: (a) rupture or cardiac tamponade, (b) renal or visceral ischemia, (c) age, and (d) site of primary intimal tear (arch> descending> ascending).[12]

This chapter focuses on the long-term results of surgical treatment with emphasis on survival, causes of late death, and reoperation, as reported in several studies (Table 9–1). Recommendations for follow-up, the controversy of medical versus surgical therapy for patients with acute type B dissections, and the issues of aortic valve repair versus replacement and concomitant arch replacement for arch tears will also be discussed.

TERMINOLOGY

Clear understanding of the different classification systems of aortic dissection is necessary in order to interpret intelligently the reported clinical data. There is now general agreement that the classification of aortic dissection should be predicated solely on whether or not the ascending aorta is involved, *irrespective of the site of primary intimal tear and regardless of the distal extent of the dissection* (Fig. 9–1). This assessment is based on the observation that the biologic behavior of dissections pivots to a large extent on whether or not the ascending aortic is involved.[4,7–9] Thus, dissections with ascending aortic involvement are termed type A (Stanford),[14,25] proximal,[8] ascending,[20] or type I/II (DeBakey)[15,26,27]; those without ascending aortic involvement are classified as type B (Stanford), distal (Massachusetts General Hospital), descending (University of Alabama), or type III (DeBakey). DeBakey type I dissections extend to the descending thoracic or abdominal aorta, whereas type II are limited to the ascending aorta; type IIIa dissections are limited to the descending thoracic aorta, and type IIIb include involvement of the abdominal aorta.

Involvement of the ascending aorta can be discerned more readily and more accurately than the site of tear and extent of distal pathology utilizing computerized tomography (CT) or magnetic resonance imaging (MRI) scans,[28,29] transesophageal echocardiography,[28,30] or angiography. The type of dissection then largely dictates the optimal treatment and the surgical approach (sternotomy and total cardiopulmonary bypass for type A vs. medical therapy or left thoracotomy with partial cardiopulmonary bypass for type B).[4]

INDICATIONS, GOALS, AND STRATEGY OF SURGICAL TREATMENT

The goal of surgical treatment in acute dissection is to prevent the most common causes of death, namely, intrapericardial rupture and tamponade (80%–90%), extrapericardial rupture, acute aortic valve regurgitation, or coronary artery compromise (type A dissections), and intrathoracic rupture (type B).

As noted above, emergency surgical intervention is the treatment of choice in essentially all patients with acute type A dissections. The few contraindications that exist may include very advanced age or other severe debilitating or terminal illnesses.[31] Even major neurologic deficit (stroke) preoperatively constitutes only a relative contraindication to operation, because full neurologic recovery and satisfactory long-term results are possible.[32] At Stanford[4,31] and other centers,[11,20,21] urgent operation is also the treatment of choice for selected (but not all) patients with acute type B dissections even if uncomplicated, especially for patients with Marfan's syndrome or with sizable localized false aneurysms of the descending thoracic aorta.[4,10,31] In addition to those noted above for type A patients, other contraindications for early surgical intervention include severe concomitant cardiac, pulmonary, or cerebral disease. It should be noted that the philosophy of universal medical management—reserving operation solely for acute type B patients who do not

TABLE 9–1. SURVIVAL, CAUSES OF LATE DEATH, AND REOPERATION IN PATIENTS WITH AORTIC DISSECTION

Series	Number of Patients	Type	Survival (%)	Causes of Death (%)	Reoperation (%)
DeBakey et al 1982[15] (Baylor)	527	A = 195 B = 332	57 (5 y) 32 (10 y) 8 (20 y)	Ao rupture = 29 Sudden = 7 MI & CVA = 22	I: 30 II: 14 IIIa: 16 IIIb: 38
Doroghazi et al 1984[18] (MGH)	160	ACA = 43 ChA = 25 AcB = 78 ChB = 14	50 (5 y) 35 (10 y) D/C pts: 76 (5 y) D/C pts: 10 (10 y)	A: AoD = 73 B: AoD = 53	
Haverich et al 1984[13] (Stanford)	135	AcA = 57 ChA = 39 AcB = 16 ChB = 23	82± 4 (5 y) 64± 6 (10 y)	A: Sudden = 18 Rupture = 18 B: Sudden = 32 Rupture = 8	13± 4 (5 y) 23± 6 (10 y) Linearized rate = 3.1/pt-y
Svensson et al 1990[17] (Baylor)	690	A = 381 (82 acute) DTAo = 195 (39 acute) TAA = 194 (34 acute)	All pts. 57 (5 y) 27 (10 y) Recent series- A: 79 (3 y) B: 71 (3 y)		9 (5 y) 22 (10 y)
Glower et al 1991[16] (Duke)	163	I = 50 (90% acute) II = 16 (38% acute) III = 69 (50% acute) medical = 51 surgical = 18	I: 29 (10 y) II: 46 (10 y) III: 29 (10 y)	Rupture = 18 Sudden = 24 Other CV = 38	23

Legend: A = type A, B = type B, AcA = acute type A, ChA = chronic type A, AcB = acute type B, ChB = chronic type B, DTAo = descending thoracic aorta, TAA = thoracoabdominal aorta, I = DeBakey type I, II = DeBakey type II, III = DeBakey type III, Ao = aortic, MI = myocardial infarction, CVA = cerebrovascular accident, AoD = aortic dissection, pt-y = patient-year, CV = cardiovascular, D/C pts = discharged patients.

Figure 9–1. Examples of different types of aortic dissection, demonstrating the functional classification system that is now generally accepted. The examples in panels **A, C,** and **F** are all type A (type I [**A**] or II [**C**], proximal, or ascending) because the ascending aorta is involved. Note that the primary intimal tear can be located in the ascending aorta (labeled "1", panel **A**), transverse arch (labeled "2", panels **A, C**) or proximal descending thoracic aorta (labeled "3", panels **A, F**). The examples in panels **B** and **D** are type B dissections (synonymous with type III, descending, or distal) because the ascending aorta is not involved, regardless of whether the tear is in the descending aorta (**B**) or arch (**D**). Isolated arch dissections without retrograde or anterograde propagation (panel **E**) are rare. (*Reproduced with permission from Miller DC. Surgical management of aortic dissections: indications, perioperative management, and long term results. In: Doroghazi RM, Slater EE, eds.* Aortic Dissection. *New York: McGraw-Hill; 1983: 196.*)

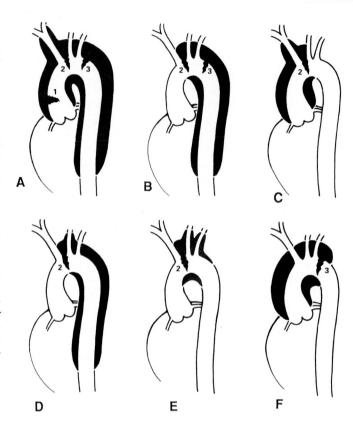

respond to medical treatment—produces the paradoxical situation where the indications for surgery represent the identical factors that portend increased surgical risk. Not surprisingly, this policy results in very high surgical mortality rates (75%–85%).[18]

The generally accepted surgical approach has been to perform a limited resection of the most diseased aortic segment, including excision of the intimal tear if exposed.[4,8,10,12,15–17,31] Preservation of the aortic valve has been possible in most patients (82% of acute type A patients in the Stanford series[12]), with excellent long-term results and no significant increase in the need for late AVR or reoperation[13]; however, AVR (frequently resorting to a composite valve graft) should always be performed in patients with Marfan syndrome or severe annuloaortic ectasia.[4,10,12,3,15–17] Separate AVR and graft replacement of the ascending aorta can be performed if the valve cannot be satisfactorily resuspended in the absence of dilated sinuses of Valsalva. Concomitant arch repair is performed if the arch is ruptured, but the surgical risk is higher. Elective simultaneous hemiarch replacement (using circulatory arrest) to resect the arch tear is appropriate in selected patients.[31]

Finally, it should be emphasized that early aggressive thoracic aortic repair remains the mainstay of therapy for patients with peripheral vascular complications (renal, visceral, or limb ischemia) due to aortic dissection because it alleviates peripheral end-organ ischemia in most instances, obviates the need for peripheral vascular procedures (aortic fenestration or direct revascularization), and reduces the likelihood of early death due to rupture of the thoracic aorta.[33,34]

EARLY RESULTS OF SURGICAL TREATMENT

The early results of surgical treatment have improved significantly over the years, as reported below. In the 20 years (1963–1982) of surgical experience at Stanford,[12] the overall surgical mortality rate was $23 \pm 3\%$ of 175 consecutive patients with aortic dissections (69% type A, 58% acute), but was substantially lower after 1977. The mortality rate in the more recent patients with acute type A dissection was $7 \pm 5\%$, in those with chronic type A it was $11 \pm 7\%$, in those with acute type B it was $13 \pm 12\%$, and in those with chronic type B dissection it was $11 \pm 11\%$ (Fig. 9–2) ($\pm 70\%$ confidence limits). Postoperative paraplegia occurred in 4% of type B patients.

In the series of 527 patients with dissections that DeBakey and associates[15] treated surgically between 1954 and 1982, 63% had type III (type B) dissections and only 27% underwent surgery within 2 weeks (acute). The overall surgical mortality was 39%, but some improvement was noted in the later part of the series, as was the case at Stanford. The mortality rates of 27%, 15%, and 19% for patients with type I, II, and III dissections treated before 1970 fell to 20%, 8%, and 16%, respectively, after 1970. The incidence of paraplegia or paraparesis was 4%, 0%, 6%, and 11%, respectively, for types I, II, IIIa, and IIIb. These rates did not change after 1970 when the various procedures previously used, such as systemic hypothermia, shunts, and left-atrial-to-femoral cardiopulmonary bypass or femorofemoral cardiopulmonary bypass were abandoned.

The Massachusetts General Hospital[18] series of 160 patients admitted with dissections between 1963 and 1978 included 108 patients treated surgically and 52 treated medically. An additional 21 patients (12% of the total) died either undiagnosed or prior to institution of definitive therapy and were excluded from analysis. There were 43 acute type A patients (34 treated surgically, with the remaining excluded from operation due to major neurologic deficit, failure to make the correct diagnosis, or patient refusal), 25 chronic type A (all treated surgically), 78 acute type

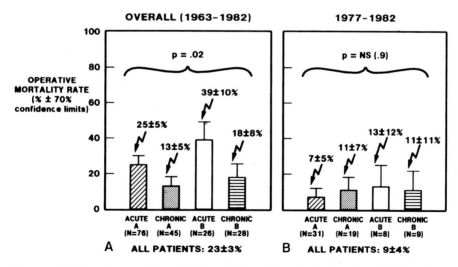

Figure 9–2. Operative mortality rates for patients with acute or chronic aortic dissections between 1963 and 1982 at Stanford. As shown in panel (**A**), the results improved over time, with the current operative risk being $7 \pm 5\%$ ($\pm 70\%$ confidence limits) for patients with acute type A dissections and $13 \pm 12\%$ for those with acute type B dissections. Before 1976, (panel **A**), the overall mortality rate was $31 \pm 5\%$, compared with (**B**) the more recent risk (1977–1982) of $9 \pm 4\%$. (*Reproduced with the permission of the American Heart Association from Miller DC, Mitchell RS, Oyer PE, et al. Circulation. 1984;70(suppl I):157.*)

B (43 treated surgically), and 14 chronic type B patients (6 treated surgically). The indications for surgical intervention for individuals with acute type B dissections were rupture, localized false aneurysm, distal ischemia, and intractable pain or hypertension. Surgical (or 30-day) mortality was 16 of 34 (47%) for acute type A patients treated surgically, 4 of 9 (44%) for acute type A patients treated medically, 9 of 25 (36%) for chronic type A patients (all treated surgically), 21 of 43 (49%) for acute type B patients treated surgically, 7 of 35 (20%) for acute type B patients treated medically, 1 of 5 (20%) for chronic type B patients treated surgically, and 0 of 8 (0%) for medically treated chronic type B patients. The authors concluded that the acuity of the dissection (chronic vs. acute) was the most significant factor influencing survival and that the number of complications (rupture, tamponade, neurologic deficit, or end-organ ischemia) had the strongest adverse effect on survival. They did not identify differences in outcome based on type of dissection or mode of treatment, with the exception of an apparent improved early survival rate for patients with acute type B dissections who were treated medically. Unfortunately, multivariate statistical analysis was not employed. The surgical mortality rate for surgically treated patients with acute type B dissections was much higher than that reported in the Stanford[12] and DeBakey and associates[15] experience, reflecting the Massachusetts General Hospital policy of reserving surgery for patients who developed life-threatening complications (rupture and renal or visceral ischemia). Indeed, the surgical mortality rate for patients who failed to respond to medical therapy due to redissection or inability to control blood pressure (rather than due to persistent pain) was 80%.

In Glower and colleagues report from Duke,[16] 163 patients with aortic dissection (1975–1988) were reviewed. Importantly, 28 of these individuals with previous cardiac or aortic operation, intraoperative (iatrogenic) dissection, or death prior to any treatment were excluded. Fifty type I patients (90% acute) and 16 type II patients (38% acute) were treated with ascending aortic replacement, with surgical mortality rates of 26% and 14%, respectively. Sixty-nine patients had type III dissections; 51 (73% acute) were treated medically and 18 (50% acute) surgically; the 30-day mortality rates were 18% and 62%, respectively. Five out of 8 patients who were operated on for aortic rupture died, but no deaths or paraplegia occurred in those operated on for aortic expansion.

The largest and most recently updated experience is Crawford and associates' personal series[17] of 690 consecutive patients with aortic dissection operated upon between 1956 and 1989. It should be noted, however, that only 22% of these cases had acute dissections. The surgical mortality rate improved considerably over time (comparing before vs. after 1986): For patients with acute dissections, it fell from 33% ($n = 45$), 45% ($n = 22$), and 47% ($n = 15$) for types I/II, IIIa, and IIIb to 5% ($n = 37$), 6% ($n = 17$), and 5% ($n = 14$), respectively. For patients with chronic dissections the rate fell from 12% ($n = 98$), 17% ($n = 60$) and 10% ($n = 60$) to 8% ($n = 121$), 4% ($n = 96$) and 5% ($n = 100$), respectively. The incidence of paraplegia was 7% for patients with acute or chronic dissection undergoing resection of a segment of the descending thoracic aorta (comparable to the 4% at Stanford[12]), 24% for patients undergoing Crawford type I thoracoabdominal aortic (TAA) replacement (most of the descending aorta and suprarenal abdominal aorta), and 36% for Crawford type II TAA replacement (the entire thoracoabdominal aorta from the left subclavian artery to the aortic bifurcation). In this and other reports,[35–37] Crawford and his colleagues demonstrated that the incidence of spinal cord injury was not reduced significantly by spinal fluid drainage, monitoring of somatosensory evoked potentials, intercostal artery reimplantation, or distal perfusion (with cardiopulmonary bypass or shunt).

LONG-TERM SURVIVAL

A simplified approach to analyzing the long-term results of surgical treatment of patients with aortic dissections is to examine survival rates. In the Stanford series of 135 surgery survivors,[13] the actuarial survival rates were 82 ± 4% at 5 years and 64 ± 6% at 10 years (Fig. 9–3). There were no significant differences in long-term survival in the four patient subsets based on type and acuity of dissection; however, comparison with computer-simulated, matched general populations revealed lower survival rates of patients with acute type A dissections, but not for acute type B patients. Using a multivariate Cox model, earlier surgical era, remote myocardial infarction (MI), preoperative renal dysfunction, and stroke were the only significant, independent predictors of late death. Long-term survival was not related to dissection type or acuity, site of intimal tear (or whether or not it was resected), distal extent of dissection, concomitant AVR or coronary artery bypass graft, previous operation, Marfan's syndrome, or preoperative paraplegia. Importantly, in type A patients 18% of late deaths were due to rupture, another 18% were "sudden" (many of which were possibly due to rupture), and 32% were due to other cardiovascular causes (stroke, MI, or congestive heart failure [CHF]). In the type B patients, 8% of late deaths were due to rupture, 32% were sudden, and 32% were due to miscellaneous cardiovascular causes.

In the DeBakey and associates series,[15] the overall 5-, 10-, and 20-year survival rates for all patients were 57%, 32%, and 5%, respectively (Fig. 9–4). There appeared to be a trend favoring higher rates in patients with types I and II (type A) dissections compared with those with type III (type B) dissections. These figures are comparable to the Stanford results,[13] since they included surgical deaths. Using Cox multivariate analysis, the authors identified that the risk of perioperative and late death was higher in the elderly, and in patients with preoperative angina, CHF, or stroke, and (unlike the Stanford experience) in patients with acute dissections. The most common cause of late death was subsequent development and rupture of the aorta, accounting for 29% of all late deaths. An additional 7% of late deaths were sudden, and 22% were due to MI and stroke. Of note, subsequent aneurysms occurred in 45% of patients with uncontrolled hypertension, but in only 17% of those with good blood pressure control, which underscores the importance of careful medical follow-up of these patients indefinitely after surgery.

In the Massachusetts General Hospital series,[18] the overall 5-year survival rate for discharged patients was 76%, comparable to the results at Stanford and Baylor. Most late deaths (73% in proximal dissection and 53% in distal dissection) could be attributed to the dissection *per se*. There was no difference in late survival between subgroups of discharged patients according to type, acuity, and mode of treatment; unfortunately, actuarial survival data are provided for combined patient groups (i.e., all acute (A and B) vs. all chronic (A and B) patients, all type A (acute and chronic) vs. all type B patients, and all medical vs. all surgical patients, thus limiting the usefulness of this analysis.) Life expectancy of patients with all types of dissections treated medically or surgically was inferior to that of age-matched control populations, except for the subset of medically treated type B patients (perhaps reflecting the greater age and increased prevalence of associated diseases compared with that in patients with type A dissections).

The Duke long-term results[16] paralleled those from Stanford and Baylor, with long-term (9–10 year) survival rates of 29%, 46%, and 29% for patients with type I, II, and III dissections, respectively (Fig. 9–5). Glower and colleagues also documented that late death was largely due to aortic rupture (18%), sudden causes (24%), or other

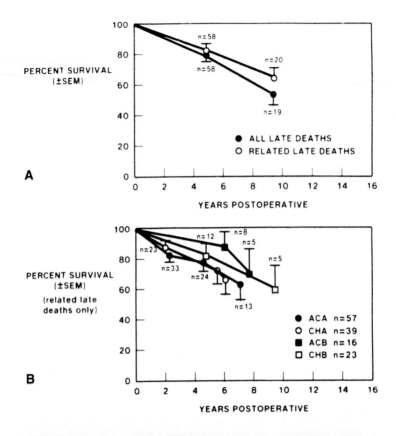

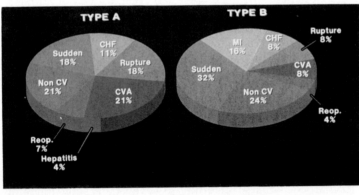

Figure 9–3. (A) Actuarial survival curves depicting all late deaths (closed circles) and deaths that were known or presumed to be related to the aortic dissection. **(B)** Late patient survival subdivided according to type and acuity of dissection. (ACA = acute type A; ACB = acute type B; CHA = chronic type A; CHB = chronic type B). **(C)** Comparative depiction of the cause of late death for the type A and B subgroups. CVA = cerebrovascular accident; CV = cardiovascular; reop = reoperation-related death. (*Reproduced with the permission of the American Heart Association from Haverich A, Miller DC, Scott WC, et al. Acute and chronic aortic dissections: determinants of long term outcome for operative survivors. Circulation. 1985;72 (suppl 2):II26.*)

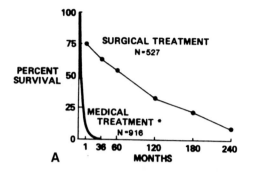

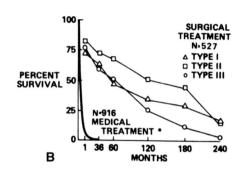

Figure 9–4. (**A**) Survival curves comparing medical and surgical treatment during a period of 20 years in 527 patients with dissecting aneurysms of the aorta. (**B**) Survival curves comparing medical and surgical treatment in the same series of patients according to type. (*Reproduced with the permission of Mosby-Year Book, Inc. from DeBakey ME, McCollum CH, Crawford ES, et al. Dissection and dissecting aneurysms of the aorta: Twenty year follow-up of five hundred twenty-seven patients treated surgically.* Surgery. *1982;92:1129.*)

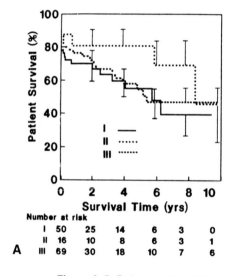

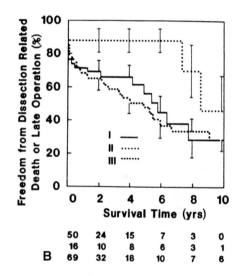

Figure 9–5. Patient survival (**A**) and freedom from dissection-related death or late operation (**B**) for type I, type II, and type III aortic dissections. (*Reproduced with the permission of JB Lippincott Co. from Glower DD, Speier RH, White WD, et al. Management and long term outcome of aortic dissection.* Ann Surg. *1991;214:34.*)

cardiovascular disease (38%).[16] For patients with type I and II dissections, only arch tear and TAA dissection were significantly related to long-term mortality (univariate analysis); for type III patients, various preoperative complications (MI, shock, renal or visceral ischemia), older age, and aortic rupture were independent predictors of death in the multivariate analysis. Proximal or distal extent of the dissection, arch tear, and mode of therapy were not significant independent predictors of late mortality.

In Crawford and colleagues' most recent report,[17] the overall 5- and 10-year survival rates were 57% and 41%, respectively, with corresponding complication-free survival rates of 42% and 21% (Fig. 9–6). For patients operated on recently, the overall 3-year actuarial survival rate was 79% for patients with type A dissections and 71% for those with type B dissections. Late death was due to rupture in 23% of type A and 13% of type B patients. Multivariate analysis revealed that several factors significantly influenced long-term survival. For type A patients, female gender, absence of CHF,

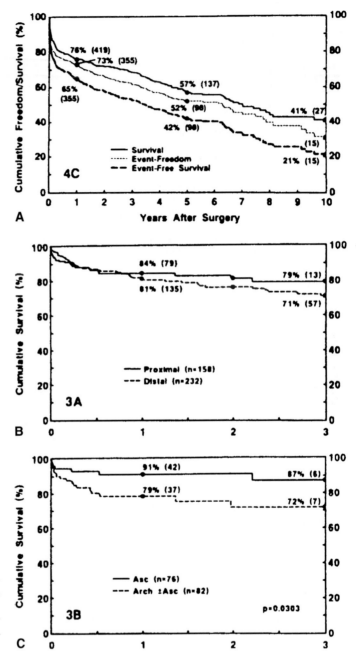

Figure 9–6. (**A**) Cumulative freedom from specific event-free survival for all 690 patients. (**B**) Three-year survival for proximal and distal dissections. (**C**) Three-year survival in patients with proximal dissections according to extent. Asc = ascending aorta; Arch ± asc = aortic arch and/or ascending aorta. (*Figure continues*)

postoperative cardiac dysfunction or renal failure, a lesser extent of aortic replacement (ascending vs. arch ± ascending), and the absence of residual aneurysm were associated with an enhanced likelihood of survival. For patients with type B dissections, a lesser extent of aortic resection (partial vs. total descending thoracic aorta vs. TAA replacement) was associated with improved survival probability, in addition to female gender and absence of preoperative renal dysfunction or hypertension.

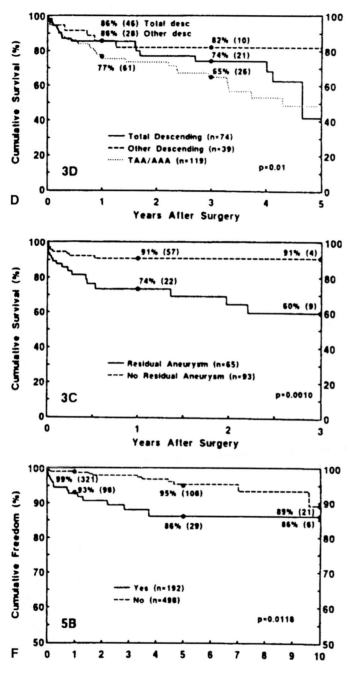

Figure 9–6. (*continued*) (**D**) Five-year survival in distal dissections according to the extent of aorta replaced. Desc = total descending thoracic aorta; Other desc = other than total descending thoracic aortic replacement; TAA/AAA = thoracoabdominal or abdominal aorta. (**E**) Three-year survival in patients with proximal dissections according to the presence of residual aneurysm elsewhere. (**F**) Ten-year freedom from fatal rupture according to residual aneurysmal disease remote from the original operation. (*Reproduced with the permission of the American Heart Association from Svensson LG, Crawford ES, Hess KR, et al. Dissection of the aorta and the dissecting aneurysms: improving early and long term surgical results.* Circulation. *1990;82(suppl 4):IV-34-IV-36.*)

REOPERATION

The causes of late death noted above demonstrate that in addition to various cardiovascular events (e.g., MI, CHF, stroke), rupture of another segment of the thoracic or abdominal aorta (which was also possibly responsible for many of the sudden deaths) was the most important cause of late mortality. This also potentially represents a preventable problem if careful medical follow-up and serial surveillance computed tomography or magnetic resonance imaging of the remainder of the aorta identify progressive aortic pathology before rupture occurs so that reoperation can be performed judiciously in selected patients.

At the outset, it should be emphasized that two categories of reoperations can be clearly distinguished.[38] The first—*treatment failure*—refers to procedures necessary to rectify problems related to the initial procedure. The initial operation was either incomplete (e.g., inadequate resection of the dissected aorta, failure to replace the aortic root in Marfan's syndrome) or failed postoperatively (e.g., development of anastomotic pseudoaneurysm, progressive aortic insufficiency after aortic valve resuspension, or structural valve failure of an implanted valve prosthesis). The second category—*late aortic sequelae*—includes reoperations that became necessary to address the pathologic evolution of the underlying disease process (e.g., to replace a distal aneurysmal segment of aorta noted to be progressively enlarging during follow-up). It is hoped that treatment failure reoperations will become less frequent in the future and that those for treating late aortic sequelae can be performed more commonly in a timely fashion before catastrophic rupture or death occur.

The actuarial incidence of reoperation in the Stanford series[13] was $13 \pm 4\%$ and $23 \pm 6\%$ at 5 and 10 years, respectively, with a linearized rate of 3.1% per patient-year (Fig. 9–7). The independent, significant predictors of higher likelihood of reoperation were younger age, site of tear (arch > descending > ascending) and (rather inexplicably), cardiac tamponade. Interestingly, Marfan's syndrome; the type, acuity, and extent of dissection; and whether or not the tear was resected were not independently associated with any increased risk of reoperation. It should be noted, however, that the actuarial rate of reoperation was higher in patients with Marfan's syndrome and in those who did not have resection of the primary intimal tear (but these variables did not achieve significance in the multivariate analysis, in part, due to the younger age of the Marfan's patients and the small number of patients in these subgroups). Regarding AVR, preservation of the native aortic valve was possible in 79% of patients with acute type A and 54% of those with chronic type A dissections. Long-term results were satisfactory. At three years, $77 \pm 7\%$ of patients without AVR were free of reoperation compared with $84 \pm 9\%$ of patients who had undergone concomitant AVR (p = not significant); moreover, the patients with aortic valve preservation who later required AVR (all of whom had Marfan's syndrome or annuloaortic ectasia) were operated on early in the Stanford experience, and thus represented an example of treatment failure. Data from the Stanford-Duke database investigation[39] showed that aortic valve resuspension had no significant effect on long-term survival. Furthermore, the incidence of late AVR (i.e., AVR for residual valve disease or redo AVR) did not differ between patients who had AVR, aortic valve resuspension, or those who required no aortic valve procedure at the time of the initial operation. Therefore, based on current information, it seems prudent to attempt to salvage the native aortic valve whenever possible, especially since the adverse effect of late complications associated with any type of valve substitute were probably not yet reflected by these data since the mean follow-up interval was only 4 years.

The site of primary intimal tear was an independent predictor of increased risk of reoperation. Patients with arch, ascending or descending aortic tears had a $27 \pm 13\%$ (after only 1 year), $21 \pm 7\%$ (at 7 years), and $29 \pm 17\%$ (10 years) probability of reoperation. In 10 of 12 (83%) discharged patients (6 type A, 6 type B), the tear was not resected during the original operation; 4 of these 10 patients (40%) subsequently required partial or complete arch replacement.

In the Duke series,[16] 13% of patients required reoperation, (17% of type I or II patients, with the freedom from reoperation rate being $87 \pm 6\%$ and $60 \pm 15\%$ at 5 and 10 years, respectively; 12% of patients with type III dissections). Aortic valve

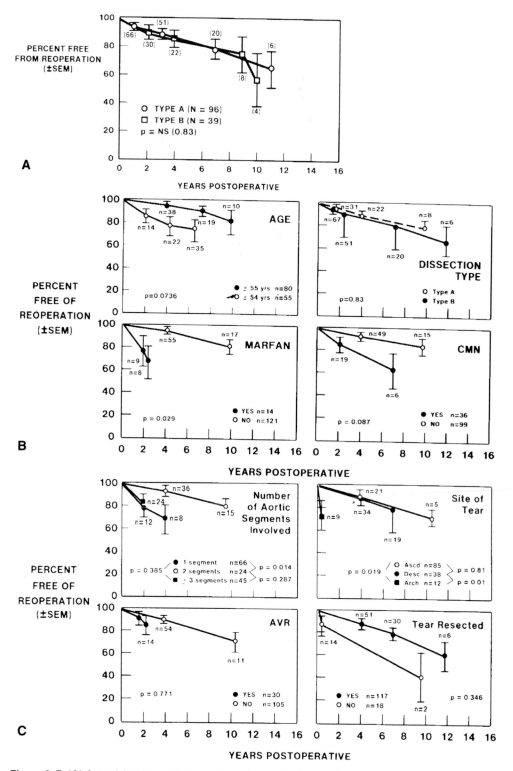

Figure 9–7. (A) Actuarial estimate of reoperation rate in patients after discharge who were treated surgically for either acute or chronic dissections at Stanford. **(B)** and **(C)** Representative univariate examples illustrating the clinical effect of various risk factors on the likelihood of late reoperation. The only significant, independent parameters were younger age, arch tear, and cardiac tamponade. CMN = cystic medial necrosis; AVR = aortic valve replacement. (*Reproduced with the permission of the American Heart Association from Haverich A, Miller DC, Scott WC, et al. Acute and chronic aortic dissections: determinants of long term outcome for operative survivors. Circulation. 1985;72(suppl 2):II26.*)

resuspension was performed in 17 patients; none required subsequent AVR. In contrast, patients with type I or II dissections who required initial AVR or who had no aortic valve procedure had a 30% probability of subsequent AVR at 10 years. Furthermore, primary repair of type I or II dissection without graft replacement was associated with a high incidence of subsequent composite aortic valve–ascending aortic replacement (2 of 8). Of the type III patients who required reoperation, 6 were initially treated medically and later developed rupture or progressive aneurysm formation, and 2 were initially surgically treated. One had a false aneurysm of the proximal anastomosis (late treatment failure), and the other suffered progression of descending thoracic dissection (late aortic sequelae).

In the Crawford and colleagues series,[17] 44 of 690 patients required late reoperation (Fig. 9–8). The univariate independent determinants of reoperation were earlier surgical era (before 1986), previous ascending aortic procedure, and lesser extent of aortic replacement. As demonstrated in the Duke series,[16] patients who only had an aortoplasty procedure (no graft replacement) were most prone to reoperation, followed by those who had ascending aortic replacement with or without valve resuspension, distal tubular graft, proximal composite valve graft, and separate valve graft. All patients with composite grafts who required reoperation had had a Bentall procedure (6 of 55); reoperation was necessary for either aortic or coronary ostial anastomotic dehiscence. On the other hand, none of the 17 patients who had composite aortic valve-graft procedures utilizing full thickness aortic buttons for

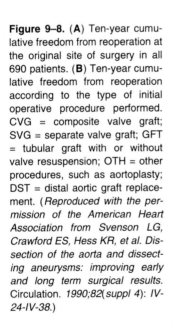

Figure 9–8. (A) Ten-year cumulative freedom from reoperation at the original site of surgery in all 690 patients. **(B)** Ten-year cumulative freedom from reoperation according to the type of initial operative procedure performed. CVG = composite valve graft; SVG = separate valve graft; GFT = tubular graft with or without valve resuspension; OTH = other procedures, such as aortoplasty; DST = distal aortic graft replacement. (*Reproduced with the permission of the American Heart Association from Svenson LG, Crawford ES, Hess KR, et al. Dissection of the aorta and dissecting aneurysms: improving early and long term surgical results. Circulation. 1990;82(suppl 4): IV-24-IV-38.*)

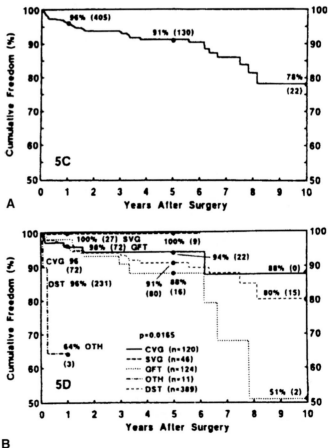

mortality rates approaching 5% to 10% in such patients, early operation may actually carry a lower overall mortality risk compared with medical therapy and may confer some degree of protection against late aortic sequelae. The Stanford policy has therefore been to offer early operation to such patients.[31,40]

Concomitant Arch Replacement in Patients with Acute Arch Tear

When aortic leak, frank rupture, or gross aneurysmal dilatation involves the transverse arch, there is no alternative to arch replacement, despite the associated high mortality risk. Conversely, ongoing debate continues regarding the advisability of "elective" concomitant arch replacement in patients with an acute type A or B dissection due to a primary intimal tear located in the arch, that is, in those patients where there is no compelling reason to replace the arch at the time of initial ascending or descending thoracic aortic repair.

In the Stanford series,[12] the primary intimal tear was located most frequently in the ascending aorta, but it was in the transverse arch in 13% (22 of 175) of patients, one-half of whom had retrograde propagation involving the ascending aorta (e.g., type A), and the other half having only distal propagation (e.g., type B). The site of intimal tear was an independent predictor of higher surgical mortality, with arch tear being associated with the highest risk. For patients with acute type A dissections, the surgical mortality rate was 22% if the tear was in the ascending aorta, but 50% if it was an arch tear. For acute type B patients, the surgical mortality rate was 75% if the primary tear was in the transverse arch compared with 32% for descending tears. Furthermore, patients with arch tears had the highest probability of reoperation ($27 \pm 13\%$ within the first year), which was significantly higher than that in those with ascending ($21 \pm 7\%$ at 7 years, $P = 0.019$) or descending tears ($29 \pm 17\%$ at 10 years, $P = 0.01$). Focusing on discharged patients only, the tear was not resected during the initial operation in 83% of patients with an arch tear (10 of 12, 6 type A, 6 type B). Four of these 10 patients (40%) subsequently required partial or complete aortic arch replacement; however, in the multivariate analysis, long-term survival was not influenced by the site of the tear or whether it was actually resected.[13]

This issue was further explored in another Stanford-Duke database investigation.[42] There were 52 patients with dissections resulting from a primary tear located in the transverse arch, 47 of whom were treated surgically (surgical mortality rate: 55%). There were 26 patients with acute type A dissections, 7 with chronic type A, 7 with acute type B, and 7 with chronic type B dissections. Concomitant arch repair was omitted in 22 patients with acute dissection, with a 30-day mortality rate of 41% (p: not significant vs. arch repair). Multivariate analysis confirmed that concomitant arch replacement had no significant bearing on survival, although there was a trend favoring improved survival after concomitant arch repair in patients with acute type A dissections, especially those younger than 55 years[38,40,42] (Fig. 9–11). Older age, number of dissection-related complications, and presence of other medical diseases were independent predictors of overall (early or late) mortality. These data do not conclusively resolve the issue (likely β error due to the small numbers) but do suggest that concomitant elective arch repair should be considered only in selected younger, low-risk patients with arch tears when the ascending or proximal descending thoracic aorta is being replaced. This can be accomplished, in most cases, by hemiarch replacement within 15 to 20 minutes of circulatory arrest at 20° to 22°C hypothermia.[31,38,42] This technique facilitates a more secure distal anastomosis and is considerably less extensive than complete arch replacement, which is required much less frequently, for example, in cases of extensive destruction or rupture of the arch.

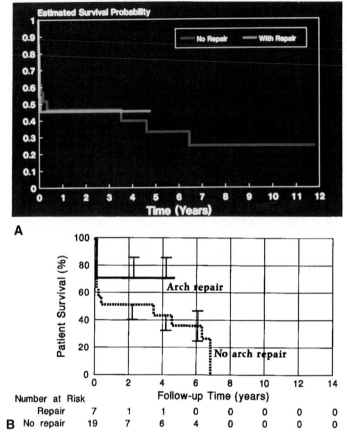

Figure 9–11. (A) Actuarial survival curves (± standard error of the estimate) for all patients in the Stanford-Duke database study, with dissections due to an acute arch tear, according to whether or not concomitant arch repair was performed. **(B)** Similar curves for patients with acute type A dissections. The trend favoring concomitant arch repair did not attain statistical significance. (*Figure continues*)

Furthermore, elective concomitant arch replacement should probably only be considered in surgical centers experienced in the treatment of such patients.[38,40,42–50]

This view is also supported by Crawford and associates[48] 1992 report of 82 patients with acute type A dissection who underwent ascending aortic replacement. Of these, 26 (32%) had concomitant arch replacement with a surgical mortality rate of 31%, and 54 had isolated ascending aortic replacement (surgical mortality rate: 17%). The primary intimal tear was in the ascending aorta in most (72%) cases; only 11% of patients had arch tears. Of those with arch tears, 9 underwent concomitant arch replacement (surgical mortality rate: 25%, which is comparable to that reported in other contemporary series). Multivariate analysis demonstrated that concomitant arch replacement and earlier surgical era were the strongest independent predictors portending a higher likelihood of surgical death. The estimated current (1989) risk for isolated ascending replacement was only 3%, and a moderate 16% for concomitant arch replacement.[48] The predictive accuracy of this statistical model was confirmed prospectively in 1990. Furthermore, the authors noted that 70% of patients were free from late reoperation for distal aortic false aneurysm and no late reoperations were necessary in the 9 patients who had the arch tear included in the resection (even though the site of tear was not identified to be a significant risk factor for either death or reoperation in this study).

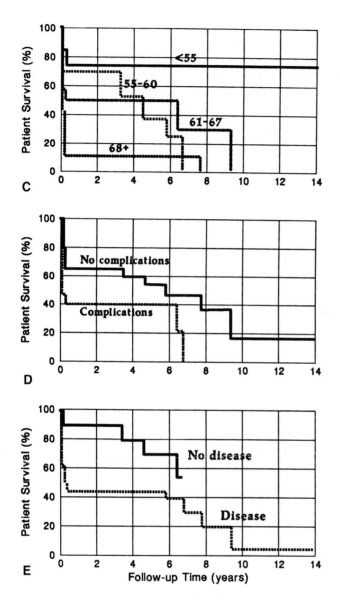

Figure 9–11. (*continued*) Survival probabilities adjusted for the three independent, incremental risk factors of early or late death: (**C**) Age, (**D**) number of dissection-related complications, and (**E**) presence of other medical problems (bottom). Patients under 55 years of age appeared to have a better prognosis. (*Reproduced with the permission of Mosby-Year Book Inc. from Yun KL, Glower DD, Miller DC, et al. Aortic dissection due to transverse arch tear: is concomitant arch repair warranted?* J Thorac Cardiovasc Surg. *1991;102:359,366.*)

SUMMARY

Patients with acute type A or with acute type B dissections presenting with or developing complications should be treated by emergency operation, which generally consists of graft replacement of the most diseased portion of the thoracic aorta. Low-risk patients with acute type B dissections (and all patients with Marfan's syndrome) should be considered for emergency operation, even if they do not have substantial complications. During surgery for acute type A dissection, the aortic valve should be repaired, if possible, but it should be replaced (composite valve graft, open end-to-end technique) in all patients with Marfan's syndrome or annuloaortic ectasia. Concomitant arch replacement should be performed if the arch is ruptured or grossly dilated, and should be electively considered in younger, low-risk patients with otherwise uncomplicated dissections due to arch tears, because the increment in surgical risk (depending on the experience of the surgical group) may be outweighed by the potential reduction in late reoperation and death.

The significant improvement in surgical results in recent reports must not divert attention from the fundamental fact that surgical management of aortic dissection is ony palliative, because the remaining aorta is permanently at risk of (false) aneurysm formation and late rupture. Therefore, close, indefinite follow-up of all patients with dissections, strict control of hypertension, treatment with beta blockers and/or calcium antagonists (even if normotensive), and, most importantly, serial imaging of the aorta with CT or MRI scans or TEE are imperative. Timely reoperation should be performed if there is documented progressive dilatation of the aorta, particularly when a localized false aneurysm is identified (>6 cm), or when symptoms occur. Since the surgical mortality rates are unlikely to fall further in the future, such meticulous postoperative surveillance, coupled with efforts to increase awareness of aortic dissection in all health care personnel in order to make the correct diagnosis earlier and more often, will hopefully result in improved overall patient recovery rates.

Acknowledgment
We thank Ms. Phoebe Taboada for her excellent assistance in the preparation of this manuscript.

REFERENCES

1. Sorenson HR, Olsen H: Ruptured and dissecting aneurysms of the aorta: incidence and prospects of surgery. *Acta Chir Scand.* 1964;128:644–650.
2. Pate JW, Richardson RL, Eastidge CE: Acute aortic dissections. *Am Surg.* 1976;42:395–404.
3. Bickerstaff LK, Pairolero PC, Hollier LH, et al. Thoracic aortic aneurysms: a population based study. *Surgery.* 1982;92:1103–1108.
4. Miller DC: Surgical management of aortic dissections: indications, perioperative management, and long-term results. In: Doroghazi RM, Slater EE, eds. *Aortic Dissection.* New York: McGraw-Hill Book Co.; 1983:193–243.
5. Jamieson WRE, Munro AI, Miyagishima RT, et al. Aortic dissections: early diagnosis and surgical management are the keys to survival. *Can J Surg.* 1982;25:145–149.
6. Miller DC: When to suspect aortic dissection: what treatment? *Cardiovasc Med.* 1984;9:811–818.
7. Acute aortic dissection. *Lancet.* 1988;827–828. Editorial.
8. DeSanctis RW, Doroghazi RM, Austen WG, et al. Aortic dissection. *New Engl J Med.* 1987;317:1060–1967.
9. Eagle KA, DeSanctis RW: Aortic dissection. *Curr Probl Cardiol.* 1989;14:225–278.
10. Crawford ES: The diagnosis and management of aortic dissection. *JAMA.* 1990;264:2537–2541.
11. Ergin MA, Galla JD, Lansman S, et al. Acute dissection of the aorta: current surgical treatment. *Surg Clin North Am.* 1985;65:721–741.
12. Miller DC, Mitchell RS, Oyer PE, et al. Independent determinants of operative mortality for patients with aortic dissections. *Circulation.* 1984;70(suppl I):I-153–164.
13. Haverich A, Miller DC, Scott WC, et al. Acute and chronic aortic dissections—determinants of long-term outcome for operative survivors. *Circulation.* 1985;72(suppl II):II-22–34.
14. Miller DC, Stinson EB, Oyer PE, et al. Operative treatment of aortic dissections. *J Thorac Cardiovasc Surg.* 1979;78:365–382.
15. DeBakey ME, McCollum CH, Crawford ES, et al. Dissection and dissecting aneurysms of the aorta: twenty-year follow-up of five hundred twenty-seven patients treated surgically. *Surgery.* 1982;92:1118–1134.
16. Glower DD, Speier RH, White WD, et al. Management and long-term outcome of aortic dissection. *Ann Surg.* 1991;214:31–41.

aortitis in 34. Marfan syndrome was present in 80 (5%) patients. There were 572 (38%) patients who were asymptomatic regarding their aneurysm. Ruptured aortic aneurysms were present in 61 (4%) patients.

SURGICAL TREATMENT

Successful repair of a thoracoabdominal aortic aneurysm was reported in 1955 by Ethridge and colleagues, who used a homograft.[7] Initial methods of treatment involved placement of a graft proximally and distally in an end-to-side fashion spanning the length of the aneurysm, with subsequent oversewing of the aneurysmal sac distal to the proximal anastomosis and proximal to the distal anastomosis. Side branch grafts were sutured from the aortic graft to the visceral arteries. The morbidity from these procedures was considerable, and the surgical mortality was 26%.[8,9]

A simplified technique was introduced in 1973 by the senior author (ESC) that resulted in a dramatic reduction of both morbidity and mortality.[10] Treatment consisted of the graft inclusion technique with direct branch vessel reattachment to openings made in the graft. The details of this particular approach have been extensively documented elsewhere.[11–17] The overwhelming majority of operations in this current series were performed by simple proximal aortic cross-clamping along with control of hemodynamic effects by pharmacologic agents. A variety of modalities, however, were employed in certain groups of patients in an attempt to evaluate the effect of therapeutic intraoperative techniques upon the incidence of spinal cord ischemia and its associated neurologic deficits and on postoperative renal dysfunction. Techniques to evaluate spinal cord ischemia have included the use of temporary distal aortic perfusion using cardiofemoral bypass with and without somatosensory evoked potential monitoring,[18] cardiopulmonary bypass with profound hypothermia and circulatory arrest,[19] and cerebrospinal fluid drainage.[20] Attempts at renal preservation have included perfusion of the renal arteries with cold (4°C.) Ringer's lactate solution and direct warm oxygenated blood.[21]

RESULTS OF TREATMENT

Very few reports have appeared in the literature addressing the short-term, much less the long-term, results of treatment of an even moderately sized series of patients treated surgically with thoracoabdominal aortic aneurysms.[22–28] In 1986, we reported upon the survival of 604 patients who underwent surgery of the thoracoabdominal aorta. At that time, 400 (66%) were alive some 3 months to 20 years following operation. The early mortality rate was 8.9% (540 patients), and there were 151 late deaths. Using the Kaplan-Meier method, the estimated survival rate for the entire group was 60% (± 3%) at 5 years and 32% (± 6%) at 10 years. Variables predictive of risk of late death in that early series of patients were rupture, renal dysfunction, extent of aneurysm (group II), dissection, old age, heart disease, cerebrovascular disease, chronic obstructive pulmonary disease, hypertension, and poor renal function. The median age was 65 years, and gender distribution was 68% male and 32% female. The incidence of aortic dissection was 17%. These factors, including the general distribution of extent of aortic replacement and other significant characteristics of the patient population, have remained surprisingly similar through the years.

In the total experience of 1,509 patients who underwent thoracoabdominal aortic operation by the authors, there were 1,386 (92%) early (30-day) survivors. Preopera-

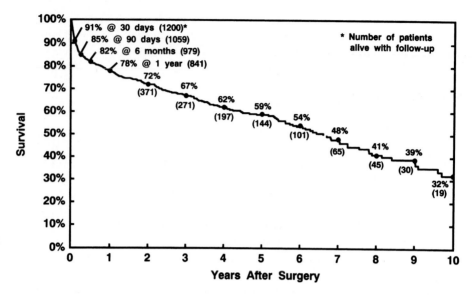

Figure 10–2. Long-term survival in all 1,509 patients estimated using the Kaplan-Meier method. (*Reproduced with permission from Crawford ES, De Natale RW. Thoracoabdominal aortic aneurysm: observations regarding the course of the disease. J Vasc Surg. 1986;3:578–582.*)

tive variables predictive of an early death included rupture, old age, and the preoperative presence of severe pulmonary, cardiac, and renal disease. These preoperative variables predictive of an early death were present equally, regardless of the cause of the aortic aneurysm or the extent of disease and replacement. Consequently, the early survival rates among these groups were essentially equal. Long-term survival determined using the Kaplan-Meier curve is shown in Figure 10–2.

DISEASE EXTENT

The extent of aortic involvement requiring repair or replacement has been extremely variable; however, four general patterns have emerged. The division of patients for purposes of evaluation into four basic groups based on extent of disease involvement and resection was described previously[1] and has been referred to as the Crawford classification.

Group I consists of those patients with involvement of most of the descending thoracic and upper abdominal aorta. Disease in group II patients involves most of the descending thoracic aorta and most, or all, of the abdominal aorta. Group III patients includes those whose disease involves the distal descending thoracic aorta and varying segments of abdominal aorta. Patients in group IV have disease that involves most, or all, of the abdominal aorta, including the segment from which the visceral vessels arise. Of the 1,509 patients treated, group I included 378 (25%) patients; group II, 442 (29%); group III, 343 (23%); and group IV, 346 (23%) (Fig. 10–3).

Early mortality was not significantly different in the various extents of aortic replacement (group I, 7%; II, 10%; III, 10%; IV, 6%). Visceral arterial reattachment naturally was more common in groups II, III, and IV (98%, 93%, and 76%) and less commonly required in group I (35%). Specifically, renal artery reattachment followed a similar pattern (group I, 8%; II, 91%; III, 84%; IV, 88%). Likewise, distal perfusion adjuncts were commonly employed in groups I and II (24%, 26%) and were required

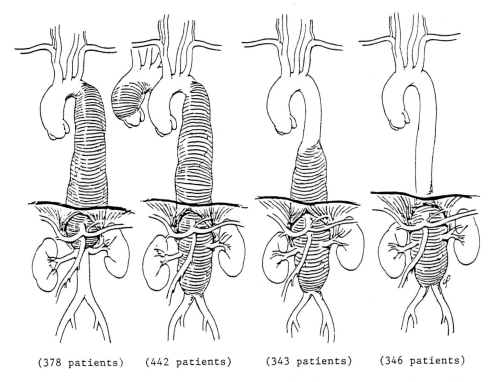

(378 patients)   (442 patients)   (343 patients)   (346 patients)

Figure 10–3. Distribution of 1,509 patients with thoracoabdominal aortic aneurysm by extent of disease.

less frequently in groups III and IV (10%, 5%). Postoperative neurologic deficits (paraparesis or paraplegia) were significantly more prevalent in patients requiring extensive resections (group II, 31%) versus those with more limited disease (groups I, 15%; III, 7%; IV, 4%). Late survival was not affected by the extent of replacement.

Aortic Dissection

Aortic dissection presents a more complicated diagnostic and therapeutic challenge to the surgeon than disease that does not involve dissection.[29–32] In the overall group of 1,509 patients, aortic dissection was present in 276 patients (18%), whereas nondissection pathology was present in 1,233 (82%). Thirty-nine (3%) patients were treated for acute dissection and 237 (16%) patients for chronic aortic dissection. The presence or absence of dissection significantly affected early mortality ($P = .0024$). Early mortality was similar for patients with nondissection and chronic dissection (8% and 7%, respectively), whereas 9 of 39 patients with acute aortic dissection (23%) were early deaths. The effect on long-term survival of patients with and without aortic dissection is shown in Figure 10–4. Throughout the entire experience, patients routinely have undergone a comprehensive examination of the aorta, usually by computed tomography scanning or total aortic aortography, and, most recently, magnetic resonance imaging to document all aortic aneurysmal disease at the time of first operation. Subsequently an aggressive approach to resect all dilated segments where the aorta exceeded twice the normal diameter, particularly in patients at low risk for surgery, was undertaken. With the aorta considered in its entirety, aneurysmal disease of nontreated segments of the aorta has been a significant deleterious factor associated with both late rupture ($P < .0004$) and late death ($P < .0173$).

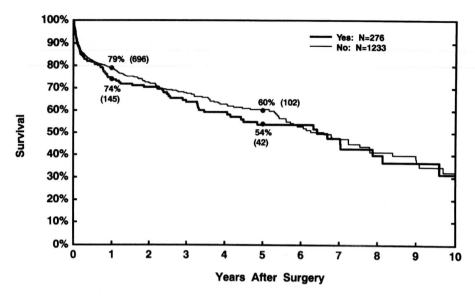

Figure 10–4. Estimated effect of aortic dissection on long-term survival calculated using the Kaplan-Meier method. (*Reproduced with permission from Crawford ES, De Natale RW. Thoracoabdominal aortic aneurysm: observations regarding the course of the disease.* J Vasc Surg. *1986;3:578–582.*)

Chronic Obstructive Pulmonary Disease

The preoperative presence of chronic obstructive pulmonary disease (COPD) in our patients moderately affected early survival following thoracoabdominal aortic aneurysm resection ($P = .0043$). There were 603 patients with COPD and 906 patients without. Early mortality in patients with COPD was 11% and was 7% without. The long-term influence of the presence of preoperative COPD is shown in Figure 10–5. Despite the very early effect upon survival, the long-term effects upon mortality appear to be rather minimal. We have found no single variable regarding preoperative pulmonary function that correlates with a prohibitive risk for either respiratory failure or death. Over and above the clinical diagnosis of chronic pulmonary disease, the instantaneous forced expiratory flow after 25% of the forced vital capacity (FEF25), forced expiratory volume (1 sec) (FEV_1), arterial partial pressure of carbon dioxide ($Paco_2$) have been identified as the most useful predictors of early death and the need for mechanical ventilation for periods exceeding 48 hours.[33] We continue to feel that pulmonary function tests, including spirometry testing and arterial blood gas analysis, are indicated as part of routine preoperative evaluation. In the presence of reversible restrictive disease, the initiation of preoperative bronchodilator therapy has been helpful.

Rupture

The presence or absence of rupture at the time of surgical intervention had a profound effect on early survival, and this effect carried through in a rather dramatic fashion upon long-term survival (Fig. 10–6). Rupture was present in 61 (4%) patients, whereas 1,448 (96%) patients were operated upon without rupture. Interestingly, rupture did not significantly vary with the extent of disease (I, 4%; II, 3%; III, 5%; IV, 5%). Early mortality was 8% without rupture and 18% with rupture ($P = .0040$). Renal failure requiring hemodialysis and postoperative neurologic deficits (paraparesis or paraplegia) were both markedly increased in patients with aortic rupture (36% vs. 17% and 26% vs. 15%, respectively). Long-term survival was dramatically affected at 5

11

Longevity of Aortofemoral Bypass Grafts

David C. Brewster, MD, and Jeffrey C. Cooke, MD

Aortoiliac occlusive disease is a common cause of symptomatic arterial insufficiency of the lower extremities. Narrowing or occlusion of the infrarenal aorta and iliac arteries, most often centered on the aortic bifurcation, occurs to varying degrees in almost all patients suffering from lower extremity occlusive disease who are in need of surgical revascularization. In many patients, obliterative disease in the aortoiliac segment is the most important contributor to the hemodynamic compromise responsible for ischemic symptoms.

In the four decades since Jacques Oudot replaced a thrombosed distal aorta with an arterial homograft in 1950, great advances in the surgical management of aortoiliac occlusive disease have been made. Direct methods of anatomic aortic reconstruction remain the most successful, and aortobifemoral grafting has emerged as the predominant method of dealing with aortoiliac occlusive disease.[1,2] With proper patient selection and preparation, and a carefully performed procedure, a beneficial result with low patient risk may almost always be anticipated. Indeed, resolution of the intractable symptoms of this disease by aortobifemoral grafting represents one of the most successful and gratifying aspects of vascular surgery.

This chapter will focus on the long-term results of aortofemoral bypass grafts done for aortoiliac occlusive disease, summarizing reported experience in terms of late outcome that may be expected in current clinical practice. Late graft patency rates will be examined, as well as various factors that may significantly influence long-term function of aortofemoral grafts. Since graft patency is only one determinant of clinical outcome, particularly in patients with multilevel occlusive disease, limb salvage rates and the success of proximal aortic reconstruction in relieving distal ischemic symptoms will also be reviewed. Finally, the important considerations of early and late mortality and the frequency of late complications of aortofemoral grafts will be analyzed.

LONG-TERM GRAFT PATENCY

In general, early and late patency of aortobifemoral bypass grafts performed for repair of aortoiliac occlusive disease is excellent. Results compiled from a number of major

TABLE 11–1. AORTOFEMORAL BYPASS STUDIES

Author	Date	Number of Patients	5 Years	10 Years	15 Years	20 Years
Nevelsteen et al[3]	1991	869	82	74	70	
Naylor et al[4]	1989	484	87			
Szilagyi et al[5]	1986	1,186	77	76	73	68
Sladen et al[6]	1986	100	84	78		
Poulias et al[7]	1985	500	87	78		
Crawford et al[8]	1981	949	87	79	70	56
Jones and Kempczinski[9]	1981	100	89			
Martinez et al[10]	1980	355	88	78		
Perdue et al[11]	1980	359	90			
Brewster and Darling[1]	1978	241	88	75		
Mulcare et al[12]	1978	104	94			
Malone et al[13]	1975	180	82	66		

series of aortofemoral grafts are shown in Table 11–1. In general, these show an expected patency rate of approximately 85% to 90% at 5 years, 75% at 10 years, 70% at 15 years, and 60% at 20 years.[1,3–13] However, these figures are applicable only in a broad sense, as the variability in long-term graft patency from series to series is often influenced by significant differences in patient characteristics within each study group. Such differences reflect the varying frequency of factors known to affect the longevity and late results of aortofemoral grafts, including the extent and distribution of aortoiliac disease, existence and possible progression of distal obliterative lesions, variety of different prosthetic grafts utilized, and the incidence of various atherosclerotic risk factors. Therefore, it is important to examine long-term results with such factors in mind.

Factors Affecting Long-Term Patency

Distribution of Disease

The distribution and extent of disease in the aortoiliac segment is important in determining the natural history of the occlusive process as well as the symptoms that result from it. This in turn may influence the method of surgical reconstruction selected and can significantly affect late graft patency.

Localized aortoiliac disease (Type I), with occlusive lesions confined to the distal aorta and common iliac vessels, is relatively infrequent, occurring in approximately 10% of our surgical candidates.[1] This incidence, of course, is reflective of those patients with symptoms serious enough to warrant surgical consideration. As other "less invasive" methods of treatment become more accepted, (i.e., endovascular transluminal balloon angioplasty, atherectomy, stenting, etc.), angiography may be more liberally used at an earlier stage in the disease process, thus increasing the incidence of relatively localized occlusive disease.[14]

Patients with Type I disease are typically younger, with a lower incidence of diabetes, hypertension, and other comorbid disease processes due to systemic arteriosclerosis.[15,16] Due to the localized nature of the disease, the potential for collateral pathway formation is great, and by definition infrainguinal runoff is good. Patients with this disease pattern therefore almost always undergo operation for claudication alone in an elective setting. Hence, the initial results of proximal aortic grafting are usually excellent. In addition, long-term observation has indicated that such patients are less likely to have progression of their occlusive disease,[17–19] and, therefore, long-term graft patency and functional results are usually better maintained compared with patency in patients with more widespread disease initially.

The vast majority of patients who present for aortoiliac operation have more diffuse occlusive disease. Although the atherosclerotic occlusive process is usually segmental and, therefore, amenable to effective surgical intervention, it is a widespread process that often involves multiple segments of the arterial tree.[20] Approximately 20% to 25% of patients will have a type II pattern, with occlusive lesions confined largely to the abdominal vessels but extending to involve the external iliac artery and occasionally the common femoral artery. Most frequent are patients exhibiting widespread occlusive disease both above and below the inguinal ligament (Type III). Such patients with multilevel disease constitute approximately two-thirds of our own surgical candidates,[1] and 50% to 66% of most surgical series.[3,5,8,13] Patients with multilevel disease are typically older; more commonly male (about 6:1 ratio); and much more likely to have diabetes, hypertension, and atherosclerotic disease involving coronary, cerebral, and/or visceral arteries.[16] Progression of the disease process over time is also more likely than in Type I patients.[19] The majority of patients with multilevel disease manifest symptoms of more advanced ischemia, such as rest pain or tissue necrosis, and operation is therefore often performed for limb salvage rather than simply for relief of claudication. All of these factors quite naturally can be expected to adversely affect long-term graft patency and clinical outcome.

Distal Occlusive Disease

The existence of multilevel disease in the majority of patients undergoing aortofemoral graft reconstruction makes the extent of infrainguinal occlusive disease an important factor in late results. Most often, disease in the outflow vasculature involves stenosis or occlusion of the superficial femoral artery (SFA), but coexistent obliterative lesions of the profunda femoris may occur in up to 15% of patients or involve the popliteal or tibial vessels.[13,21,22] In the presence of compromised SFA runoff, unimpeded outflow via the deep femoral artery is universally recognized and acknowledged to be of vital importance to the long-term success of inflow reconstruction.[1,5,8,13,17,23,24] Correction of any orificial profunda disease by profundaplasty using the tip of the inflow graft, or more formal endarterectomy with or without patching, is a key factor in the long-term success of such procedures.[1–3,14,23–27] It is important to assess the profunda by preoperative arteriography, and intraoperatively by inspection, palpation, and gentle exploration with probes. In our experience, a satisfactory profunda system should accept at least a 4-mm probe proximally, and passage of a noninflated embolectomy catheter should be possible for at least 20 cm.[1,2,16,27] Such criteria generally indicate a well-developed profunda system that will function satisfactorily as an outflow tract and collateral pathway to the lower leg. Although some authors propose that profundaplasty performed in patients with an occluded SFA but without a pathologic orificial stenosis of the profunda ("functional" profunda stenosis) is beneficial,[28] most evidence shows that it is not.[29]

More controversial is the influence of associated SFA occlusive disease alone on aortofemoral graft patency. Some investigators have reported negligible influence of the SFA on graft patency. Hill and colleagues[30] studied 56 patients with claudication alone for a mean of 3.3 years, and found no effect of SFA involvement on aortofemoral graft patency. Similar conclusions were reached by Martinez and coworkers following review of 376 consecutive patients undergoing aortobifemoral bypass grafts at the Cleveland Clinic during the 10-year period from 1967 to 1977.[10] This conclusion is also supported by studies that show that flow rates in the external iliac are similar whether SFA occlusion is present or not, suggesting the capacity of the profunda system to compensate for SFA occlusion.[24] However, other authors feel that SFA occlusion has a definite adverse effect upon the long-term patency of aortofemoral grafts.[3,9,13,31] Rutherford and associates[32] showed a reduction of patency from 90% to 76% when SFA occlusion existed. Harris and colleagues[33] identified a marked decrease in the patency of aortofemoral grafts in patients who had occluded femoropopliteal arteries versus those with patent outflow occurring as early as the first year. At 5 years this difference was even greater, with a 97% patency for those with patent outflow versus 65% without. Additionally, as testament to the effect of SFA occlusion, a significantly improved late patency of aortofemoral grafts was noted at 1 and 5 years in those who had a concomitant outflow bypass versus those who did not.[33]

Graft Selection

Although the standard fabric prosthetic grafts constructed from Dacron or Teflon that were used during the initial era of aortofemoral reconstruction have generally performed well, in recent years a wide variety of aortic prosthetic grafts have become available to the vascular surgeon. Numerous modifications in graft material (Dacron vs. polytetrafluoroethylene (PTFE), methods of fabrication (knitted vs. woven, external velour vs. double velour, porosity differences), and addition of various biologic coatings (collagen, albumin) to the graft have been devised.

Such alterations have been proposed with the hope of improving the performance and characteristics of the graft, usually in terms of patency, durability, healing and incorporation within host tissue, resistance to infection, reduced blood loss through the graft, and improved handling qualities. Various claims concerning the benefits of one type over another have been made, though it is often difficult to discern science from salesmanship. Past studies done to evaluate the differences frequently lacked adequate control to allow an accurate conclusion to be drawn. One attempt by Robicsek and coworkers to help clarify this situation involved the use of "half-and-half" grafts of woven and knitted Dacron.[34] Implanting a bifurcated Dacron graft constructed with one limb woven and the other knitted allowed these surgeons to directly compare patency of the two limbs. Although approximately half of their 158 patients underwent replacement for aneurysm, at an average 5.5 years follow-up no significant difference was found in patency between the two limbs. In our experience, the use of woven or knitted Dacron graft material is dictated by the clinical situation without prejudice concerning patency. Our preference in aortofemoral grafting has largely been for knitted Dacron grafts, due mostly to their flexibility and ease of handling and suturing—factors that are particularly helpful when a difficult profunda anastomosis is necessary. However, newer manufacturing techniques have begun to blur the former distinct differences in mechanical properties and characteristics between knitted and woven Dacron grafts, making such considerations less important in current practice.

Whether internal or external velour surfaces or a combination of the two is beneficial remains unproven. Although porosity and incorporation by the host remain desirable features, the successful use of PTFE grafts in other locations has made these considerations questionable. The bifurcated PTFE graft, introduced in 1982, has had too limited use in the United States to allow meaningful evaluation of its long-term reliability. Studies by Burke and colleagues of PTFE use in the hypoplastic aortic syndrome suggested improved patency results compared with Dacron grafts,[35] but statistical significance was not achieved. High-porosity grafts sealed with protein matrix substances, fibrin glue, or other materials show promise for improvement in host tolerance and lower thrombogenicity, but are too new to allow comment on long-term results. Clearly, both PTFE and biologically coated prosthetics do limit blood loss and facilitate the procedure by obviating the need for preclotting of the graft, but all such grafts are generally more expensive than a conventional fabric prosthesis, and any improved performance is unproven.

One may currently conclude that, in general, no single large-caliber graft is clearly superior and that long-term patency is more closely related to proper surgical methods of graft implantation and limitation of disease progression than to the specific graft employed.

Irrespective of the exact type of graft material and fabrication, use of a proper size graft is important, realizing that flow rate through the graft limbs affects patency. An excessively large-diameter graft in a limb may result in a decreased flow rate through the graft. This phenomenon was seen in the early era of revascularization when surgeons often used grafts too large for the size of the outflow tract vessels, resulting in sluggish flow and excessive deposition of laminar pseudointima, which may promote subsequent thrombosis of the prosthesis. Additionally, this deposited material often has a propensity to fragment or dislodge. For treating occlusive disease, a 16 × 8 mm bifurcated graft is now most often used, although a 14 × 7 mm (or even smaller) prosthesis is used without hesitation when appropriate, as is frequently the case with some female patients. The limb size of these grafts will most closely approximate the femoral arteries of patients with occlusive disease, particularly, the size of the profunda femoris. In addition, many Dacron prosthetic grafts have a tendency to dilate 10% to 20% when subjected to arterial pressure.[36] Selection of smaller graft size can help compensate for this dilatation.

Anastomotic Configuration

Although the technique of aortic graft insertion has been fairly well standardized, some differences in methods still remain and are quite controversial. For example, the issue of whether an end-to-end proximal aortic anastomosis is superior to an end-to-side configuration is still debated and unresolved. End-to-end anastomosis is clearly indicated in patients with coexistent aneurysmal disease or complete aortic occlusion up to the renal arteries. In addition, it is preferred by many vascular surgeons for routine use in most cases for several reasons. First, it is theoretically more sound from a hemodynamic standpoint, producing less turbulence, better flow characteristics, and less chance of competitive flow with still patent host iliac vessels. Second, application of partially occluding tangential clamps for construction of an end-to-side anastomosis often carries a higher risk of dislodging intra-aortic debris that may embolize to the pelvis or extremity. Finally, an end-to-end anastomosis generally reduces the possibility of kinking of the graft limbs, and greatly facilitates subsequent tissue coverage and reperitonealization over the prosthesis, all of which may contribute to fewer late graft complications. All of these considerations have led to better long-term patency of grafts done with end-to-end proximal anastomosis in many reported series, although none have been controlled or prospective.[1,12,16,37,38]

The end-to-side anastomosis may be advantageous in certain anatomic patterns of disease.[2] These include the presence of accessory renal arteries from the lower aorta, the desire to preserve a patent inferior mesenteric artery, or occlusive disease confined largely to the external iliac artery that precludes retrograde flow into the pelvis with end-to-end graft insertion, and the potential adverse consequences thereof. Presently, both proximal anastomotic methods have experienced and skilled vascular surgeons as advocates. Regardless of the method, the principle of placing the graft high in the aorta, relatively close to the renal arteries, is very important. This area is almost always less involved with the occlusive process, and less likely to have problems with future disease progression.

Although the distal anastomosis of the graft may occasionally be accomplished at the level of the external iliac artery in the pelvis, it is almost always preferable to carry the graft to the femoral level. Surgical exposure is usually better and anastomosis technically easier. Most importantly, exposure at the femoral level provides the surgeon with the opportunity to examine and ensure adequate outflow through the profunda femoral artery. Reported experience has shown an increased late failure rate of aortoexternal iliac grafts compared with grafts carried down to the femoral level for correction of occlusive disease.[1,39,40] With modern surgical care, the anticipated higher rate of infection in grafts carried to the groin has not been borne out.

Smoking

Although most of the factors that ultimately decide the fate of the graft are not under the control of the patient, one of the most important is. Use of tobacco is clearly the greatest risk factor for the development and progression of atherosclerotic occlusive disease.[41]

Persistent cigarette smoking has also been shown to have a detrimental effect upon the success of arterial revascularization procedures. Myers and coworkers, in a retrospective review of 217 patients, found that a patient who smoked more than five cigarettes a day after the bypass, had a threefold increase in the likelihood of occluding their aortofemoral graft.[42] This result was irrespective of patient age, gender, or severity of disease. Greenhalgh and colleagues[43] prospectively followed 64 patients for 5 years who underwent arterial reconstruction, measuring their carboxy-hemoglobin and lipid levels. Twelve of the grafts failed during that period, with the only difference between the patients with a failed graft and those with a patent graft being significantly higher carboxyhemoglobin levels in the group whose grafts failed. This suggested that the vast majority of patients who had graft failure continued to smoke cigarettes. Several other studies[44-46] overwhelmingly show that smoking after arterial revascularization severely increases the risk of graft failure and, therefore, needs to be strictly curtailed if the best long-term patency is to be achieved.

SYMPTOM RELIEF

A patent aortofemoral graft in patients with relatively localized aortoiliac disease (Types I and II) quite logically leads to highly successful functional results in terms of relief of ischemic symptoms and salvage of limbs with more advanced preoperative ischemic impairment. Due to the well-established good long-term patency rates of aortofemoral grafts and the documented lower incidence of distal disease progression in patients with occlusive disease initially confined to the aortoiliac segment, long-term functional results in patients with Type I or II disease patterns are generally well maintained.

However, because of the presence of more widespread multilevel disease in the majority of patients who are considered candidates for aortofemoral grafts, even a technically successful proximal operation with sustained patency may not always improve distal circulation sufficiently to attain satisfactory relief of lower extremity ischemia. Hence, in patients with multilevel disease, it is important to consider functional outcome in addition to the traditional criteria of late graft patency in assessing long-term results.

TABLE 11–2. CLINICAL OUTCOME OF AORTOFEMORAL GRAFTS IN PATIENTS WITH MULTILEVEL DISEASE[a]

Postoperative Symptom Status	Percentage of Patients	
Good Result	74	
Total Relief		24
Improved		50
Unsatisfactory Result	26	
Unimproved		18
Worse		8
	100	100

[a] From Brewster et al[27]

Reports of patients with multilevel disease treated in a conventional fashion by an initial inflow procedure have documented that approximately 25% to 33% of such patients may have an unsatisfactory clinical result from proximal revascularization alone.[10,12,13,19,27,30,47–49] In such patients, clinically important, persistent ischemia due to uncorrected distal disease requires subsequent distal arterial reconstructive procedures in 10% to 25% of patients.[8,10,12,27,33,40,50] Data from review of our own experience[27] are representative of this important point (Table 11–2). Although 74% of patients with multilevel disease were classified as improved following aortofemoral grafting alone, 26% were judged to have an unsatisfactory outcome from inflow correction only. Of the 74% of patients deemed improved, only 24% had total relief of ischemic symptoms, and 50% were still restricted by varying degrees of claudication. When analyzed in terms of the original indications for operation, 82% of patients with only claudication were improved, but only 35% were completely free of symptoms. Ten percent of these patients ultimately underwent an additional distal bypass due to the continued severity of their claudication disability. If results of aortofemoral grafts in patients with multilevel disease assessed by hemodynamic parameters rather than simply subjective symptom relief, long-term functional results appear even more disappointing.[19,32,49]

LIMB SALVAGE

The subset of patients undergoing aortoiliac bypass for limb salvage generally do worse than those with claudication alone. This result generally reflects a more extensive pattern of disease seen in these patients. Limb salvage is achieved in 75% to 98% of those with gangrene or ulcers in the first 5 years.[3,13,27,50–52] However, approximately one-third of these patients require additional distal bypass to maintain the ischemic limb.[27,50]

Diabetics have a poorer limb salvage rate compared with nondiabetics, probably reflecting the extent to which microangiopathy and large-vessel occlusive disease act concomitantly to threaten loss of limb.[51] No single predictor exists to determine which patients require distal revascularization, but those manifesting severe necrosis or infection of the forefoot are the ones that the clinician must recognize to be in the high-probability group. With such advanced ischemic symptoms, serious consideration should be given to simultaneous inflow and outflow revascularization at the time of initial surgical intervention. Even if aortofemoral grafting alone is sufficient to salvage the limb, almost all patients still have residual claudication symptoms.[27]

LATE MORTALITY

Despite significant reduction in perioperative mortality rates, with some experienced health centers reporting 30-day death rates of only 1% to 2% following aortofemoral grafts, late survival of these patients continues to be compromised. The cumulative long-term survival rate for patients undergoing aortoiliac reconstruction continues to be 10 to 15 years less than that anticipated for a normal age- and sex-matched population. Overall, approximately 20% to 30% of patients will be dead within 5 years of operation, and 50% to 60% by the 10-year interval.[3,5,8,53] As expected, the majority of late deaths are attributable to coronary artery disease and its sequelae. The important influence of the extent of disease is once again emphasized, as patients with more localized aortoiliac disease, who have a lower incidence of coronary disease, systemic arteriosclerosis, diabetes, and other risk factors, appear to have a much more favorable long-term prognosis that approaches that of a normal population at risk.[10,53]

LATE COMPLICATIONS

Reflecting the advances in surgical technique and perioperative anesthetic and supportive care, which have collectively achieved significantly reduced early operative mortality, major early complications of direct aortic surgery are seen relatively infrequently and occur in approximately 5% to 10% of patients.[2] Bleeding requiring reoperation or acute limb ischemia secondary to graft thrombosis or distal thromboembolism are each encountered in 1% to 2% of patients. Acute postoperative renal failure is currently quite unusual after elective operation due to recognition of the importance of adequate fluid administration during the operation, intraoperative optimization of cardiac function, and avoidance of declamping hypotension. Bowel and spinal cord ischemia remain serious problems but fortunately are relatively rare occurrences. Nonfatal myocardial infarction develops in 3% to 5% of patients, often with little hemodynamic consequence. Significant pulmonary insufficiency is unusual in contemporary practice in the absence of severe preoperative chronic lung disease.

Despite the generally good durability of aortofemoral grafts, the progressive nature of atherosclerotic disease and other degenerative factors continue to result in late complications of even technically successful reconstructive procedures. The frequency of late complications is largely dependent upon the length of follow-up, but by 10 years approximately 15% of patients may be expected to experience problems related to the initial graft procedure.

Graft Occlusion

Graft occlusion remains the most common late complication of aortofemoral grafts performed for aortoiliac occlusive disease. By far the most frequent occurrence is thrombosis of one limb of an aortobifemoral bifurcated prosthesis. Although the exact incidence varies from series to series, thrombosis may occur in 5% to 10% of patients within the first 5 years following primary operation and in 15% to 30% of patients surviving in excess of 10 years.[1,3,5,8,12,13] The great majority of late occlusions of the graft limb are attributable to progressive occlusive disease or perianastomotic intimal hyperplasia involving the femoral anastomosis. Most of these patients have a chronically occluded SFA, and the progressive obliterative process compromises profunda runoff and eventually leads to occlusion of the graft limb.[54] Other less common causes of graft limb occlusion include thrombosis of a femoral anastomotic aneurysm, thromboembolism from a proximal source, various hypercoagulable states, or episodes of low cardiac output secondary to a variety of acute systemic illnesses.

In our review, the average interval from original graft insertion to thrombosis of one limb of the prothesis was 33.8 months.[54] The resulting extremity ischemia is often more severe than that occurring prior to the primary operation, and frequently urgent surgical intervention is required to alleviate limb-threatening symptoms. Restoration of graft limb patency may often be successfully accomplished by catheter thrombectomy, but often a mechanical stripper may be required to ensure complete removal of adherent fibrothrombotic debris.[54,55] Once inflow is re-established, some form of profundaplasty is generally required to provide reliable outflow.[26,54,55] If the profunda is felt inadequate, addition of a distal bypass may be required to attain adequate perfusion of the extremity and maintain secondary patency of the inflow graft.[54]

If thrombectomy is not successful in restoring good flow through the occluded graft limb, a femorofemoral graft from the contralateral patent graft limb is often the next best choice for redo revascularization. Actual replacement of the occluded graft limb via direct transabdominal or retroperitoneal approach is rarely necessary for unilateral graft limb failures, as other methods of restoring inflow and correcting outflow problems work equally well and carry less morbidity and mortality risk. Proximal aortic disease or problems at the aortic anastomosis are infrequently the cause of failure of one limb of a bifurcation graft. If proximal abnormalities are indeed present, failure of the entire graft usually results. In these circumstances, direct replacement of the entire prosthesis, and construction of a more proximal new aortic anastomosis, is required. If total redo aortofemoral grafting is felt too difficult or excessively risky for the patient, alternative reconstructive choices include axillobifemoral bypass or the use of alternative inflow sites, including the supraceliac aorta, descending thoracic aorta, or even the ascending aorta.[56]

Anastomotic False Aneurysm

These aneurysms have an incidence of 3% to 5% following aortofemoral graft insertion and most often occur at the femoral anastomosis.[5] Although numerous factors may contribute to anastomotic pseudoaneurysms, degenerative changes within the host arterial wall leading to dehiscence of a portion of the intact suture line appear most common. Predisposing factors include excessive graft tension, inadequate shallow suture bites of the arterial wall, or a thin-walled or endarterectomized artery. Late graft dilatation may promote formation of an anastomotic aneurysm, probably creating areas of alternating tension within a suture line. Because of the preponderance of femoral pseudoaneurysms, the end-to-side configuration and mechanical stresses across the groin crease are likely contributing factors as well. Infection may occasionally be responsible and must always be considered as a possible cause. Sometimes such an infection may be quite occult, particularly when due to certain microorganisms, such as *Staphylococcus epidermidis,* and the clinical picture is difficult to differentiate from the typically bland appearing anastomotic aneurysm due to noninfectious causes.[57]

In a review by Satiani, the mean interval between primary operation and the diagnosis of an anastomotic aneurysm was 42 months.[58] Recognition of a femoral pseudoaneurysm is usually straightforward with development of an obvious palpable pulsatile mass that is occasionally tender. Even if the diagnosis is readily apparent, an arteriogram and/or computed tomography scan is generally advisable to help plan surgical correction and particularly to evaluate other anastomotic sites for similar problems. For instance, Schellack and colleagues reviewed 41 patients with a femoral anastomotic aneurysm after aortobifemoral grafting and found that 70% had bilateral femoral pseudoaneurysm and 17% had associated proximal aortic false aneurysm.[59] Retroperitoneal anastomotic aneurysms are usually difficult to palpate and often escape detection until symptoms or complications occur, or they are discovered by radiologic screening.

Although frank rupture of a femoral anastomotic pseudoaneurysm is unusual, these lesions may cause distal ischemia by *in-situ* thrombosis or dislodgment of mural thrombus. Retroperitoneal false aneurysms appear more prone to rupture or erosion into adjacent bowel and may cause symptoms by compression on adjacent structures. For instance, development of hydronephrosis secondary to ureteral obstruction may be the first clue to graft or anastomotic complications.[60] Because of the potential for such complications, most anastomotic aneurysms should be repaired when detected, even if asymptomatic.

Graft Infection

Graft infection following aortofemoral prosthetic graft procedures remains the most feared late complication of such surgery, with formidable morbidity and mortality rates up to 75% in some series when treating extensive graft infections. Fortunately, with current surgical methods and use of prophylactic antibiotics, the incidence of graft infection is only 1% to 2%.[1,5] In all series, the inguinal portion of an aortofemoral graft is most commonly involved. Important contributing factors include (1) multiple vascular procedures; (2) postoperative wound healing difficulties, such as hematoma, seroma formation, or lymphatic leaks; and (3) emergency operation.

Although most graft infections are recognized more than a year after graft implantation, it is generally believed that most graft infections are attributable to contamination at the time of primary operation.[2] Several studies have implicated the importance of bacteria in inguinal lymph nodes in the pathophysiology of subsequent graft infection. Late graft infections due to bacteremic implantation on the luminal surface of functioning grafts may occasionally occur.

The diagnosis and management of infected aortofemoral grafts is complex and beyond the scope of this review. In general, excision of the infected graft is almost always required and revascularization via remote uncontaminated routes, or use of autogenous tissue reconstructive methods, are often necessary to maintain limb viability. Although the entire prosthesis must often be removed, more localized excision of only involved portions of the graft may sometimes be feasible and appropriate.

Aortoenteric Fistula

Such fistulas and subsequent gastrointestinal hemorrhage are a final, infrequent, but often devastating late complication, with a continued high incidence of death or limb loss despite efforts at treatment. Communication between the proximal graft anastomosis and the third or fourth portion of the overlying duodenum is most common, but erosion of the graft body or limb into adjacent small or large bowel may occur as well. In this latter situation of paraprosthetic graft erosion, massive bleeding does not occur as no direct communication of the graft and bowel lumens exists, and most patients manifest the clinical picture of graft infection.

Such secondary aortoenteric fistula formation or enteric erosion may occur as a result of several mechanisms. If the adjacent bowel is improperly separated from the graft and anastomosis, fibrotic adherence and subsequent bowel wall erosion may occur. Indeed, the incidence of aortoenteric fistula formation appears to be higher following end-to-side aortic anastomosis than in end-to-end anastomosis because of the greater difficulty in covering an end-to-side anastomotic configuration with retroperitoneal tissues and in avoiding contact with the bowel.[1,16,37] Another mechanism of aortoenteric fistula or erosion involves initial development of an aortic anastomotic pseudoaneurysm due to either mechanical factors or infection, with later erosion of this pulsating false aneurysm into adjacent bowel.

As with primary cases of graft infection, treatment decisions are difficult and complex. Standard management principles generally require removal of the graft, closure of the infrarenal aortic stump, repair of the gastrointestinal tract defect, and extra-anatomic revascularization. Although some recent reports have cited successful results of *in-situ* replacement with a new anatomic prosthetic graft if local contamination is minimal, routine adoption of this method remains unproven. Despite advances in treatment, death and limb loss still occur in up to 50% of these patients; mortality is often related to continued sepsis, multiorgan system failure, or disruption of the aortic stump closure.

REFERENCES

1. Brewster DC, Darling RC. Optimal methods of aortoiliac reconstruction. *Surgery.* 1978;84:739–748.
2. Brewster DC. Direct reconstruction for aortoiliac occlusive disease. In: Rutherford RB, ed. *Vascular Surgery,* 3rd ed. Philadelphia: WB Saunders Co; 1989:667–691.
3. Nevelsteen A, Wouters L, Suy R. Aortofemoral Dacron reconstruction for aortoiliac occlusive disease: a 25 year survey. *Eur J Vasc Surg.* 1991;5:179–186.
4. Naylor AR, Ah See AK, Engeset J. The morbidity and mortality after aortofemoral grafting for peripheral limb ischemia. *J R Coll Surg Edinb.* 1989;34:215–218.
5. Szilagyi DE, Elliott JP Jr, Smith RF, et al. A thirty-year survey of the reconstructive surgical treatment of aortoiliac occlusive disease. *J Vasc Surg.* 1986;3:421–436.
6. Sladen JG, Gilmour JL, Wong RW. Cumulative patency and actual palliation in patients with claudication after aortofemoral bypass. Prospective long-term follow-up of 100 patients. *Am J Surg.* 1986;152:190–195.
7. Poulias GE, Polemis L, Skoutas B, et al. Bilateral aorto-femoral bypass in the presence of aorto-iliac occlusive disease and factors determining results: experience and long term follow up with 500 consecutive cases. *J Cardiovasc Surg.* 1985;26:527–538.
8. Crawford ES, Bomberger RA, Glaeser DH, et al. Aortoiliac occlusive disease: factors influencing survival and function following reconstructive operation over a twenty-five year period. *Surgery.* 1981;90:1055–1067.
9. Jones AF, Kempczinski RF. Aortofemoral bypass grafting: a reappraisal. *Arch Surg.* 1981;116:301–305.
10. Martinez BD, Hertzer NR, Beven EG. Influence of distal arterial occlusive disease on prognosis following aortobifemoral bypass. *Surgery.* 1980;88:795–805.
11. Perdue GD, Smith RB III, Veazey CR, et al. Revascularization for severe limb ischemia. *Arch Surg.* 1980;115:168–171.
12. Mulcare RJ, Royster TS, Lynn RA, et al. Long-term results of operative therapy for aortoiliac occlusive disease. *Arch Surg.* 1978;113:601–604.
13. Malone JM, Moore WS, Goldstone J. The natural history of bilateral aortofemoral bypass grafts for ischemia of the lower extremities. *Arch Surg.* 1975;110:1300–1306.
14. Brewster DC. Clinical and anatomic considerations for surgery in aortoiliac disease and results of surgical treatment. *Circulation.* 1991;83(suppl I):I-42–I-52.
15. Cronenwett JL, Davis JT Jr, Gooch JB, et al. Aortoiliac occlusive disease in women. *Surgery.* 1980;88:775.
16. Darling RC, Brewster DC, Hallett JW Jr, et al. Aortoiliac reconstruction. *Surg Clin North Am.* 1979;59:565.

17. Moore WS, Cafferata HT, Hall AD, et al. In defense of grafts across the inguinal ligament: an evaluation of early and late results of aorto-femoral bypass grafts. *Ann Surg.* 1968;168:207–214.

18. Staples TW. The solitary aortoiliac lesion. *Surgery.* 1968;64:569–576.

19. Mozersky DJ, Sumner DS, Strandness DE. Long-term results of reconstructive aortoiliac surgery. *Am J Surg.* 1972;123:503–509.

20. DeBakey ME, Lawrie GM, Glaeser DH. Patterns of atherosclerosis and their surgical significance. *Ann Surg.* 1985;201:115–131.

21. Haimovici H. Patterns of arteriosclerotic lesions of the lower extremity. *Arch Surg.* 1967;95:918–933.

22. Veith FJ, Gupta SK, Wengerter KR, et al. Changing arteriosclerotic disease patterns and management strategies in lower-limb-threatening ischemia. *Ann Surg.* 1990;212:401–412.

23. Morris GC Jr, Edwards W, Cooley DA, et al. Surgical importance of the profunda femoris artery: analysis of 102 cases with combined aortoiliac and femoropopliteal occlusive disease treated by revascularization of deep femoral artery. *Arch Surg.* 1961;82:32–37.

24. Bernhard VM, Ray LI, Militello JP. The role of angioplasty in the profunda femoris artery in revascularization of the ischemic limb. *Surg, Gynecol, Obstet.* 1976;142:840–844.

25. Edwards WH, Jenkins JM, Mulherin JL, et al. Extended profundaplasty to minimize pelvic and distal tissue loss. *Ann Surg.* 1990;211:694–702.

26. Malone JM, Goldstone J, Moore WS. Autogenous profundaplasty: the key to long-term patency in secondary repair of aortofemoral graft occlusion. *Ann Surg.* 1978;188:817–823.

27. Brewster DC, Perler BA, Robinson JG, et al. Aortofemoral graft for MLD: predictors of success and need for distal bypass. *Arch Surg.* 1982;117:1593–1600.

28. Berguer R, Higgins RF, Colton LT. Geometry, blood flow, and reconstruction of the deep femoral artery. *Am J Surg.* 1975;130:68–73.

29. Rutherford RB, Jones DN, Martin MS, et al. Serial hemodynamic assessment of aortobifemoral bypass. *J Vasc Surg.* 1986;4:428–435.

30. Hill DA, McGrath MA, Lord RSA, et al. The effect of superficial femoral artery occlusion on the outcome of aortofemoral bypass for intermittent claudication. *Surgery.* 1980;87:133–136.

31. Charlesworth D. Simultaneous proximal and distal reconstruction. In: Bergen JJ, Yao JST, eds. *Aortic Surgery.* Philadelphia and London: WB Saunders; 1989:373.

32. Rutherford RB, Jones DN, Martin MS, et al. Serial hemodynamic assessment of aortobifemoral bypass. *J Vasc Surg.* 1986;4:428–435.

33. Harris PL, Cave Bigel DJ, McSweeney L. Aortofemoral bypass and the role of concomitant femorodistal reconstruction. *Br J Surg.* 1985;72:317–320.

34. Robicsek F, Duncan GD, Daugherty HK, et al. "Half and half" woven and knitted Dacron grafts in the aortoiliac and aortofemoral positions: seven and one-half years follow-up. *Ann Vasc Surg.* 1991;5:315–319.

35. Burke PM, Herrmann JB, Cutler BS. Optimal grafting methods for the small abdominal aorta. *J Cardiovasc Surg.* 1987;28:420–426.

36. Nunn DB, Carter MM, Donohue MT, et al. Postoperative dilation of knitted Dacron aortic bifurcation graft. *J Vasc Surg.* 1990;12:291–297.

37. Dunn DA, Downs AT, Lye CR. Aortoiliac reconstruction for occlusive disease: comparison of end-to-end and end-to-side proximal anastomosis. *Can J Surg.* 1982;25:382–384.

38. Pierce GE, Turrentine M, Stringfield S, et al. Evaluation of end-to-side v. end-to-end proximal anastomosis in aortobifemoral bypass. *Arch Surg.* 1982;117:1580–1588.

39. Crawford ES, Manning LG, Kelly TF. "Redo" surgery after operations for aneurysms and occlusion of the abdominal aorta. *Surgery.* 1977;81:41–52.

40. Baird RJ, Feldman P, Miles JT, et al. Subsequent downstream repair after aorto-iliac and aorto-femoral bypass operations. *Surgery.* 1977;82:785–793.

41. Kannel WB, Shurtleff D. The Framingham study: cigarettes and the development of intermittent claudication. *Geriatrics.* 1973;28:61.

42. Myers KA, King RB, Scott DF, et al. The effect of smoking on the late patency of arterial reconstructions in the legs. *Br J Surg.* 1978;65:267–271.

TABLE 12–3. MATCHED CONTROL STUDY OF STRAIGHT VERSUS BIFURCATED AORTIC GRAFTS[a] [b]

Late Complications	Straight n=39	Bifurcated N=39
Graft-related complications	2 (5.0%)	5 (12.5%)
New aneurysms	2 (5.0%)	2 (5.0%)
Thoracic aortic dissection		1 (2.5%)
New distal occlusive disease	1 (2.5%)	4 (10.0%)
Total	5 (12.5%)	12 (30.0%)

[a] Matched for age, gender, and year of operation. Mean follow-up was 6 years.
[b] From Castagno et al.[8]

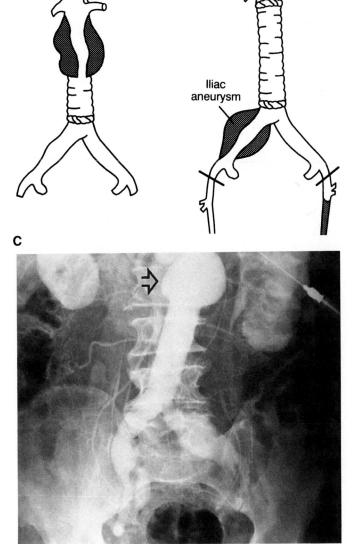

Figure 12–1. (**A**) Proximal aortic aneurysm. (**B**) Iliac aneurysm or distal occlusive disease. (**C**) A new aortic aneurysm (arrow) above the original aortic tube graft occurs in about 5% of AAA patients in long-term follow-up.

Figure 12–2. Cumulative incidence of graft-related complications in patients undergoing tube versus bifurcated Dacron grafts for abdominal aortic aneurysms, matched for age and year of operation, Rochester, Minnesota, 1951–1984. (*Reproduced with permission from Calcagno D, Hallett JW, Ballard DJ, et al. Late iliac artery aneurysms and occlusive disease after aortic tube grafts for abdominal aortic aneurysm repair. Ann Surg. 1991; 214:733–736.*)

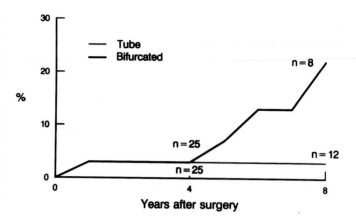

10% of patients with bifurcated grafts. All of these vascular and graft-related problems were more likely to occur at relatively late dates, ranging from 5 to 15 years (Fig. 12–4). Survival of patients undergoing tube versus bifurcated Dacron grafts was similar at 8 years (50% vs. 45%, respectively) (Fig. 12–5).

TRENDS IN TUBE GRAFTING

There has been a general trend toward using more straight grafts for AAA repair. In reporting a 20-year experience of over 1,000 AAA patients at the Massachusetts General Hospital, Darling and Brewster mentioned that only 5% of the AAAs in the early part of their experience were treated with a tube graft compared with at least 20% at the end of the period.[10] In a 25-year experience with 920 consecutive AAA repairs, Crawford and colleagues reported that straight tubes were used in 60% of patients and bifurcated grafts in 40%.[11] In their specific report of a 16-year experience with tube graft replacement for AAA, Evans and Hayes used the straight grafts in 46% of 332 elective AAA repairs.[4] In the more recent Canadian multicenter prospec-

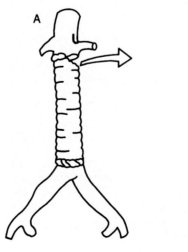
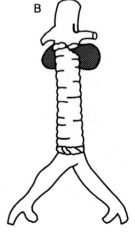

Figure 12–3. Aortic suture-line disruption of pseudoaneurysm affects about 5% of AAA patients with tube grafts. (**A**) Proximal anastomotic rupture. (**B**) Proximal anastomotic pseudoaneurysm.

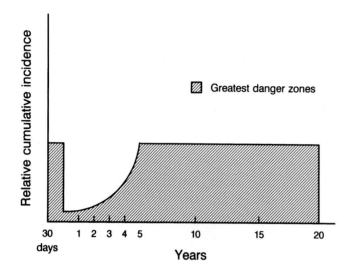

Figure 12–4. Graft-related complications usually occur within 30 days of initial operation or after 5 years. New aneurysms are also usually detected between 5 and 15 years.

tive trial of elective AAA repairs, Johnson and Scobie reported the following distribution of grafts in 666 patients: tube grafts in 38.5%, bi-iliac grafts in 30.7%, iliac–femoral grafts in 6.5%, and bifemoral grafts in 24.3%.[12] Finally, Olsen and colleagues reported that in their series of 656 patients the use of tube grafts increased from 14% in 1979 to 63% by 1988.[13]

The trend toward more tube grafts for AAA repair appears to occur for several reasons. First, a tube graft can simplify surgical dissection and time. Second, long-term follow-up indicates a low likelihood of patients developing subsequent iliac aneurysm or occlusive disease. Third, limiting the graft to the aneurysmal aorta avoids any complications of more extensive pelvic dissection for aortoiliac grafts or groin incisions for aortofemoral grafts that may be complicated by infection.

TECHNICAL TIPS FOR TUBE GRAFTS

The technical advantages and disadvantages of aortic tube grafts are still debated. Advocates emphasize minimal aortoiliac dissection in treating the significant aneurysm. On the other hand, critics point out the difficulties of working with a calcified

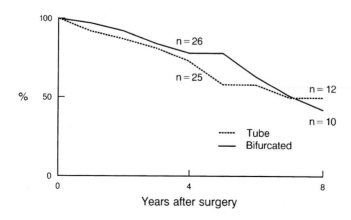

Figure 12–5. Percentage of patients that survive surgery for tube versus bifurcated Dacron grafts for abdominal aortic aneurysms, matched for age and year of operation, Rochester, Minnesota, 1951–1984. (*Reproduced with permission from Calcagno D, Hallett JW, Ballard DJ, et al. Late iliac artery aneurysms and occlusive disease after aortic tube grafts for abdominal aortic aneurysm repair. Ann Surg. 1991; 214:733–736.*)

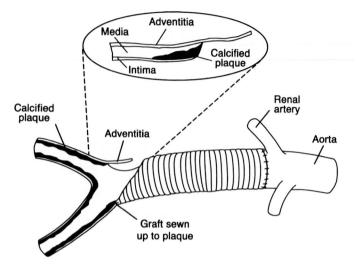

Figure 12–6. A tube graft can be safely secured to a calcified aortic bifurcation by (1) first, trimming the posterior calcified aortic rim with heavy cardiac valve scissors and (2), sewing the graft anastomosis to the endarterectomized aortic adventitia flushly against (not through) the calcified aortic cuff.

aortic bifurcation and their concerns for late iliac aneurysmal or occlusive disease progression.

The following technical tips will assist with tube graft replacement. First, aortoiliac dissection should be minimized to expose only enough proximal aorta and iliac arteries for safe clamping. The aorta and the iliac arteries do not need to be completely encircled. In fact, iliac venous injury is minimized by simply dissecting the iliac arteries on their medial and lateral surfaces for safe application of a vascular clamp. Second, if the common iliac arteries are severely calcified, clamps may be applied more safely to the internal and external iliac arteries. The proximal external iliac arteries are often relatively soft. Even if the internal iliac arteries are calcified, clamp injury to the hypogastric arteries is usually less devastating than clamp application to a calcified common iliac artery. Third, a calcified aortic bifurcation can be managed safely by trimming the plaque with heavy cardiac valve scissors. Instead of trying to penetrate this plaque with the suture needle, one can simply sew the graft to the adventitia adjacent to the calcified plaque, a technique that experienced surgeons have advocated over the years. By sewing the graft up to and flush with the calcified plaque, intimal flap dissection of the aortic bifurcation or common iliac arteries is rarely a problem (Fig. 12–6).

LONG-TERM GRAFT SURVEILLANCE

Long-term graft surveillance makes sense when one considers the risk of subsequent aneurysmal or graft-related complications. However, many aneurysm patients still elude close long-term follow-up. Since most graft-related problems and new aneurysms do not appear until sometime between 5 and 15 years after the initial operation, cost-effective graft imaging should focus on this time period. Edwards and colleagues detected para-anastomotic aortic aneurysms in 10% of 138 patients examined by ultrasound after grafting for an AAA.[14] The incidence of such aneurysms in their series was a worrisome 27% at 15 years. Most were detected late (7–28 years after surgery).

Reasonable recommendations include a simple annual evaluation of cardiovascular symptoms plus a focused physical examination, including blood pressure and all peripheral pulses. It seems reasonable to image the graft at 1 year after implantation with ultrasound that includes the abdominal aortic area as well as the femoral and popliteal arteries. A chest x-ray can adequately detect any significant thoracic aneurysm at that point. The appropriate timing for subsequent graft imaging is debatable. Imaging the graft at intervals of every 2 to 3 years is likely to detect most significant problems. Patients who have had a graft for more than 5 years and have not had any postoperative graft surveillance should be encouraged to have either an ultrasound or computed tomographic scan to check both the graft and adjacent arteries. Current duplex ultrasound equipment allows for excellent visualization of both the proximal abdominal aorta and the aortoiliac graft segments. Computed tomographic scanning can be reversed for patients where ultrasound has not clearly visualized these areas or where clearer delineation of any suspected graft complication is needed.

SUMMARY

Straight tube grafts for repair of abdominal aortic aneurysms provide excellent late patency with minimal risk of subsequent iliac aneurysm development. Any significant development of new aneurysms or graft-related complications is likely to occur relatively late, usually between 5 and 15 years after surgery. These problems can usually be detected by the combination of a periodic physical examination, chest x-ray, and ultrasound. Computed tomographic or magnetic resonance scanning should be used selectively for long-term graft evaluation.

Acknowledgment
The author gratefully acknowledges the editorial assistance of Gail Prechel.

REFERENCES

1. Snellen JP, Terpstra OT, VanUrk H. The use of a straight tube graft decreases blood loss and operation time in patients with an abdominal aortic aneurysm. *Neth J Surg*. 1984;36:45–47.
2. Glickman MH, Julian CC, Kimmins S, et al. Aortic aneurysm: to tube or not to tube. *Surgery*. 1982;9:603–605.
3. Nash T. Abdominal aortic aneurysm: experience with the use of the straight tube method of treatment. *Med J Aust*. 1975;2:85–88.
4. Evans WE, Hayes JP. Tube graft replacement of abdominal aortic aneurysm. *Am J Surg*. 1988;156:199–121.
5. Provan J, Fialkov JA, Amerli FM, et al. Is "tube" prosthetic repair of abdominal aortic aneurysm followed by postoperative dilation of the common iliac arteries? *Can J Surg*. 1990;33:394–397.
6. Plate G, Hollier LH, O'Brien PC, et al. Recurrent aneurysms and late vascular complications following repair of abdominal aortic aneurysms. *Arch Surg*. 1985;120:590–594.
7. Kurland LT, Molgaard CA. The patient record in epidemiology. *Sci Am*. 1981;245:54–63.
8. Calcagno D, Hallett JW, Ballard DJ, et al. Late iliac artery aneurysms and occlusive disease after aortic tube grafts for abdominal aortic aneurysm repair. *Ann Surg*. 1991;214:733–736.
9. Hallett JW, Calcagno D. Long-term results of straight and bifurcated aortic grafts for abdominal aortic aneurysm repair: a population-based experience. In: Greenhalgh RM, Hollier LH, eds. *The Maintenance of Arterial Reconstruction*. London: W B Saunders Co; 1991.
10. Darling RC, Brewster DC. Elective treatment of abdominal aortic aneurysms. *World J Surg*. 1980;4:661–667.
11. Crawford ES, Saleh SA, Babb JW, et al. Infrarenal abdominal aortic aneurysm: factors

influencing survival after operation performed over a 25-year period. *Ann Surg.* 1981;193:699–709.

12. Johnston KW, Scobie TK. Multicenter prospective study of nonruptured abdominal aortic aneurysms. I. Population and operative management. *J Vasc Surg.* 1988;7:69–81.

13. Olsen PS, Schroeder T, Agerskov K, et al. Surgery for abdominal aortic aneurysms: a survey of 656 patients. *J Cardiovasc Surg.* 1991;32:636–642.

14. Edwards JM, Teefey SA, Zierler RE, et al. Intra-abdominal para-anastomotic aneurysms after aortic bypass grafting. *J Vasc Surg.* 1992;15:344–353.

13

Factors Influencing the Long-Term Results of Aortic Aneurysm Surgery

Jack L. Cronenwett, MD

The principal indication for repair of abdominal aortic aneurysms (AAA) is the prevention of rupture to prolong life. Only occasionally do these aneurysms thrombose, embolize, cause local symptoms, or harbor infection that requires surgical treatment independent of rupture. Thus, the ultimate success of AAA surgery is best judged in terms of complication-free long-term survival. During the past 20 years, substantial improvements have been made in reducing early mortality after aneurysm surgery. Most health centers now report rates less than 5% of perioperative mortality after elective infrarenal AAA repair, with even lower mortality in low-risk patients.[1-6] Many factors, including surgical experience, anesthesia technique, hemodynamic monitoring, and postoperative intensive care, have contributed to this progressive reduction in operative mortality. Current efforts are focused on the identification of those higher risk patients who require preoperative modification of their risk factors or those cases that may not benefit from AAA repair. This process involves the careful delineation of cardiac, pulmonary, and renal dysfunction that are known to adversely affect short-term survival after AAA repair.[6]

Although surgeons have appropriately focused on early postoperative mortality after AAA repair, the ultimate benefit of this treatment depends on long-term survival. Since many patients are subsequently followed by their primary physician after AAA repair, it is much more difficult for individual vascular surgeons to appreciate their long-term results. Now that perioperative mortality has been reduced to an appropriately low level, however, it is important to ensure that AAA repair meets the ultimate goal of improved long-term survival. Accordingly, the purpose of this chapter is to review the long-term results of aortic aneurysm surgery, including the incidence of late complications, the long-term survival, and factors that adversely affect long-term survival that should influence the initial decision to operate.

LATE COMPLICATIONS

Fortunately, the complication rate after discharge following AAA repair is very low. When these repairs involve only the aorta or the aorta and iliac arteries, the development of pseudoaneurysms is unusual. After a 3-year mean follow-up of 2,126 patients with aortic anastomoses, Szilagyi and associates found that the incidence of aortic pseudoaneurysms was 0.2%.[7] Similarly, of 1,605 patients with iliac anastomoses, the incidence of pseudoaneurysms was only 1.2%.[7] If the aortic reconstruction is extended to the femoral arteries, the incidence of pseudoaneurysms increases, similar to that observed in occlusive disease, to approximately 3% after a mean interval of 3.5 years.[7] Although the development of aortoiliac pseudoaneurysms is unusual, these do require repair, since approximately one-third of such patients will present with rupture and experience a substantially higher mortality rate (67%) than patients who undergo elective repair (8% mortality).[8] The difficulty in detecting aortoiliac pseudoaneurysms has led some authors to recommend periodic computed tomographic scans of these patients at 2- to 3-year intervals after surgery.[9] Recently, based on ultrasound screening of 138 patients at various times after AAA repair, pseudoaneurysms were detected in 1% of patients after 8 years, but in 20% of patients after 15 years.[10] Although survival for this duration after AAA repair is unusual, screening for abdominal pseudoaneurysms appears to be more appropriate in patients who survive more than 10 years.

Like pseudoaneurysms, infection of grafts placed for AAA repair is rare unless these grafts incorporate a femoral anastomosis. In large series of patients, the incidence of aortoiliac graft infection is estimated to be 0.3% to 0.7%, usually presenting 3 to 4 years after AAA repair.[2,11] Somewhat more frequent is the development of aortoenteric fistulas after AAA repair. These nearly always involve the duodenum, are usually associated with the proximal graft suture line, and present with gastrointestinal hemorrhage.[12] Less common is graft infection without suture line involvement, or erosion of other segments of intestine. Overall, the incidence of these fistulas is estimated to be 0.9%, and they usually occur 5 years after graft implantation.[12] Fortunately, the incidence of both aortoiliac graft infection and aortoduodenal fistulas is low, since these complications are associated with high mortality rates.

Thrombosis of an aortoiliac graft limb after AAA repair is distinctly unusual, unless significant aortoiliac occlusive disease exists at the time of aneurysm repair. In such cases, graft thrombosis usually occurs early in the postoperative period and requires graft extension to the femoral level. Thus, most large series reporting long-term follow-up of AAA surgery do not even mention this complication.[1,2,10] Depending on the length of patient survival, additional subsequent procedures may be required if significant occlusive disease develops in the distal iliac arteries. However, this appears to be extraordinarily rare in patients who do not initially present with such symptoms at the time of AAA repair.

Thus, after hospital discharge from AAA surgery, only 2% to 3% of patients will ever experience late complications of this repair. Unfortunately, these complications are severe and often fatal if they occur. They have been avoided largely due to the elimination of silk suture, the use of prophylactic perioperative antibiotics, careful closure of viable tissue between the aortic graft and duodenum, and preoperative assessment of iliac occlusive disease with extension of the graft to the femoral level as required.

LONG-TERM SURVIVAL

Based on five series published during the past 10 years, the 5-year survival rate of more than 3,000 patients was 70% after successful AAA repair.[1-5] Corresponding 10-

TABLE 13–1. LONG-TERM SURVIVAL AFTER SUCCESSFUL AAA REPAIR

Author	Year	n	Median Age (yrs)	Survival Rate (%) 5-yr	10-yr	15-yr
Crawford et al[1]	1981	737	66	63	38	18
Hollier et al[2]	1984	1,066	68	68	41	—
Søreide et al[3]	1982	310	—	75	—	—
Vohra et al[4]	1990	286	70	60	—	—
Olsen et al[5]	1991	656	69	83	—	—
Weighted mean		3,055		70	40	18

Excluded <30-day postoperative survival.

and 15-year life expectancy rates were 40% and 18%, respectively (Table 13–1). There was no clear trend toward improved survival rates over the interval of these studies, although the most recent (1991) report had the highest (83%) 5-year survival rate.[5] These cases represented a mixture of patients undergoing surgery electively or urgently or because of ruptured abdominal aneurysms. All of the patients had survived at least 30 days after surgery. Thus, the early postoperative mortality rates must be added to these figures to determine the overall expected survival after 5 years. However, these survival rates after successful surgery are useful, because they most directly address the question of whether such patients have excessive long-term mortality rates compared with an age-matched, United States control population. The answer to this question varies between reported series, probably reflecting underlying differences in patient population. Hollier and colleagues found that the observed survival rate of 1,087 AAA patients was only 85% and 70% of that expected in an age-matched control population after 5 and 10 years, respectively.[2] However, both Søreide and associates and Olsen, and colleagues found no difference between the observed and expected survival rates of their patients after successful aneurysm repair.[3,5] To understand these differences, it is important to examine the factors influencing long-term survival.

FACTORS INFLUENCING LONG-TERM SURVIVAL

Not surprisingly, systemic complications of atherosclerosis were responsible for most late deaths after AAA repair in these predominantly elderly, male patients. A compilation of three large series indicated that late mortality was due to cardiac complications in 44%, rupture of another aneurysm in 12%, and stroke in 9% (Table 13–2).[1,2,13] Thus, vascular complications accounted for 65% of the late deaths following AAA repair in these series. This dramatic result has focused attention on cardiovascular risk factors present at the time of initial surgery that could be modified to improve outcome, or that might accurately predict long-term survival, and hence, facilitate operative decision making.

Obviously, the most important factor influencing long-term survival in any population is patient age. This is certainly true for patients after AAA repair.[1,14] In the current United States population, women survive 3 to 5 years longer than men, on the average, but the life expectancy for a 70-year-old is greater than 10 years for either sex (Table 13–3).[15] It is important to be aware of these data for accurate estimation of expected survival after AAA repair.

TABLE 13–2. LATE CAUSES OF DEATH AFTER AAA REPAIR BY PERCENTAGE

Cardiac	44
Cancer	15
Rupture of other aneurysm	11
Stroke	9
Pulmonary	6
Other	15
Total (*n* = 962)[a]	100

[a] Weighted mean of three large series.[1,2,13]

Most authors have not found a difference between the long-term survival rates of patients who were operated upon electively versus those with ruptured AAAs after they survived the initial surgery.[3–5] In part, this may reflect a selection process, because patients with the most severe associated disease die in the early postoperative period, especially among those with ruptured aneurysms. At least one report indicates an improved long-term survival after initially surviving aneurysm rupture, no doubt related to this election process.[3] However, in another series, patients with ruptured AAAs had somewhat worse long-term survival rates than those who underwent elective surgery, even after accounting for differences in early postoperative mortality.[1] Overall, AAA rupture does not appear to be an important determinant of long-term survival after initially successful surgery.

A number of other variables have been analyzed to determine their possible effect on long-term survival after successful AAA surgery. Concerning possible gender differences, Crawford and coworkers found that men and women had identical long-term survival rates.[1] However, based on the expected longer survival for women in the United States population, this suggests that the outcome for women after AAA repair is slightly worse than men compared with their respective controls. More importantly, however, these authors found that atherosclerotic heart disease significantly worsened long-term survival after AAA surgery. At 5 years, the observed survival rate was 84% in patients without heart disease, significantly better than the 54% observed in patients with known atherosclerotic heart disease.[1] Hypertension also reduced 5-year survival rates after AAA repair, from 84% to 59%, comparable to that in patients with atherosclerotic heart disease.[1] Hollier and colleagues confirmed that hypertension and heart disease significantly worsened the long-term survival rate after AAA repair.[2] Among patients with these risk factors, the 5-year mortality rate from myocardial infarction alone was 11.7%, three times higher than the 3.7%

TABLE 13–3. EXPECTED SURVIVAL (YEARS) BASED ON CURRENT YEARS[a]

Age	Men	Women
50	26	31
55	22	27
60	18	23
65	15	19
70	12	15
75	9	12
80	7	9
85	5	6

[a] United States population, 1988.[15]

incidence of myocardial infarction in AAA patients without these risk factors. When analyzing patients with both hypertension and heart disease, the 5-year observed survival rate was only 58%, compared with an expected survival rate in the control population of 81%.[2] Importantly, among AAA patients without hypertension or heart disease, the 5-year observed survival rate was 75%, statistically equivalent to the expected 78% survival rate for age- and sex-matched control subjects. Hollier and colleagues found that hypertension influenced mortality by increasing death from stroke and other aneurysm rupture but not by increasing the incidence of myocardial infarction, which was a separate risk factor related to underlying atherosclerotic heart disease.[2]

When analyzing their overall results, the Mayo Clinic group found that the survival of patients younger than 60 years of age was much worse than expected, whereas elderly patients (>70 years of age) had survival much more similar to age-matched controls.[2,14] This suggested that the maximum benefit of correcting underlying heart disease or hypertension would be observed in patients who are younger at the time of initial presentation. Since these patients tend to die from heart disease some years after AAA repair, it is important to emphasize careful follow-up to detect any deterioration of cardiac status. This result also indicates that aortic aneurysmal disease is an important marker for systemic (especially cardiac) atherosclerosis. In their analysis of preoperative risk factors, Olsen and coworkers found that atherosclerotic heart disease, hypertension, peripheral arterial disease, and impaired renal function all contributed to excessive long-term mortality after initially successful AAA repair.[5]

Based on these results, AAA patients without overt heart disease or hypertension appear to have long-term survival comparable to an age-matched control population. This conclusion is also supported by a population-based study of patients undergoing elective AAA repair in Olmstead County, Minnesota. In this study, Roger and associates reported an 8-year survival rate of 59% in patients without overt cardiac disease after AAA repair, statistically similar to an expected survival rate of 68%.[16] However, in patients with suspected or overt coronary artery disease (CAD), the observed 8-year survival rate was only 34% compared with an expected survival rate of 61% in the normal population (P<.01). After 8 years, the cumulative incidence of cardiac events in AAA patients who initially did not have overt CAD was only 15%, significantly less than the 61% event rate in AAA patients who initially had suspected or overt CAD (P<.01).[16] Using a multivariate analysis, these authors found that uncorrected CAD was the most significant variable associated with late mortality in patients after AAA repair, nearly doubling the risk of death. Increased age and a history of stroke were also associated with reduced long-term survival but were much less important predictors than CAD.[16] In this particular study, hypertension was not an independent risk factor. These authors emphasized the need for aggressive life-long management of CAD in patients undergoing AAA repair.

PREDICTING LONG-TERM RESULTS AFTER AAA REPAIR

The above results lead to the inescapable conclusion that survival after AAA repair is optimal in patients without associated heart disease. A number of preoperative tests, including stress-thallium and dipyridamole-thallium scintigraphy (DTS), and radionuclide-determined ejection fraction, have been proposed to identify patients at high surgical risk prior to AAA repair. Recent studies suggest that these same modalities can accurately predict long-term survival in such patients. Kazmers and coworkers demonstrated that AAA patients with an ejection fraction above 35% had an 85% 2-year survival rate significantly better than the 55% survival rate among AAA patients with an ejection fraction less than or equal to 35% (P<.01).[17] Although preoperative ejection fraction predicted long-term survival, it did not influence early postoperative mortality in this report. Patients with an ejection fraction above 50% had even better long-term survival, whereas patients with a previous myocardial infarction, previous vascular surgery, or those above the age of 70 had worse late survival.[17] Cutler and colleagues have recently analyzed the ability of DTS to predict long-term survival following vascular surgery.[18] They found that redistribution on the DTS scan was the strongest predictor of early postoperative cardiac events, and that fixed defects were not predictive. In their analysis of late cardiac events, however, a persistent (fixed) defect was the strongest predictor of late cardiac morbidity and mortality, and the size of this defect correlated with long-term survival. Interestingly, redistribution on the DTS scan was not a good predictor of long-term survival in this experience.[18]

MODIFYING LONG-TERM SURVIVAL AFTER AAA REPAIR

Based on the knowledge that long-term survival following AAA repair is most influenced by CAD, which is known to be prevalent in AAA patients, one must ask whether patients with CAD should undergo coronary artery bypass graft (CABG) surgery prior to AAA surgery in order to improve long-term survival. Hertzer and associates at the Cleveland Clinic have reported their experience using routine coronary arteriography and aggressive coronary revascularization in appropriate patients prior to AAA surgery.[19] Among 236 elective AAA patients who survived surgery, the overall 5-year survival rate was 72%. Among patients with normal coronary arteries, this rate was 79%, equivalent to the 5-year survival rate of 75% in patients with severe CAD who had undergone preoperative CABG. This was also similar to the 71% 5-year survival rate observed in AAA patients with advanced but well-compensated-for CAD, but much greater than the 29% 5-year rate observed in 10 AAA patients with severe uncorrectable CAD who underwent AAA repair.[19] Fewer diseased coronary arteries, good ventricular function, and complete myocardial revascularization were important predictors of improved survival after CABG plus AAA repair. These authors concluded that selective use of CABG prior to AAA repair substantially improved survival rates of patients with significant CAD.

Although the Cleveland Clinic results show comparable long-term survival rates in patients with normal coronary arteries versus those with severe CAD and preoperative CABG before AAA repair, there was no true control group. The 10 patients with severe uncorrected CAD who fared poorly were, in fact, surgically unreconstructible and presumably had much more severe CAD. This is not an optimal control group. Not surprisingly, there has not been a randomized study to ascertain the value of prophylactic CABG for enhancing late survival after AAA repair. In fact, although CABG can relieve cardiac symptoms, it has only been shown to improve survival rates in patients with left main coronary artery disease, or three-vessel disease.[20] In this regard, surgeons from the Mayo Clinic compared the late survival of 485 patients who successfully recovered from elective AAA repair, in whom CAD had been investigated and treated selectively, based on clinical symptoms and preoperative cardiology evaluation.[14] Of these patients, 41% had untreated CAD, and 10% had undergone prior CABG. The 5-year survival rate of 83% observed in patients with no CAD was actually better than the 76% rate for an age-matched control population.

The 66% 5-year survival rate for patients with CAD appeared less than the 73% expected rate for this group. Similarly, patients with CAD plus previous CABG had a 5-year survival rate of 66% compared with a predicted rate of 78%. Although these differences were not statistically significant, they suggest excessive late mortality in patients with CAD. Interestingly, younger patients (those in their 60s and 70s) had the worst long-term outcome when compared with their expected survival, whereas elderly patients (those in their 80s and 90s) actually had improved survival compared with an age-matched control population.[14] These authors concluded that selective management of CAD on the basis of cardiac symptoms provides good late survival in patients more than 70 years old, but that younger patients had worse prospects for survival and might benefit from more aggressive intervention to treat underlying CAD.

Although it is clear that long-term survival after AAA repair is adversely influenced by CAD, it has not been proven that prophylactic CABG surgery prior to AAA repair will alter this survival. When considering this approach, one must remember that the mortality associated with CABG itself may exceed 10% in some patient subgroups, especially elderly patients.[20] In fact, the best time to intervene in these patients may not be prior to their AAA surgery, but rather subsequent to it, if their CAD becomes clinically apparent. Obviously this approach requires diligent clinical follow-up.

OTHER ANEURYSMS PRESENTING DURING FOLLOW-UP

Aneurysmal disease of the aorta is known to be a multifocal problem. In a review of more than 1,500 patients treated for aortic aneurysms, Crawford and Cohen found that 12.6% had multiple aneurysms.[21] More than half of the patients with thoracic aneurysms had other aortic involvement, and fully 12% of patients with AAAs had thoracic aneurysms. This frequency is undoubtedly biased by the unique referral practice that has attracted patients with multiple aneurysms to this health center. However, other large series have also emphasized the effect of other aneurysms on the long-term results of AAA surgery. Plate and colleagues found that 5.4% of patients developed complications due to other aneurysms at a mean interval of 5 years after their initial AAA repair.[9] These were predominantly true aneurysms, most frequently involving the thoracic aorta, abdominal aorta, or iliacfemoral arteries. Importantly, less than 4% of patients presenting with rupture of a secondary aneurysm survived this complication, emphasizing the importance of surveillance for other aneurysms in patients after AAA repair. Although chest x-ray and careful physical examination will detect many aneurysms, selective computed tomographic scanning may be appropriate for the thoracic, aortic, and iliac regions in patients who are difficult to examine or those with tortuous thoracic aortas on chest x-ray. When these aneurysms present simultaneously with the initial AAA, combined sequential repair of the larger followed by the smaller aneurysm provides the best chance for long-term survival.[21,22] Hypertension significantly increased the incidence of other aneurysms following AAA repair and emphasizes the need for frequent surveillance in this subgroup.[9] Despite optimum treatment, patients with multiple aortic aneurysms have a significantly worse 5-year survival than that of comparable patients with only AAAs (40% compared with 65%).[22] It appears that this survival difference relates to worse perioperative survival rates due to more extensive surgery in patients with multiple aneurysms, rather than to worse survival after successful surgery.

THORACOABDOMINAL ANEURYSMS

Although far fewer thoracoabdominal aneurysms are treated than infrarenal aortic aneurysms, the long-term outcome after successful thoracoabdominal aneurysm surgery appears similar to that after AAA repair. In the largest individual series, Crawford and associates reported a 60% 5-year survival rate in 605 such patients.[23] These authors noted that advanced age, aneurysm rupture, renal dysfunction, extent of the aneurysm, and dissection were all factors that significantly reduced long-term survival. Similar to patients with multiple aortic aneurysms, the lower long-term survival of patients with thoracoabdominal aneurysms compared with those for patients with infrarenal AAAs appears to be related to the initially higher perioperative mortality in patients with more extensive aneurysms. Based on the existing data, it does not appear that multiple or more extensive aneurysms *per se* are an additional, independent marker for decreased long-term survival after initially successful surgery.

SUMMARY

Refinements in patient care, operative techniques, cardiac evaluation, and selective preoperative cardiac intervention have reduced perioperative mortality rate of AAA repair to less than 5%. Subsequent outcome in these patients is best assessed by long-term survival, since late complications of AAA surgery are infrequent, although often fatal. Since most late deaths after AAA repair are due to systemic complications of atherosclerosis, the most controversial current question relates to the wisdom of prophylactic CABG prior to AAA repair in order to prolong long-term survival. The wisdom of this approach, compared with careful cardiac follow-up and subsequent intervention for appropriate symptoms, remains to be tested in a randomized trial. Careful follow-up for the late, future development of other aneurysms is also important in these patients. Aortic aneurysmal disease is an important marker of additional cardiac risk, which, if not corrected preoperatively, must be carefully followed to ensure satisfactory long-term survival.

REFERENCES

1. Crawford ES, Saleh SA, Babb JW III, et al. Infrarenal abdominal aortic aneurysm. Factors influencing survival after operation performed over a 25-year period. *Ann Surg.* 1981;193:699–709.
2. Hollier LH, Plate G, O'Brien PC, et al. Late survival after abdominal aortic aneurysm repair: influence of coronary artery disease. *J Vasc Surg.* 1984;1:290–299.
3. Søreide O, Lillestøl J, Christensen O, et al. Abdominal aortic aneurysm: survival analysis of four hundred thirty-four patients. *Surgery.* 1982;91:188–193.
4. Vohra R, Reid D, Groome J, et al. Long-term survival in patients undergoing resection of abdominal aortic aneurysm. *Ann Vasc Surg.* 1990;4:460–465.
5. Olsen PS, Schroeder T, Agerskov K, et al. Surgery for abdominal aortic aneurysms. A survey of 656 patients. *J Cardiovasc Surg.* 1991;32:636–642.
6. Johnston KW, Scobie TK. Multicenter prospective study of nonruptured abdominal aortic aneurysms. I. Population and operative management. *J Vasc Surg.* 1988;7:69–81.
7. Szilagyi DE, Smith RF, Elliot JP, et al. Anastomotic aneurysms after vascular reconstruction: problems of incidence, etiology, and treatment. *Surgery.* 1975;78:800–816.
8. Treiman GS, Weaver FA, Cossman DV, et al. Anastomotic false aneurysms of the abdominal aorta and the iliac arteries. *J Vasc Surg.* 1988;8:268–273.

9. Plate G, Hollier LA, O'Brien P, et al. Recurrent aneurysms and late vascular complications following repair of abdominal aortic aneurysms. *Arch Surg*. 1985;120:590–594.
10. Edwards JM, Teefey SA, Zierler RE, et al. Intraabdominal paraanstomotic aneurysms after aortic bypass grafting. *J Vasc Surg*. 1992;15:344–353.
11. Szilagyi DE, Smith RF, Elliot JP, et al. Infection in arterial reconstruction with synthetic grafts. *Ann Surg*. 1972;176:321–333.
12. Bunt TJ. Synthetic vascular graft infection. II. Graft-enteric erosions and graft-enteric fistulas. *Surgery*. 1983;94:1–9.
13. Hertzer NR. Fatal myocardial infarction following abdominal aortic aneurysm resection. Three hundred forty-three patients followed 6–11 years postoperatively. *Ann Surg*. 1980;192:667–673.
14. Reigel MM, Hollier LH, Kazmier FJ, et al. Late survival in abdominal aortic aneurysm patients: the role of selective myocardial revascularization on the basis of clinical symptoms. *J Vasc Surg*. 1987;5:222–227.
15. U.S. Department of Health and Human Services, Public Health Service Centers for Disease Control. Vital Statistics of the United States, 1988. National Center for Health Statistics, Vol. II, Section 6, pp 11.
16. Roger VL, Ballard DJ, Hallett JW Jr, et al. Influence of coronary artery disease on morbidity and mortality after abdominal aortic aneurysmectomy: a population-based study, 1971–1987. *J Am Coll Cardiol*. 1989;14:1245–1252.
17. Kazmers A, Cerqueira MD, Zierler RE. The role of preoperative radionuclide ejection fraction in direct abdominal aortic aneurysm repair. *J Vasc Surg*. 1988;8:128–136.
18. Cutler BC, Leppo JA, Hendel R. Dipyridamole thallium scintigraphy predicts long-term survival following vascular surgery. *J Vasc Surg*. 1992 (in press).
19. Hertzer NR, Young JR, Beven EG, et al. Late results of coronary bypass in patients with infrarenal aortic aneurysms. The Cleveland Clinic study. *Ann Surg*. 1987;205:360–367.
20. Kennedy JW, Kaiser GC, Fisher LD, et al. Clinical and angiographic predictors of operative mortality from the collaborative study in coronary artery surgery (CASS). *Circulation*. 1981;63:793–802.
21. Crawford ES, Cohen ES. Aortic aneurysm: a multifocal disease. *Arch Surg*. 1982;117:1393–1400.
22. Gloviczki P, Pairolero P, Welch T, et al. Multiple aortic aneurysms: the results of surgical management. *J Vasc Surg*. 1990;11:19–28.
23. Crawford ES, Crawford JL, Safi HJ, et al. Thoracoabdominal aortic aneurysms: preoperative and intraoperative factors determining immediate and long-term results of operations in 605 patients. *J Vasc Surg*. 1986;3:389–404.

14

Patency Characteristics
of Descending Thoracic
Aortofemoral Bypass

Walter J. McCarthy, MD, William R. Flinn, MD,
William H. Pearce, MD, W. D. McMillan, MD, and
James S. T. Yao, MD, PhD

Arterial bypass from the descending thoracic aorta to the femoral level has been contemplated for several different indications. Patients who have failed multiple attempts at transabdominal aortic bypass may have successful reconstruction in this fashion. Rarely, an individual whose retroperitoneum has been previously dissected or irradiated would be better served with arterial reconstruction that avoids the infrarenal aorta. Perhaps the most numerically important group of patients to be considered for this repair are those who have previously had an infected intra-abdominal aortic graft removed for sepsis. In the years after their recovery with an axillary femorofemoral repair or axillary popliteal bypass, these patients may experience multiple extra-anatomic graft occlusions. Conversion to thoracic aortofemoral bypass surgery may be the solution to this problem. Debating the exact surgical indications or technical approach for this bypass is not within the boundaries of the present report, instead we will present what is known about the long-term patency of these grafts.

Comments on the actual durability of descending thoracic aortofemoral bypass would have been largely anecdotal before 1985. In fact, the first surgical cases performed at Northwestern University beginning in 1982 were followed with considerable interest, as their patency potential was unknown. After several other operations failed, these early patients were treated using this technique as a last hope for long-term limb salvage. In concept, these bypasses seemed very likely to succeed. Inflow for the graft from the descending thoracic aorta is very seldom impeded by any atherosclerotic or aneurysmal degeneration (Fig. 14–1). There is almost never a hemodynamic impediment to inflow. The bypass graft used is of large diameter and passes through intercavity plains without significant motion during body movement (Figs. 14–2, 14–3). Only bypass graft outflow at the femoral level is potentially complicated. This region may be severely diseased or may develop stenosis during the years following an initially successful operation. Thus, it was no surprise when

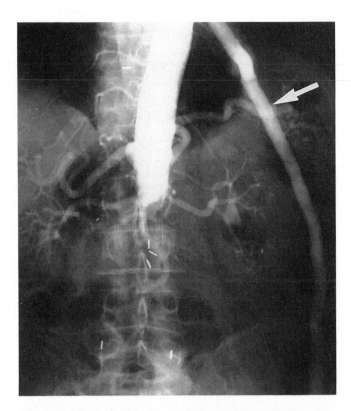

Figure 14–1. The unusually good patency afforded by this extra-anatomic bypass may be explained by the relatively large (10- or 12-mm) bypass graft used (arrow). In addition, the graft passes through intercavitary tunnels where little motion is transmitted during active body movement.

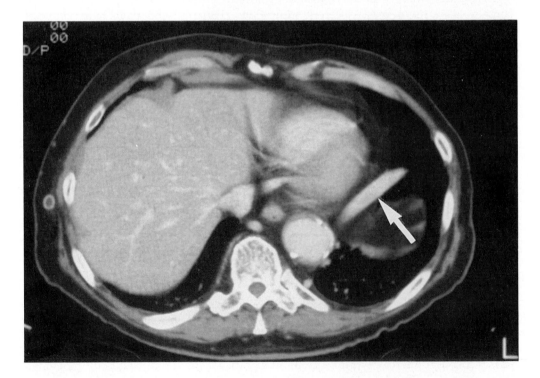

Figure 14–2. With the technique employed at Northwestern, a graft is tunneled over the dome of the left diaphragm (arrow) after being anastomosed end-to-side to the descending thoracic aorta.

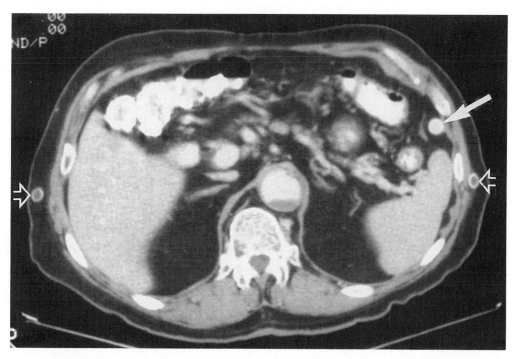

Figure 14–3. The Northwestern technique routinely uses passage of the bypass graft along the anterior axillary line to the left groin in the retroperitoneum (solid arrow). This places the graft anterior to the spleen and kidney. Previously placed, now thrombosed, axillary popliteal 8-mm bypass grafts can be appreciated bilaterally (open arrows).

additions to the literature containing significant numbers of patients began to appear in 1985, that patency reports were very good. It is of interest when reviewing all the published reports of this operation to note that in the 23 years following the first operation in 1956, there were 25 reported cases in the literature. From 1985 to the present time, approximately 150 additional operations have been chronicled and followed sufficiently for report over only 7 years (Table 14–1).[1–28]

PATENCY OF EARLY OPERATIONS

The first reported bypass using the descending thoracic aorta for inflow to the femoral vessels was completed by Lester R. Sauvage on June 7, 1956. He later reported this work with coauthors Stevenson and Harkins in the September 1961 *Annals of Surgery*.[1] The patient was a 47-year-old ranch hand who had undergone aorta–bi-iliac grafting with an aortic homograft placed below the renal arteries 6 months previously. Because of the scarring around the failed earlier surgical site, it was decided to use the descending thoracic aorta, which was exposed with a midline incision extending through the fourth interspace. The bypass graft consisted of two aortic homografts sewn together for sufficient length and tunneled directly through the diaphragm adjacent to the esophageal hiatus. The operation was completely successful, and the patient returned to work and normal physical activity. However, he presented 20 months later with failure of the right side of his reconstruction and soon after had complete bypass graft thrombosis requiring a unilateral hip disarticulation. Several months thereafter the patient died of complications following a cerebral vascular

TABLE 14–1. PATENCY FEATURES FROM REPRESENTATIVE PAPERS

Author	Year	City	Journal	Number of Patients	Mean Follow-up	Patency
Stevenson et al[1]	1961	Seattle	*Ann Surg*	1	20 mo	Occluded at 20 mo
Blaisdell et al[2]	1961	San Francisco	*Am J Surg*	1	4 wks	Died with patent graft at 4 wks
Robicsek et al[3]	1967	Charlotte	*Ann Thor Surg*	1	6 mo	100%, 6 mo
Reichle et al[4]	1970	Philadelphia	*Ann Surg*	1	4½ yrs	100%, 4.5 yrs
Nunn and Kamal[5]	1972	Jacksonville	*Surgery*	3	Not given	Not given
Froysaker et al[6]	1973	Oslo	*J Cardiovasc Surg*	6	22 mo	83%, 2 yrs
Finseth and Abbott[7]	1974	Boston	*Ann Surg*	1	15 mo	100%, 15 mo
Jarrett et al[8]	1975	Boston	*Arch Surg*	2	Not given	Not given
Cevese and Gallucci[9]	1975	Padua, Italy	*J Cardiovasc Surg*	6	30 mo	100%, 3 yr
Buxton et al[10]	1976	Melbourne	*Med J Aust*	1	24 mo	100%, 2 yr
Lakner and Lukacs[11]	1983	Budapest	*J Cardiovasc Surg*	2	15 mo	100%, 1 yr
Rosenfeld et al[12]	1985	Philadelphia	*J Vasc Surg*	9	36 mo	88%, 3 yr
Haas et al[13]	1985	New Orleans	*Am Surg*	3	19 mo	100%, 18 mo
Feldhaus et al[14]	1985	Omaha	*Ann Thor Surg*	18	Not given	85%, 5 yr
Enon et al[15]	1985	Angers, France	*J Chir*	3	Not given	Not given
Schultz et al[16]	1986	Omaha	*Surgery*	15	37 mo	80%, 5 yr
McCarthy et al[17]	1986	Chicago	*Arch Surg*	13	22 mo	92%, 2 yr
di Marzo et al[18]	1987	Omaha	*Vasc Surg*	5	Not given	Not given
Hussain[19]	1988	Toledo	*Int Surg*	8	36 mo	75%, 1°; 100%, 2°
Schellack et al[20]	1988	Atlanta	*J Cardiovasc Surg*	3	21 mo	100%
Bradham et al[21]	1989	Charleston	*J South Carolina Med Assoc*	2	None	At discharge
Bowes et al[22]	1990	Danville, PA	*J Cardiovasc Surg*	26	53 mo	86%, 42 mo
O'Brien et al[23]	1991	Galway, Ireland	*Ir Med J*	1	None	At discharge
Branchereau et al[24]	1991	Marseille	*Ann Vasc Surg*	10	14 mo	55%, 1°; 100%, 2°
Kalman et al[25]	1991	Toronto	*J Cardiovasc Surg*	6	17 mo	100%
Criado et al[26]	1992	Chapel Hill, NC	*J Vasc Surg*	16	24 mo	83.3%, 2 yr
Branchereau et al[27]	1992	Marseille	*Eur J Vasc Surg*	27	26.3 mo	72.6%, 2°, 2 yr
McCarthy et al[28]	1992	Chicago	*J Vasc Surg*	21	44 mo	86%, 48 mo

accident, and an autopsy was performed. The homograft seemed intact, although thrombosed, and patency failure was attributed to progressive bilateral disease in his outflow vessels. Thus, the primary patency of this repair was 20 months with failure due to outflow disease. This pattern is consistent with current findings, but in the present day might have been modified by attempts at femoropopliteal reconstruction.

The next documented case was performed at the San Francisco Veterans Administration Hospital on September 6, 1960. This operation was reported by F. William Blaisdell and associates in the *American Journal of Surgery* in October 1961.[2] The patient, a 66-year-old man, had previously undergone removal of an infected aorta–bi-iliac graft that had been placed to treat an aneurysm. A second aortoexternal iliac graft was in position when, 4 weeks later, it too degenerated from sepsis with aortic rupture. The patient had his second aortic graft removed, and with the obvious presence of an intensely septic intra-abdominal aorta, the thoracic region was selected for inflow. After reprepping the patient, and in the presence of severe ischemia of the lower trunk, an anterior lateral approach was used through the eighth intercostal space. Fourteen-millimeter Dacron graft material was passed posteriorly in the region of the twelfth rib and tunneled to the left groin. A femorofemoral graft was then placed to supply the right leg. The patient did well, and for several weeks showed signs of good distal perfusion. However, a low-grade fever persisted from the time of surgery, and eventually he became irreversibly septic and died of septic shock with a patent graft 4.5 weeks after the thoracic operation. Autopsy revealed intra-abdominal sepsis but no sign of infection along the extra-anatomic bypass. The authors were impressed by this bypass, feeling that "bypass graft from the thoracic aorta to the femoral arteries via an extraperitoneal tunnel is a satisfactory way of maintaining the distal circulation." It is of interest that publication of this case report came several years before Blaisdell published details of the first axillary femorofemoral bypass.

SERIES OF OPERATIONS

After the first two operations were reported in 1961, additional sporadic patency feedback became available, including a report by Robicsek and associates[3] and another by Reichle and colleagues,[4] with initial success and patency after 6 months and 4.5 years, respectively. In 1972, Nunn and Kamal published the report of three successful operations done in Jacksonville, Florida, but did not include any significant follow-up.[5] It was not until Froysaker and coworkers compiled work done in Oslo that reasonable follow-up on more than one case was available.[6] The Norwegian group reported no surgical mortality with six patients and an 83% 2-year patency with a mean follow-up of 22 months. Cevese and Gallucci of the University of Padua echoed these results with six patients, all of whose grafts were patent within a 30-month mean follow-up.[9] In 1985, a flurry of papers allowed the beginning of standard Life Table analysis. Rosenfeld and colleagues,[12] Feldhaus and associates,[14] and Schultz and coworkers[16] each contributed significantly to the patency information available and concurred with each other, demonstrating greater than 80% successful graft function in the 3- to 5-year sector.

In the 1990s, three papers have already become available detailing more than 20 patients, and with each, conventional Life Table analysis is included.[22,26,27] Table 14–1 delineates the important patency features from 28 representative papers since the first publication in 1961. Only recently has this literature exhibited graft function with cumulative Life Table patency methods, so this author has summarized what is available from each paper for tabulation. Criado and colleagues also attempted to organize patency information, compiling a Life Table cumulative patency summary of 124 bypasses available at the time of their paper's publication.[26] From this aggregate analysis, at 1 year with 105 grafts at risk, the cumulative patency was 98.3%. With 64 grafts at risk after 24 months, the patency had fallen to 88%. This rate declined to 70.4% in the 54- to 60-month interval, with 16 grafts at risk. These numbers may be several points lower than the 77% to 90% 5-year patency reported for standard aortofemoral grafting in the many series available.[27,29] This must, of course, be considered with the recognition that most of the thoracofemoral bypasses have been completed as reoperative rather than primary surgical procedures.

From its conception in 1956, bypass from the descending thoracic aorta to the femoral region has been marked by patency comparable to standard aortofemoral grafting. Patency flaws are usually related to progression of femoral occlusive disease and may be tempered by industrious surveillance and reoperation where necessary at that level. Patency determination has become more than anecdotal, with approximately 200 cases now reported in the world literature. With what is known, one can optimistically recommend this procedure for aortic bypass when the infrarenal aorta is undesirable for dissection.

Acknowledgments

Our research was supported in part by the Alyce F. Salerno Foundation, the Gaylord Freeman Aneurysm Research Fund, and the Veterans Administration Research Service.

REFERENCES

1. Stevenson JK, Sauvage LR, Harkins HN. A bypass homograft from thoracic aorta to femoral arteries for occlusive vascular disease: case report. *Ann Surg.* 1961;27:632–637.
2. Blaisdell FW, DeMattei GA, Gauder PJ. Extraperitoneal thoracic aorta to femoral bypass graft as replacement for an infected aortic bifurcation prosthesis: case reports. *Am J Surg.* 1961;102:583–585.
3. Robicsek F, McCall MM, Sanger PW, et al. Case reports: recurrent aneurysm of the abdominal aorta: insertion of a vascular prosthesis from the distal aortic arch to the femoral arteries. *Ann Thor Surg.* 1967;3:549–552.
4. Reichle FA, Tyson RR, Soloff LA, et al. Salmonellosis and aneurysm of the distal abdominal aorta: case report with a review. *Ann Surg.* 1970;171:219–228.
5. Nunn DB, Kamal MA. Bypass grafting from the thoracic aorta to femoral arteries for high aortoiliac occlusive disease. *Surgery.* 1972;72:749–755.
6. Froysaker T, Skagseth E, Dundas P, et al. Bypass procedures in the treatment of obstructions of the abdominal aorta. *J Cardiovasc Surg.* 1973;14:317–321.
7. Finseth F, Abbott WM. One-stage operative therapy for salmonella mycotic abdominal aortic aneurysm. *Ann Surg.* 1974;179:8–11.
8. Jarrett F, Darling RC, Mundth ED, et al. Experience with infected aneurysms of the abdominal aorta. *Arch Surg.* 1975;110:1281–1286.
9. Cevese PG, Gallucci V. Thoracic aorta-to-femoral artery by-pass. *J Cardiovasc Surg.* 1975; 16:432–438.
10. Buxton B, Simpson L, Johnson N, et al. Descending thoracic aortofemoral bypass for distal aortic reconstruction after removal of an infected Dacron prosthesis. *Med J Aust.* 1976;2: 133–136.
11. Lakner G, Lukacs L. High aortoiliac occlusion: treatment with thoracic aorta to femoral arterial bypass. *J Cardiovasc Surg.* 1983;24:532–534.
12. Rosenfeld JC, Savarese RP, DeLaurentis DA. Distal thoracic aorta to femoral artery bypass: a surgical alternative. *J Vasc Surg.* 1985;2:747–750.
13. Haas KL, Moulder PV, Kerstein MD. Use of thoracic aortobifemoral artery bypass grafting as an alternative procedure for occlusive aortoiliac disease. *Am Surg.* 1985;51:573–576.

14. Feldhaus RJ, Sterpetti AV, Schultz RD, et al. Thoracic aorta-femoral artery bypass: indications, technique, and late results. *Ann Thor Surg.* 1985;40:588–592.
15. Enon B, Chevalier JM, Moreau P, et al. Revascularisation des membres inferieurs a partir de l'aorte thoracique descendante. *J Chir.* 1985;122:539–543.
16. Schultz RD, Sterpetti AV, Feldhaus RJ. Thoracic aorta as source of inflow in reoperation for occluded aortoiliac reconstruction. *Surgery.* 1986;100:635–644.
17. McCarthy WJ, Rubin JR, Flinn WR, et al. Descending thoracic aorta-to-femoral artery bypass. *Arch Surg.* 1986;121:681–688.
18. di Marzo L, Feldhaus RJ, Schultz RD. Surgical treatment of infected aortofemoral grafts: a fifteen-year experience. *Vasc Surg.* 1987;21:229–236.
19. Hussain SA. Descending thoracic aorta to bifemoral by-pass graft without laparotomy. *Int Surg.* 1988;73:260–263.
20. Schellack J, Fulenwider JT, Smith RB III. Descending thoracic aortofemoral-femoral bypass: a remedial alternative for the failed aortobifemoral bypass. *J Cardiovasc Surg.* 1988;29: 201–204.
21. Bradham RR, Locklair PR Jr, Grimball A. Descending thoracic aorta to femoral artery bypass. *J South Carolina Med Assn.* 1989;June:283–286.
22. Bowes DE, Youkey JR, Pharr WP, et al. Long term follow-up of descending thoracic aorto-iliac/femoral bypass. *J Cardiovasc Surg.* 1990;31:430–437.
23. O'Brien D, Waldron RP, McCabe JP, et al. Descending thoracic aorto-bifemoral bypass graft: a safe alternative in the high risk patients. *Ir Med J.* 1991:84:58–59.
24. Branchereau A, Espinoza H, Rudondy P, et al. Descending thoracic aorta as an inflow source for late occlusive failures following aortoiliac reconstruction. *Ann Vas Surg.* 1991:5: 8–15.
25. Kalman PG, Johnston KW, Walker PM. Descending thoracic aortofemoral bypass as an alternative for aortoiliac revascularization. *J Cardiovasc Surg.* 1991;32:443–446.
26. Criado E, Johnson G Jr, Burnham SJ, et al. Descending thoracic aorta-to-iliofemoral artery bypass as an alternative to aortoiliac reconstruction. *J Vasc Surg.* 1992;15:550–557.
27. Branchereau A, Magnan P-E, Moracchini P, et al. Use of descending thoracic aorta for lower limb revascularization. *Eur J Vasc Surg.* 1992;6:255–262.
28. McCarthy WJ, McGee GS, Lin WW, et al. Axillary to popliteal bypass provides successful limb salvage after removal of infected aortofemoral grafts. *Arch Surg.* 1992; 127:974–978.
29. Nevelsteen A, Wouters L, Suy R. Aortofemoral Dacron reconstruction for aortoiliac occlusive disease: a 25-year survey. *Eur J Vas Surg.* 1991;5:179–186.

15

Endarterectomy for Iliofemoral Occlusive Disease:

Ten-Year Follow-Up

Toshio Inahara, MD

Unilateral iliofemoral occlusive disease is unique in that its segmental distribution allows for a choice from several methods of vascular reconstruction. Initially, alternative methods were devised for less invasive procedures to effect limb salvage or to minimize undue risk. The concept of a crossover femorofemoral graft to salvage the contralateral limb was first reported by Freeman and Leeds[1] in 1952. In 1960, McCaughn and Kahn[2] reported two iliopopliteal crossover grafts. Vetto's two reports in 1962[3] and 1966[4] brought to attention the elective application of the crossover graft as an alternative to the aortofemoral graft. Axillofemoral graft was introduced by Blaisdell and Hall[5] in 1963. In 1977, Crawford and colleagues[6] described the unilateral aortofemoral or iliofemoral bypass for reoperation on previous aortic procedures. Piotrowski and associates[7] recommended the elective use of an aortobifemoral bypass in preference to unilateral iliofemoral grafts.

The purpose of this article is to present another alternative method of reconstruction, a direct reconstruction developed by Wylie and coworkers[8] in 1951, namely, endarterectomy, which preceded any extra-anatomic bypass procedures. Subsequently, the eversion technique of endarterectomy was developed in 1962 by Inahara[9] specifically to restore the long segment of the external iliac and common femoral arteries to avoid the problems of a difficult exposure, vessel injuries, and the repairs of longitudinal arteriotomies.

From 1966 to the present, 79 patients have undergone endarterectomy for unilateral iliofemoral occlusive disease by this method. To provide a minimum follow-up of 10 years on the outcome of this procedure, the series reviewed here encompasses a period of 16 years from February, 1966 to February, 1982 involving 37 patients and 42 limbs.

The incidence of unilateral iliofemoral occlusive disease was less common than that of bilateral aortoiliac or aortoiliofemoral occlusive disease. During the same 16-year period, 37 patients (42 limbs) were treated for unilateral disease, 83 patients were treated by bilateral aortoiliac endarterectomy, 212 by bilateral aortoiliofemoral endarterectomy, and 9 by aortobifemoral grafts. The incidence of unilateral iliofemoral disease was 10.9% in the series of inflow occlusive disease.

MATERIAL AND METHODS

From February, 1966 to February, 1982, 37 consecutive patients were treated for unilateral common, external iliac and common femoral occlusive disease, undergoing 42 primary endarterectomies. Men predominated 24 to 13. The mean ages for men and women were 75.0 and 75.5 years, respectively. The presenting symptoms were claudication in 28 (67%), rest pain in 6 (14%), and tissue necrosis in 8 (19%). Associated risk factors were characteristic of this age group with vascular disease (Table 15–1) but with a low incidence of diabetes mellitus (4 patients).

Patients were carefully evaluated for site and severity of ischemic symptoms, for level of disease, and for associated risk factors. Noninvasive vascular studies in the early years consisted of evaluation of pulses, oscillometry, and, later, Doppler indices. All patients underwent extensive arteriography and, in some, simultaneous measurement of femoral–brachial pressure gradients. Arteriography was performed via the common femoral arteries with large-bore, 17-gauge, thin-wall needles. With a pressure- or volume-controlled injector, both retrograde and anterograde arteriography were performed. With the contrast injected in the midportion of the arterial tree to be studied, the visualization was excellent for both inflow and outflow segments. The infrageniculate vessels in particular were clearly visualized due to minimal hemodilution of the contrast medium. Absence of palpable femoral pulses was not a deterrent because either the common or the profunda femoral vessels were nearly always cannulated to obtain outflow vessel visualization. Arteriograms confirmed 29 superficial femoral and/or popliteal occlusions ipsilateral to the 42 iliofemoral occlusions.

Data were entered and analyzed by the SYSTAT microcomputer program,[10,11] from which cumulative patency, survival, gender, and outflow disease risk factor rates were calculated by the Life Table method.[12] The statistical significance between Life Table curves was evaluated by the log-rank test.[13]

SURGICAL TECHNIQUE

Regional block was the anesthesia of choice: continuous epidural in 22 patients, spinal in 19, and general anesthesia in 1. Currently, continuous epidural is employed in most cases, using bupivacaine or fentanyl or a combination of both. On occasion, supple mental light general anesthesia is employed to ensure adequate ventilation and to allay apprehension. Postoperatively, the epidural injection is continued for 24 to 48

TABLE 15–1. ASSOCIATED RISK FACTORS

Angina	5
Congestive heart failure	10
Myocardial infarction	5
Prior coronary bypass graft	2
Hypertension	15
Diabetes mellitus	4
Stroke	5
Prior carotid endarterectomy	2
Tobacco abuse	24
Prior femeropopliteal graft	6

hours to control pain effectively without impairment of motor function and to provide the ancillary benefit of a sympathetic block with bupivacaine.

The surgical approach is through a lower quadrant oblique incision with a muscle-splitting retroperitoneal exposure of the iliac vessels from the aortic bifurcation to the inguinal ligament. With an additional incision in the groin, the arterial exposure is ideal. Access to the aortic bifurcation is important when the common iliac is severely diseased or occluded at its origin. When this is the case, proximal control is obtained by clamping the terminal aorta or by inserting an intra-aortic balloon catheter. Calcified common iliac artery is also best occluded with the use of a balloon catheter. The iliofemoral artery is next mobilized from the aortic bifurcation to the common femoral bifurcation. The artery must be free of any perivascular tissue because such tissue would impede the eversion of the adventitia (Fig. 15–1). Endarterectomy is performed through two arteriotomies: the first through a 3-cm arteriotomy in the distal common iliac artery; the second through the obliquely divided distal common femoral artery. It is important not to extend the arteriotomy into the external iliac artery because it invariably narrows upon closure. The common femoral artery must be divided at the bifurcation to deal with the orifice disease of the profunda and superficial femoral vessels. The common iliac artery is first endarterectomized to its

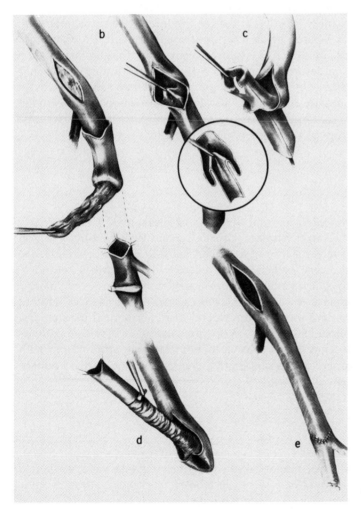

Figure 15–1. (*Reproduced with permission from* Surgery *1974; 75:772.*)

proximal limit. To avoid injuring the hypogastric artery, it is then endarterectomized blindly through the common iliac arteriotomy by guiding the tip of a Kelly clamp by palpation along the course of the vessel. Lastly, an endarterectomy is performed on the mobilized iliofemoral segment using the eversion method. Starting at its distal end, the adventitia of the common femoral artery is everted and rolled up the vessel, using a single layer of gauze for traction. The denuded core of plaque is amputated, and the adventitia is then uneverted. The remaining proximal third of the atheromatous core is gently pulled out through the common iliac arteriotomy, a process assisted by pushing the external iliac into the opening of the common iliac artery with a right-angle clamp. Retrograde eversion is continued until the entire vessel is turned inside out. With this complete exposure, the medial layer is gently abraded and peeled using the serrated edges of the Atraugrip forceps. The debrided lumenal surface should be smooth and glistening. The vessel is distended with heparinized solution to check for leaks and to identify any remaining tags. The vessel is uneverted, again distended with the same solution or from proximal arterial inflow after repair of the common iliac artery. This approach avoids torsion of the vessel before the femoral anastomosis is completed. For a small-diameter common femoral artery, a patch graft is often applied across its anastomosis to avoid suture-line narrowing.

All endarterectomies were completed without technical problems, and substitute grafts were not required. The importance of ensuring an adequate outflow tract and fashioning a nonobstructive outflow junction at the termination of the endarterectomy cannot be overemphasized. In 9 limbs, endarterectomy was extended 5 to 6 cm into the superficial femoral artery, of which 7 required vein patch angioplasties. The profunda femoral artery was endarterectomized 4 to 10 cm in 10 limbs, of which 5 required vein patch angioplasties. One profunda femoral artery was substituted with a bypass graft from the common femoral to its distal bifurcation, employing a segment of endarterectomized superficial femoral artery. Two patients with ischemic ulcers had concomitant femoropopliteal saphenous vein grafts.

EARLY RESULTS

Endarterectomy successfully restored femoral pulses in 42 limbs in 37 patients. Early complications were encountered in 5 patients. On the second postoperative day, an acute hemorrhage resulted from a rupture of a saphenous vein patch for endarterectomy of a superficial femoral artery, which was repaired without further complications. Another patient developed apnea and cardiac arrest from a presumed allergic reaction to a narcotic medication. With prompt measures, a resuscitation was without complications. A superficial wound infection developed in an abdominal incision and 2 patients developed symptomatic atelectasis. With pre-existing ischemia, 2 patients later underwent a great-toe amputation and a transmetatarsal amputation with uncomplicated healing. There were no postoperative deaths or other cardiac, pulmonary, or vascular complications.

LATE RESULTS

All patients were discharged with patent reconstructions. Patients were examined postoperatively at intervals of 2 weeks, 6 weeks, 6 months, and yearly, though some were seen less frequently. Patency of the iliofemoral endarterectomy was determined

vision, debridement is complete, and the artery is less subject to injury. The removal of the medial layer, which can be quite adherent, is safely accomplished. The principal benefit of the removal of the circular fibers of the media is that it allows the adventitial wall to expand an additional 2 mm to 5 mm in diameter. The resulting enlarged artery, we feel, contributes toward its long-term patency.

This concept is also supported by the use of a full-length autogenous vein patch graft of the iliofemoral arteries, with 100% patency to 6 years as reported by Taylor and colleagues.[14]

4. Although the anatomic reconstruction following endarterectomy maintains the linear continuity with less turbulent flow, whether restoring the hemodynamic status quo provides any beneficial effect is unknown. The presence of calcifications in the arterial wall, no matter how dense or extensive, in our experience has not been a deterrent or a contraindication for endarterectomy.

The disadvantages of endarterectomy are that the techniques are somewhat more meticulous and that, since it is infrequently performed in many centers, the procedure is not familiar to many. It is thought that this is a prolonged operation, however, the time to perform it is comparable to that for iliofemoral or axillofemoral graft placement. Our experience has shown that the eversion method of endarterectomy performed retroperitoneally is ideally suited for the treatment of unilateral iliofemoral disease and has proven to be effective, safe, and durable.

ALTERNATIVE OPERATIONS

Since the initial experiences with the extra-anatomic grafts were developed mainly for limb salvage and for high-risk patients, their application has been directed gradually toward elective procedures because of their favorable long-term results (Table 15–6).

Among more recent reports, Lamerton and associates[15] reported in 1985, 61 femorofemoral grafts in 54 high-risk patients followed to 10 years. The perioperative morbidity and mortality rate were 26% and 3.7%, respectively. With 12 late graft failures, the cumulative patency rate at 5 years was 60%. The authors continue to advocate the use of femorofemoral grafts for the highest risk patients with severe ischemia.

Kalman and coworkers[16] reported in 1987 a 10-year experience with femorofemoral grafts in 82 patients. Indications were claudication in 48% and limb threat in 52%. Perioperative morbidity and mortality rates were 13.2% and 0%, respectively. Cumulative patency rates were 80% and 67% at 1 and 3 years, respectively. The authors advocate the use of femorofemoral graft as an elective procedure if the donor vessels are normal.

The results of unilateral iliofemoral graft in 50 patients as reported in 1987 by Kalman and colleagues[17] were cumulative patency rates of 96% and 92% at 1 and 3 years, respectively. The procedure is recommended for all patients if the common iliac artery is a suitable source of inflow. In 1988, Chamm and coworkers[18] reported their experience with unilateral iliofemoral grafts. In a series of 110 patients, the cumulative patency rates were 91% and 86% at 3 and 5 years, respectively. Mortality rate was 1.9%. For bilateral disease, their aortobifemoral grafts during the same period had virtually identical patency results.

The results of a 10-year experience with axillofemoral grafts were reported in 1987 by Kalman and associates.[19] Ninety patients were treated to salvage limbs in

TABLE 15–6. RESULTS OF ALTERNATIVE PROCEDURES FOR UNILATERAL ILIOFEMORAL ARTERIAL DISEASE

		Patients or limbs	1 yr	Cumulative Patency Rates (%)			
				3 yrs	5 yrs	10 yrs	15 yrs
Femorofemoral grafts Lamerton et al[15]	1985	61			60		
Femorofemoral grafts Kalman et al[16]	1987	82	80	67			
Femorofemoral grafts Piotrowski et al[7]	1989	47	92		92		
Iliofemoral graft Kalman et al[17]	1987	50	96	92			
Iliofemoral graft Cham et al[18]	1988	110		91		86	
Iliofemoral graft Piotrowski et al[7]	1989	17	71	36			
Axillofemoral graft Kalman et al[19]	1987	90		68			
Axillofemoral graft Harris et al[20]	1990	76			85 (4 yrs)		
Aortobifemoral graft Piotrowski et al[7]	1989	32	100		89		
Iliofemoral endarterectomy Taylor et al[14]	1986	63			100 (6 yrs)		
Iliofemoral endarterectomy van den Dungen et al[21]	1991	93	94		83	65	
Iliofemoral endarterectomy Inahara[9]	1992	42			90	77	63

67%, for intra-abdominal sepsis in 21%, and for disabling claudication in 12%. Cumulative patency and limb salvage rates were 68% and 78%, respectively, at 3 years. When direct revascularization is not feasible, axillofemoral graft is recommended.

In 1990, Harris and coworkers[20] reported a 7-year experience in 76 patients with axillofemoral grafts using externally supported polytetrafluoroethylene grafts. Indications were aortic sepsis in 26% and relative indications in 74%. The perioperative mortality rate was 4.5%. Cumulative patency rates were 93% and 85% at 1 and 4 years, respectively. This was a significant improvement over their earlier series in which nonexternally supported grafts were used, for which the patency rate was 51% at 1 year. With the improved results, the authors now recommend the use of axillofemoral grafts as an alternative in elderly high-risk patients in whom aorto-bifemoral graft would have been placed.

The use of aortobifemoral grafts for unilateral iliac occlusion in 32 patients was reported in 1988 by Piotrowski and colleagues.[7] The cumulative patency rates with open superficial femoral arteries were 100% and 89% at 1 and 5 years, respectively. During the same period, cumulative patency rates for unilateral iliofemoral grafts in 17 patients were 56% and 56%, at 1 and 5 years respectively. The authors preferred the use of aortobifemoral grafts for unilateral disease unless the procedure was contraindicated by prohibitive risk.

Alternative techniques for iliofemoral endarterectomy were also reported. In 1986, Taylor and associates[14] reported 65 unilateral iliofemoral endarterectomies combined with distal femoropopliteal repairs. Endarterectomy was performed through a single arteriotomy and closed with a full-length vein or arterial patch graft. When autogenous patch graft vessels were unavailable, the eversion method of endarterectomy was preferred. Morbidity and mortality rates were 8% and 5%, respectively, with follow-up from 2 months to 6.5 years (mean 27 months). The cumulative patency rate for the open iliofemoral endarterectomy at 6 years was 100%.

In 1991, van den Dungen and coworkers[21] reported a series of 101 patients who underwent unilateral iliofemoral endarterectomy by the semiclosed method using arterial ring strippers. However, in 8, attempted endarterectomy was converted to insertion of iliofemoral grafts due to perforations, small artery size, or extensive calcification. There were no perioperative deaths. Cumulative patency rates were 87%, 83%, and 65% at 3, 5, and 10 years, respectively. With these results and minimal complications, the authors recommended the semiclosed method of endarterectomy.

The long-term results of iliofemoral endarterectomy compare favorably with other methods of revascularization and offer a broader scope of operability. Iliofemoral graft bypass requires a near normal inflow from the common iliac artery. Our routine is to carry the endarterectomy to the aortic bifurcation, as needed, to ensure adequate inflow. The semiclosed endarterectomy is a blind technique with limitations as described by the authors. With eversion endarterectomy, all procedures were completed without injury to the vessels and prosthetic grafts were not required. Calcification of the artery was not a deterrent to endarterectomy. In spite of the advanced median age of 75 years in our series, morbidity was minimal, with no mortality.

In recent years, the indications for treatment of unilateral iliofemoral disease or treatment failure of bilateral disease has progressed from the procedure of last choice, least invasive, and sparing, to that of an elective alternative choice to major aortic procedures. The early and midterm patency results of these procedures are reasonably predictive, in the range of 60% to 80% up to 5 years. It is of interest to compare the results of the various procedures, but one must be cognizant that there are many differences between series. To evaluate the final outcome, considerations must be given to such variables as indications, prior operations, patient selection, perioperative complications, effectiveness of the procedure, and long-term patency. Nevertheless, there are similarities in the pursuit of the same goal by different operations. With the availability of a diverse surgical armamentarium, the procedure best suited can be applied for each individual patient.

Acknowledgments

Special acknowledgment is made to Gary Grunkemeier, PhD and to Richard Shepard, PhD for their assistance and statistical analysis.

REFERENCES

1. Freeman NE, Leeds FH. Operations on large arteries. *Calif Med.* 1952;77:229–233.
2. McCaughn JJ Jr, Kahn SF. Cross-over graft for unilateral occlusion of the iliofemoral arteries. *Ann Surg.* 1960;151:26–28.
3. Vetto RM. The treatment of unilateral iliac artery obstruction with a transabdominal subcutaneous femorofemoral graft. *Surgery.* 1962;52:342–345.
4. Vetto RM. The femorofemoral shunt: an appraisal. *Am J Surg.* 1966;112:162–165.
5. Blaisdell FW, Hall AD. Axillary femoral artery bypass for lower extremity ischemia. *Surgery.* 1963;54:536.

6. Crawford ES, Manning LG, Kelly TF. "Redo" surgery after operations for aneurysm and occlusion of the abdominal aorta. *Surgery.* 1977;81:41–52.

7. Piotrowski JJ, Pearce WH, Jones DN, et al. Aortobifemoral bypass: the operation of choice for unilateral iliac occlusion? *J Vasc Surg.* 1988;8:211–218.

8. Wylie EJ, Kerr E, Davies O. Experimental and clinical experiences with the use of fascia lata applied as a graft about major arteries after endarterectomy and aneurysmography. *Surg Gynecol Obstet.* 1951;3:257–272.

9. Inahara T. The surgical treatment of aortoiliac atherosclerosis. *Surgery.* 1965;58:960–968.

10. Steinberg D, Colla P. *Survival: A supplementary module for SYSTAT.* Evanston, IL: SYSTAT, Inc; 1991.

11. Wilkinson L. *SYSTAT: The System for Statistics.* Evanston, IL: SYSTAT, Inc; 1991.

12. Kaplan EL, Meier P. Nonparametric estimation from incomplete observations. *J Amer Stat Assoc.* 1958;53:457–481.

13. Mantel N, Haenszel W. Statistical aspects of the analysis of data from retrospective studies of disease. *J Nat Cancer Inst.* 1959;22:719–748.

14. Taylor LM Jr, Freimanis IE, Edwards JM, et al. Extraperitoneal iliac endarterectomy in the treatment of multilevel lower extremity arterial occlusive disease. *Am J Surg.* 1986;152:34–38.

15. Lamerton AJ, Nicolaides AN, Eastcott HHG. The femorofemoral graft. *Arch Surg.* 1985;120:1274–1278.

16. Kalman PG, Hosang M, Johnston KW, et al. The current role for femorofemoral bypass. *J Vasc Surg.* 1987;6:71–75.

17. Kalman PG, Hosang M, Johnston KW, et al. Unilateral iliac disease: The role of iliofemoral bypass. *J Vasc Surg.* 1987;6:139–143.

18. Cham C, Myers KA, Scott DF, et al. Extraperitoneal unilateral iliac artery bypass for chronic lower limb ischemia. *Aust N Z J Surg.* 1988;58:859–863.

19. Kalman PG, Hosang M, Cina C, et al. Current indications for axillounifemoral and axillobifemoral bypass grafts. *J Vasc Surg.* 1987;5:828–832.

20. Harris EJ Jr, Taylor LM Jr, McConnell DB, et al. Clinical results of axillobifemoral bypass using externally supported polytetrafluoroethylene. *J Vasc Surg.* 1990;12:416–419.

21. van den Dungen JJAM, Boontje AH, Kropveld A. Unilateral iliofemoral occlusive disease: long term result of the semiclosed endarterectomy with the ring stripper. *J Vasc Surg.* 1991;14:673–677.

16

Technique and Six-Year Follow-Up on Percutaneous Transluminal Angioplasty to Treat Iliac Arterial Occlusive Disease

Peter G. Kalman, MD, FRCSC, Ken W. Sniderman, MD, FRCPC, and K. Wayne Johnston, MD, FRCSC

Percutaneous transluminal angioplasty (PTA) for the management of aortoiliac occlusive disease is a valuable option in the treatment of selected individuals and offers potential benefit to those patients who may not ordinarily be surgical candidates. The reported overall success rate for iliac PTA is generally lower than that for surgical revascularization; however, rather than being competitive with surgery, PTA should be regarded as an adjunctive modality. It is important to determine the variables that might be useful in predicting the long-term success of PTA. The objectives of this chapter, therefore, are to describe the current technique of PTA, to summarize the results for iliac PTA at the Toronto General Hospital,[1] and specifically, to identify the variables that are predictive of long-term success.

TECHNICAL ASPECTS OF ILIAC PERCUTANEOUS TRANSLUMINAL ANGIOPLASTY

A diagnostic arteriogram is performed, usually with a femoral artery puncture on the contralateral or less symptomatic side, leaving the other femoral artery available for retrograde puncture for PTA. For an ipsilateral iliac stenosis and for some contralateral iliac or proximal femoral stenoses, no further arterial puncture may be necessary since the aortic bifurcation can be crossed and the contralateral lesion approached superiorly. This approach is not recommended for proximal common iliac stenoses, since the balloon segment of the catheter will not be straight and may damage the bifurcation. Also, most occlusions should be approached ipsilaterally, as the contralateral approach does not allow much forward force to be applied at the catheter or guide wire tip.

Usual Ipsilateral Approach

Following a common femoral artery puncture, a 3-mm safety J guide wire is advanced retrograde into the iliac artery, and placed just distal to the site of the stenosis or occlusion. A No. 5 French torque catheter with a small bend close to its tip is advanced over the guide wire and is positioned just distal to the stenotic region. The guide wire is removed, the catheter flushed with heparinized saline, and the intra-arterial pressure measured. A forcible injection of contrast medium is made through the catheter in order to retrogradely opacify the stenotic segment and to create a vascular road map for subsequent guide wire and catheter manipulations.

A floppy guide wire (Bentson's) is advanced through the stenotic region, directing the guide wire with the curved catheter. If the guide wire will not advance easily through any region, the catheter is advanced to this site, the guide wire is withdrawn, and a further road map performed to demonstrate the anatomy. The guide wire is once again advanced using the curved catheter to direct it. Once the guide wire is proximal to the stenosis, the catheter is advanced over it, the guide wire is withdrawn, the catheter is flushed with heparinized saline, and the blood pressure measured. Once the lesion is traversed, an arteriogram is performed to confirm an intraluminal passage of the catheter through the lesion. On occasion, the catheter may pass within the walls of the vessel without being recognized; a balloon angioplasty performed in this circumstance may result in arterial rupture. If the catheter course is intramural, it is withdrawn and the correct route is found.

Marking the Lesion for Dilatation

The lesion must be appropriately marked for dilatation. With the central fluoroscopic beam directly over the lesion, the lesion is marked either through observation of bony landmarks or by placement of a radiopaque marker on the patient's skin.

Choosing the Correct Balloon Size

We believe that slight overdilation of a lesion results in improved PTA success; therefore, the artery just proximal to the stenotic region is measured, and a balloon is chosen that has a diameter 1 mm larger than the artery, commonly resulting in overdilation by approximately 15% to 20%. We have not encountered arterial rupture using this technique when the catheter was truly intraluminal in the stenotic segment. The usual balloon diameter is 8 to 9 mm for a common iliac artery lesion and 7 to 8 mm for an external iliac artery lesion. The length of the balloon should just exceed the length of the lesion.

Dilating a Lesion

The safety J wire is advanced through the initial catheter and positioned in the abdominal aorta, well superior to the site of dilatation. A catheter exchange is performed over the guide wire. For iliac arteries, the guide wire is left in place during PTA to ensure that the catheter tip will not traumatize the vessel wall when the balloon is inflated. The balloon segment is positioned at the lesion and is inflated under fluoroscopic guidance. The inflation characteristic is monitored, and "hour-glassing" or a "waist" is often noted in the balloon initially, with loss of the waist during balloon inflation. A 10-mL syringe with diluted contrast medium is used to inflate the balloon and is left maximally inflated for 30 seconds, then deflated, monitoring the deflation characteristic (if residual stenosis remains, the waist on the balloon will often recur; if the lesion has been dilated appropriately, the balloon will deflate symmetrically). The balloon is often reinflated gently one more time to evaluate the inflation and deflation characteristics. Of note, use of a pressure gauge is often recommended during balloon inflation because angioplasty balloon catheters have a burst pressure that should not be exceeded. However, using a 10-mL syringe for inflation, the burst pressure of these catheters cannot be exceeded. Following balloon deflation, the guide wire is removed, and the catheter flushed with heparinized saline. An arteriogram is performed to demonstrate the anatomic result of PTA. If the angioplasty has been successful, a systolic pressure gradient is once again measured on pull-back across the dilated segment.

Radiologic Management of Inadequate Percutaneous Transluminal Angioplasty or Complications

If the dilatation is considered inadequate or the angiogram demonstrates severe dissection at or distal to the dilated segment, further intervention is necessary. Occasionally, redilatation with a slightly larger diameter balloon is sufficient. However, especially with eccentric stenoses, further dilatation is not in order. This is especially true if the waist on the balloon was effaced during balloon inflation, suggesting an elastic lesion; in this case, as well as when substantial dissection has occurred, an intravascular stent may be indicated. This is easily placed because the arteriogram is reviewed before withdrawing the catheter distal to the dilated segment during pressure measurement.

Bilateral Common Iliac Stenoses

For stenoses at both proximal common iliac arteries or at the aortic bifurcation, a tandem, or "kissing" balloon technique is indicated. Two balloon catheters are placed at the aortic bifurcation extending into both iliac arteries. Balloon diameters should not exceed the expected normal diameter of the common iliac artery to ensure that iliac artery rupture does not occur. For unilateral lesions, the contralateral balloon acts as a buttress on the aortic bifurcation, permitting adequate dilatation of the stenotic region and protecting the contralateral side from displacement of plaque into it, which might cause subsequent occlusion or distal embolization. For unilateral lesions, the contralateral balloon should match the diameter of the common iliac artery, and an ipsilateral balloon should be chosen that exceeds the expected normal calibre of the common iliac artery by 1 mm. The balloons are inflated simultaneously and are monitored fluoroscopically. Following a 30-second inflation, the balloons are deflated simultaneously.

Iliac Artery Occlusions

Primary recanalization and PTA of short segmental occlusions can be performed. Previously, we dilated iliac occlusions without significant consequences; however, others considered PTA only for occlusions of less than 5 cm in length in patients who had stable symptoms for at least 3 months because of the risk of embolization of the unorganized thrombus. Recently, we have felt that it is safer to perform initial fibrinolysis in order to remove unorganized thrombus and reduce the risk of distal embolization during angioplasty. The fibrinolysis is performed from the contralateral approach over a 12- to 18-hour infusion. A channel is often opened, leaving only a stenosis for PTA.

To traverse an occlusion in an iliac artery, the angiographic catheter is initially plugged into the distal portion of the occluded segment, and an attempt is made to traverse the occluded segment using a floppy guide wire. If this is not possible, the catheter is used alone. This technique is totally blind since the thrombotic core cannot be differentiated from an intramural passage of the catheter, which explains why there is greater risk for iliac artery rupture of occluded segments than of stenotic segments after PTA. Once the occluded segment is traversed, the technique for PTA is similar to that for stenotic regions.

Adjunctive Considerations

Five thousand units of heparin is administered intra-arterially before crossing a lesion if the flow is slow, and it is not reversed with protamine following PTA. Patients are given low doses of enteric-coated aspirin (325 mg daily), beginning before angioplasty and continuing for a minimum of 3 months after angioplasty. The patient is restricted to bed rest and observed for 6 hours after the procedure for bleeding or potential ischemic complications. Selected patients are discharged home and required to rest in bed.

CRITERIA FOR SUCCESS IN PERCUTANEOUS TRANSLUMINAL ANGIOPLASTY

The factors that were considered important for predicting long-term results were recorded prospectively, and PTA was considered a success only if both clinical and vascular laboratory criteria improved[1]: improvement of clinical grade by at least one level (i.e., asymptomatic, mild claudication, disabling claudication, ischemic night pain or rest pain, or ulceration or gangrene); improvement of vascular laboratory measurements of one or more of the following:

1. Ankle–brachial systolic pressure ratio increased by at least 0.10.
2. Monophasic Doppler frequency analysis recordings became biphasic or triphasic.
3. The Doppler pulsatility index increased by more than 20%.
4. The treadmill exercise distance at least doubled.

DATA ANALYSIS

The data were analyzed using both univariate and multivariate techniques to determine the long-term results of iliac PTA. For individual variables and subgroups (univariate analysis), survival function was estimated using the Kaplan-Meier method (cumulative percentage success rate versus follow-up time).[2] The generalized Wilcoxon (Breslow) test and the log-rank (Mantel-Cox) test were employed to test statistical differences between survival curves, and significance was assumed for a P value less than .05. A multivariate analysis of the factors associated with late success of iliac PTA was performed using the Cox proportional hazard model[3] to estimate the chances for success with all combinations of significant variables. The multiple

TABLE 16–1. COMPLICATIONS (MORBIDITY AND MORTALITY) FOR ILIAC PTA

Complication	All Iliac Cases (*n*=667)	Iliac Stenosis (*n*=584)	Iliac Occlusion (*n*=83)
Nil	92.1	92.8	86.8
Death	0.3	0.3	0.0
Hematoma (small)	2.7	2.4	4.8
Hematoma (large)	1.9	2.1	1.2
False aneurysm	0.1	0.2	0.0
Ischemia (no OR)	0.7	0.5	2.4
Ischemia (OR)	0.9	0.9	1.2
Distal emboli	0.4	0.3	1.2
Dissection or tear	0.4	0.3	1.2
Dye extravasation	0.1	0.0	1.2
Other	0.1	0.2	0.0

determinants for technical failure were analyzed using logistic regression for categoric variables.[4]

MORBIDITY AND MORTALITY

Of the 667 iliac PTAs, 2 patients died as a result of the iliac PTA: 1 following a myocardial infarction and 1 from bleeding secondary to arterial rupture, for a mortality rate of 0.3%. Complications occurred after 7.9% of PTAs and are detailed in Table 16–1. Most of the morbidity was minor in nature, and emergency surgery was necessary in only 1.0%.

FACTORS DETERMINING LONG-TERM SUCCESS

General Description of the Patient Population

Six hundred sixty-seven iliac PTAs were performed between July 1978 and July 1986 at the Toronto General Hospital. Follow-up was complete in 99% of cases and was continued until the end of the study period or until failure or death. Five cases were excluded from the analyses since their outcome could not be determined, because multilevel occlusive disease or a systemic disease precluded accurate assessment. The patient and anatomic data is summarized in Table 16–2. A technical success was achieved in 96.5% of iliac PTAs (conversely, technical failure occurred in 3.5% and occurred more frequently when PTA was performed for occlusion than for stenosis (18.1% vs. 1.4%, respectively; $P < .001$). When other variables were included into a logistic regression model, only the severity of the lesion (stenosis vs. occlusion) was related to early success or failure. Our data analysis takes this important difference in severity of lesion into account; therefore, the data is presented separately for iliac stenoses and occlusions.

TABLE 16–2. PATIENT SUMMARY OF ALL 667 CASES OF ILIAC PTA

Age	59.2 ± 9.5	
Sex	male	68.5%
	female	31.5%
Diabetes	no	90%
	yes	10%
Indication	claudication	91.3%
	salvage	8.8%
	other	3.1%
Pre-PTA ankle–brachial ratio	0.59 ± 0.18	
Post-PTA ankle–brachial ratio	0.71 ± 0.22	
Site	common iliac	56.4%
	external iliac	33.3%
	both	10.3%
Lesion severity	stenosis	87.6%
	occlusion	12.4%
Runoff	good (<50%)	60.6%
	poor (>50%)	39.4%
Previous PTA	no	90.7%
	yes	9.3%
Number of sites dilated	one	86.4%
	two	13.3%
	three	0.3%
Pressure gradient pre-PTA	41.9 ± 27.5 mm Hg	
Pressure gradient post-PTA	7.0 ± 11.0 mm Hg	
Technical failure	no	96.5%
	yes	3.5%

The overall long-term results for 667 iliac PTAs calculated by the Kaplan-Meier method are summarized in Table 16–3.

Results of Percutaneous Transluminal Angioplasty for Iliac Occlusions

The cumulative percentage of success for 82 PTAs for iliac occlusion analyzed by the Kaplan-Meier method (including the 15 cases that failed for technical reasons) is illustrated in Figure 16–1. The success rate at 1 month was 75.6 ± 4.7%, 59.8 ± 5.5% at 1 year, 52.8% ± 5.9% at 2 years, and 48.0 ± 6.3% at 3 years. Only the number of sites dilated (i.e., one site vs. two or more) was related to success of the procedure

TABLE 16–3. RESULTS OF ILIAC PTA (667 CASES) CALCULATED BY THE KAPLAN-MEIER METHOD

Time of Follow-up	Cumulative % Success (Mean ± SE)
1 mo	90.0 ± 1.2
1 yr	75.1 ± 1.8
2 yrs	64.7 ± 2.1
3 yrs	59.6 ± 2.2
4 yrs	56.0 ± 2.4
5 yrs	51.4 ± 2.9
6 yrs	49.9 ± 3.2

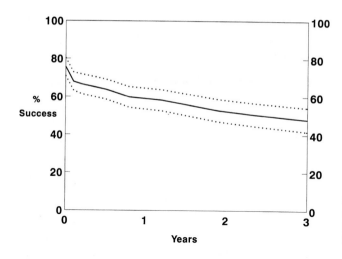

Figure 16–1. Percutaneous translu-minal angioplasty of 82 iliac artery occlusions. Success as calculated by the Kaplan-Meier method (mean ± SE plotted).

(P = .04). The initial success for PTA at one site was 80.3 ± 4.7% compared with 45.5 ± 15.0% if two or more sites were dilated.

Results for Percutaneous Transluminal Angioplasty for Iliac Stenoses

Figure 16–2 shows the long-term success of PTA for 580 iliac stenoses (584 were performed, but 4 cases were excluded because outcome could not be determined). The success rate at 1 month was 95.9 ± 0.8%, 77.2 ± 1.8% at 1 year, 66.5 ± 2.2% at 2 years, 61.2 ± 2.4% at 3 years, 57.8 ± 2.6% at 4 years, 54.0 ± 2.9% at 5 years, and 50.0 ± 3.5 at 6 years. Only 8 of the 584 attempted cases were technical failures; therefore, it is not surprising that the late results were the same, whether the technical failures were included or excluded (e.g., at 6 years 50.0 ± 3.5% if included vs. 50.7 ± 3.6% if excluded). Therefore, the technical failures were included in subsequent analyses. The following variables were related to the long-term result by Kaplan-Meier analysis:

1. indication for the PTA (P = .006)
2. site of the PTA (P = .025)
3. diabetes (P = .022)
4. runoff (P = .004)
5. pre-PTA ankle–brachial blood pressure ratio greater than 0.50 (P = .040)

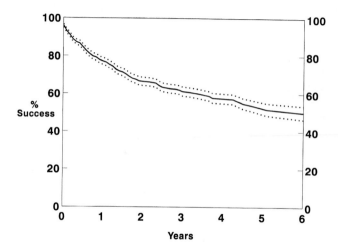

Figure 16–2. Percutaneous translu-minal angioplasty for all 580 iliac stenoses (Kaplan-Meier) (mean ± SE plotted).

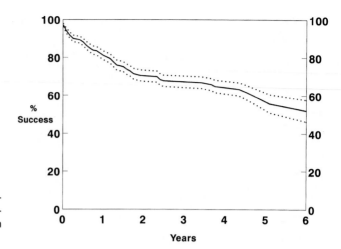

Figure 16–3. Percutaneous transluminal angioplasty of 313 common iliac stenoses (Kaplan-Meier) (mean ± SE plotted).

However, using Cox regression analysis, the indication (claudication = 1, salvage = 2), site (common iliac = 1, external iliac = 2, both = 3), and runoff (good = 1, poor = 2) were together associated with a successful outcome ($P<.001$).

In the following sections, the results are analyzed by the site of the PTA for further simplification.

Use for Common Iliac Stenoses

The success rate of PTA for common iliac stenoses at 1 month was 97.1 ± 0.9%, 81.1 ± 2.3% at 1 year, 70.6 ± 2.9% at 2 years, 67.8 ± 3.0% at 3 years, 64.9 ± 3.3% at 4 years, 60.2 ± 4.0% at 5 years, and 52.0 ± 5.7% at 6 years (Fig. 16–3). Long-term results were not predicted by any of the recorded variables.

Use for External Iliac Stenoses

The success rate of PTA for external iliac stenoses at 1 month was 95.2 ± 1.5%, 74.1 ± 3.2% at 1 year, 62.0 ± 3.8% at 2 years, 51.0 ± 4.4% at 3 years, and 48.4 ± 4.5% at 4 years (Fig. 16–4). The gender of the patient ($P = .005$) and the indication for the procedure ($P = .023$) were related to long-term success using Kaplan-Meier analysis. However, using Cox regression analysis, only patient gender was significant. The predicted

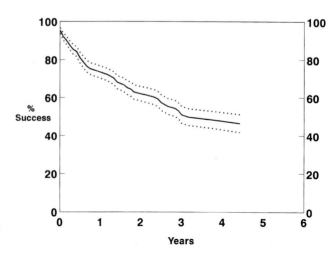

Figure 16–4. Percutaneous transluminal angioplasty of external iliac stenoses (Kaplan-Meier) (mean ± SE plotted).

IV

Five- to Ten-Year Patency Rate of Infrainguinal Reconstructions

17

The Polytetrafluoroethylene Graft for Infrainguinal Revascularization:

Long-Term Results

George E. Hajjar, MD, and
William J. Quiñones-Baldrich, MD

Infrainguinal arterial reconstruction for atherosclerotic disease remains an area of great debate among various leading authorities in the field of vascular surgery. Controversies exist regarding indications, type of intervention, source of inflow, and level of distal anastomosis. The greatest subject of controversy and debate, however, continues to be the preferential use of synthetic graft or autogenous vein as the primary conduit for revascularization.

Advocates of the autogenous vein as the primary arterial substitute cite the greater patency rate as the major advantage: 68% versus 38% for polytetrafluoroethylene (PTFE) at 5 years for below the knee anastomoses.[1] In addition, synthetic material acts as a foreign body and runs a greater risk of infection; it may also induce local vessel wall changes, causing intimal hyperplasia, which may lead to graft failure.

We and others have previously published our results with the preferential use of expanded polytetrafluoroethylene (ePTFE) for infrainguinal arterial reconstruction, with a 5-year patency rate of 57% and a limb salvage rate of 73%.[2,3] These results, along with the shorter surgery time and the relative ease of the procedure (requiring two small incisions) has prompted us to use ePTFE as the first choice arterial substitute in femoropopliteal arterial reconstruction. Most importantly, preservation of the saphenous vein for future use in more complicated distal reconstructions where synthetic arterial substitute have proven to yield poor results, seems to be the major benefit of this approach.

In this present era of vascular surgery, where various treatment modalities became available to alleviate lower limb ischemia, the therapeutic approach must be tailored to each patient's need. A good knowledge of the long-term outcome of these interventions is essential in the decision-making process.

This chapter presents our experience with infrainguinal arterial reconstruction using ePTFE, discusses the outcome, and provides long-term follow-up data for up to 10 years.

PATIENT POPULATION

At the University of California at Los Angeles Medical Center between 1978 and 1988, we performed a total of 322 infrainguinal reconstructions in 258 patients, preferentially using 6-mm ePTFE grafts. Patient characteristics were similar to those in other studies of lower limb ischemia, with males predominating (61%) and a mean age of 67 years with a range of 43 to 91 years. Similarly, cigarette smoking (82%) was the most common risk factor, followed by hypertension (60%) and diabetes mellitus (31%). Coronary artery disease was the most commonly associated disease and was clinically manifested in 47% of the patients.

INDICATION FOR SURGERY

Lower limb ischemia can be graded according to the severity of symptoms. Severe claudication (grade I, chronic limb ischemia), critical ischemia, also referred to as ischemic rest pain (grade II, chronic limb ischemia), and acute tissue loss due to ischemia (grade III, chronic limb ischemia).

The indication for revascularization in our series of patients (Table 17–1) consisted of severe claudication in 132 bypasses (41%), with 110 reconstructions to the popliteal artery above the knee and 22 to the popliteal artery below the knee. Critical ischemia, ischemic rest pain, and acute tissue loss were the indications in 190 (59%) where the procedure was performed for limb salvage. Of these, 109 grafts were placed to the popliteal artery above the knee, 53 to the popliteal artery below the knee, and 28 bypasses were performed to an infrapopliteal vessel. This last group of 28 infrapopliteal reconstructions constituted an obligatory use of ePTFE, where multiple previous reconstructions had been performed and no autogenous vein was available as substitute.

FOLLOW-UP

In postoperative follow-up, patients should be returned to the clinic, and followed for as long as possible, regardless of outcome. They should be questioned about the recurrence of symptoms, and a physical vascular assessment should be performed. An ankle–brachial index or digital plethysmography should be obtained to provide a more objective assessment. Duplex scanning has now become an important tool in following grafts noninvasively in the vascular laboratory, not only to identify failed grafts, but also to diagnose failing ones where intervention and correction of the underlying problem may prolong the patency of such grafts. We consider a drop in

TABLE 17–1. INDICATION FOR SURGERY AND SITE OF DISTAL ANASTOMOSIS IN 322 INFRAINGUINAL RECONSTRUCTIONS

Indication	Above Knee	Below Knee	Infrapopliteal
Severe claudication (132 grafts)	110 grafts	22 grafts	—
Critical ischemia (190 grafts)	109 grafts	53 grafts	28 grafts[a]

[a] Obligatory ePTFE.

the ankle–brachial index of more than 0.1 from the maximum postoperative value an indication of failure, requiring angiographic confirmation and necessary intervention.

A failed graft is any graft requiring thrombectomy at any time, even within 48 hours after surgery, or any graft that must be removed due to infection, even if the graft remains patent. However if a graft remains patent but fails to salvage a severely ischemic limb, it should not be considered graft failure, but rather failure to salvage the limb.

In our study, patients had a follow-up period that ranged from 12 to 144 months, with a mean of 66 months. A total of 42 patients, representing 48 grafts (15% of implants) were lost to follow-up. We suspected graft failure if a subjective deterioration was reported by the patient, a deterioration in the status of the limb was detected on physical examination, or a change in noninvasive studies was noted.

MORTALITY FROM INFRAINGUINAL REVASCULARIZATION

Various studies report the perioperative mortality rate (1 to 30 days) for patients undergoing infrainguinal reconstruction to range from 1.7% to 3.5% and to be due mainly to cardiac events.[4–7] The delayed mortality rate of such a patient population, however, is markedly higher and ranged from 30%[8] to 42% at 5 years[5] to 46.3%[7] to 72%[9] at 10 years. In addition, unlike the early postoperative mortality rate, the delayed mortality rate appears to be related to various factors as reported by DeWeese and Rob.[9] In their study, patients with claudication had a mortality rate of 48% at 10 years compared with 80% for patients with rest pain and 95% for patients with gangrene. Age seemed to play an important role as well. Patients 50 to 59 years of age had a mortality rate of 57% compared with 83%, 70%, 88%, and 100% for patients 20 to 49, 60 to 69, 70 to 79, and 80 to 89 years old, respectively. Patients with diabetes had a 10-year mortality rate of 92%, but it was 65% in nondiabetics. Similarly, hypertension affected the long-term mortality rate in these patients, where 83% of hypertensive patients died compared with 67% of those without hypertension.

In our series, the perioperative mortality rate was comparable to that found in other reports. A total of nine patients died within 30 days of surgery (3.4%). Eight patients died between 1 and 5 days following their bypass. The other patient died following an amputation during the same hospitalization. As expected from other studies, there was no significant difference in the mortality rate based on the indication for surgery: 2.9% for patients with claudication and 3.7% for patients with critical ischemia who underwent the operation for foot salvage.

The overall survival rate calculated by actuarial method for the patients followed was 65% at 5 years and 52% at 8 years. Most of the deaths occurred in the first and second year after surgery, with a steady lower yearly attrition rate thereafter. These rates are similar to the observations of others. DeWeese and Rob reported an attrition rate of 10%/yr for the first 5 years, then 5%/yr for the following 5 years.[9] Maini and Mannick reported that 64% of the deaths occurred in the first and second years after surgery, with the remainder equally distributed over the next third, fourth, and fifth years.[5] Such a high delayed mortality rate could be explained by the systemic nature of atherosclerosis, affecting both cerebral and coronary circulations, with most deaths due to coronary vascular disease.

It remains to be seen if the more aggressive medical and surgical management of coronary artery disease, as suggested in reports by us[2] and others[3] have indeed had an effect on the long-term survival of this select population of patients.

PATENCY

Graft patency is usually discussed in terms of primary and secondary patency. *Primary patency* refers to grafts that remain patent since implantation and do not require any additional intervention. *Secondary patency* denotes the grafts that remain open following subsequent operative or less invasive procedures, regardless of the number of interventions performed.

Synthetic graft patency rates have been related to various factors. It is generally agreed that the more distal the level of anastomosis, the lower the patency rate. Polytetrafluoroethylene grafts to the infrapopliteal segment are known to yield notoriously poor patency rates. A 12% 4-year primary patency rate was reported by Veith and colleagues in a randomized prospective trial when PTFE was used for infrapopliteal reconstructions, compared with a 70% primary patency when the distal anastomosis was to the popliteal artery.[1]

The status of the recipient vascular bed also seems to play an important role in graft patency. Prendeville and coworkers[6] reported a patency rate for ePTFE used above the knee of 80% at 30 months for patients with good angiographic runoff compared with 52% when the runoff was poor. In addition, the indication for operation was found to be significant in determining graft patency, dropping from 57% at 5 years for severe claudication to 37% at 5 years for critical ischemia. Similar results were published by Hobson and his colleagues.[10] Their patency rates at 2 years for PTFE used below the knee for limb salvage were 90% for good runoff and 45% when the runoff was considered poor.

Finally, a host of patient-dependent factors influence the long-term patency rate of an infrainguinal bypass graft. Diabetes, continued cigarette smoking, and the rate of acceleration of atherosclerosis distal to the anastomosis all have an adverse effect.

The literature is replete with short- and intermediate-term follow-up reports on the use of ePTFE grafts in peripheral vascular reconstruction, some of which are summarized in Table 17–2.

In a review of 127 femoropopliteal reconstructions using ePTFE, McAuley and his associates[11] reported an overall patency rate of 74% at 6 months, 63% at 1 year, 48% at 3 years, 40% at 5 years, and 35% at 7 years. Their early patency rate at 1 year was lower than that of others,[10,12] a fact they attributed to more heroic attempts at limb salvage since pregangrenous or gangrenous changes were present in approximately half of the patients.

Ascer and associates[12] reported on a large series of 822 PTFE grafts performed for limb salvage. The patency rate for 427 femoropopliteal reconstructions was 55% at 6 years, 79 of which were to a blind popliteal segment, with a 6-year patency rate of 72%. For infrapopliteal grafts the patency rate was 37% at 4 years. For extra-anatomic reconstructions, axillofemoral and femorofemoral bypasses, the patency rates were 83% and 75%, respectively, at 5.5 years. For the 34 axillopopliteal reconstructions using PTFE, patency rates were 74% at 1 year and 45% at 5 years.

In a 6-year prospective multicenter randomized trial, Veith and associates[1] compared autologous saphenous vein and ePTFE grafts for infrainguinal arterial reconstructions. The overall 6-year patency rate for ePTFE was 38%. For above-the-knee anastomosis the patency rate was 38%, compared with 54% when the anastomosis was below the knee. The reason for such a difference was not evident in their study. They hypothesized that uncontrolled patient-related factors possibly played a role and warned that this should not be considered firm evidence for improved graft patency with below-the-knee anastomosis.

In our experience in infrainguinal reconstruction with ePTFE, the primary

TABLE 17–2. POLYTETRAFLUOROETHYLENE GRAFT PATENCY STUDIES

Author	Study	Period (years)	Patency Rate (%)
Sterpetti et al[3]	90 PTFE above-the-knee femoropopliteal grafts	7	58.3
Hobson et al[10]	36 PTFE below-the-knee grafts for limb salvage	2	43
Sladen and Maxwell[20]	130 obligatory PTFE grafts for infrainguinal reconstruction	3	30
Gupta and Veith[21]	PTFE grafts for limb salvage	3	77 femoropopliteal 93 axillofemoral 69 axillotibral 48 to foot
McAuley et al[11]	127 PTFE grafts for femoropopliteal bypass	7	35 including early failures 55 excluding early failures
Ascer et al[12]	822 ePTFE for grafts limb salvage	6	55 fem popliteal 72 blind popliteal segment 37 infrapopliteal 80 extra-anatomic
Veith et al[1]	PTFE vs. autogenous vein grafts, multicenter randomized prospective trial	6	38 femoropopliteal 12 femorotibial
Prendeville et al[6]	114 above-the-knee ePTFE grafts for popliteal reconstructions	6	69 at 2 yrs 42 at 5 yrs
Quiñones et al[17]	322 ePTFE infrainguinal reconstructions	10	femoropopliteal 59 at 5 yrs 53 at 8 yrs infrapopliteal 22 at 3 yrs

patency rate for all femoropopliteal bypasses was 59% and 53% at 5 and 8 years, respectively. Twenty-two of our 294 femoropopliteal reconstructions were secondary attempts at revascularization. Our patency rate for primary reconstruction with ePTFE was 61.5% at 5 years and 54.5% at 8 years. The difference in patency between primary and secondary revascularization did not appear statistically significant, however, due to the low number of secondary revascularizations involved. The overall secondary patency rate achieved was 74% and 72% at 5 and 8 years, respectively (Fig. 17–1).

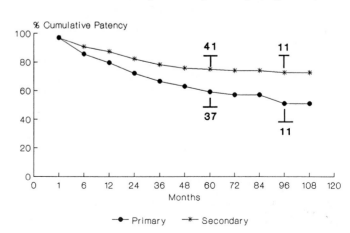

Figure 17–1. Primary and secondary patency for 294 femoropopliteal bypasses.

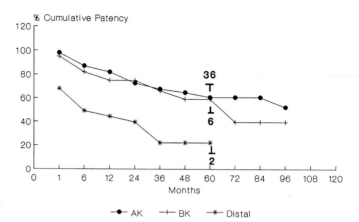

Figure 17–2. Primary patency of infrainguinal PTFE bypasses to (AK) supragenicular (*N*=219), (BK) infragenicular (*N*=75), and (Distal) infrapopliteal (*N*=28) arteries. (т, ⊥ = number of patients in that interval)

The primary patency rates for above-the-knee femoropopliteal bypasses (*N* = 219), regardless of indication, were 60.5% and 53% at 5 and 8 years, respectively. Below-the-knee reconstructions (*N* = 75), regardless of indication, had a 59% and 39% patency rate at 5 and 8 years, respectively (Fig. 17–2). When analyzing the data based on the indication for surgery, the primary patency rates of femoropopliteal reconstructions done for severe claudication (*N* = 132) at 5 and 8 years were 68.5% and 63%, respectively. For limb salvage, however, the primary patency rates for femoropopliteal reconstructions were 51% and 38% at 5 and 8 years, respectively. This is a statistically significant difference when compared with rates for grafts done for claudication (*P* < .02) (Fig. 17–3).

Taking into account the location of the disal anastomosis, PTFE grafts with an above-the-knee anastomosis performed for severe claudication had a patency rate of 68% at both 5 and 8 years. Below-the-knee femoropopliteal bypasses done for severe claudication had a similar primary patency rate of 71% at 5 years; however a significant drop to 43% was observed at the end of 8 years (Fig. 17–4). Above-the-knee femoropopliteal bypasses performed for foot salvage had a patency rate of 50% at 5 years and 40% at 8 years, whereas the patency rate for below-the-knee bypasses for the same indication was 45% at 5 years, with not enough data for the 8-year interval. For femoroinfrapopliteal bypasses (*N* = 28) the primary patency rate at 3 years was 22% (Fig. 17–5).

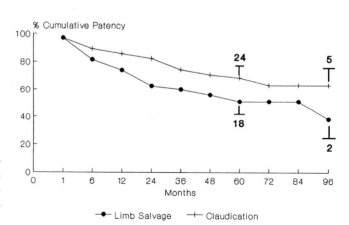

Figure 17–3. Primary patency for femoropopliteal bypasses done for disabling claudication (*N*=132) or critical ischemia (*N*=162) (*P* < .02).

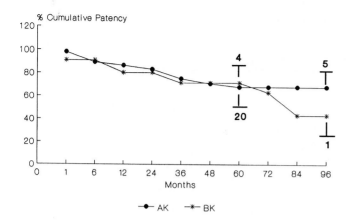

Figure 17–4. Primary patency for above-the-knee or below-the-knee femoropopliteal bypasses performed for disabling claudication.

LIMB SALVAGE

Limb salvage is an important consideration in the assessment of any surgical intervention since it is the ultimate goal for which an infrainguinal operation is performed. Limb salvage does not equate with patency and vice versa. A graft might remain patent long enough to allow tissue healing, resolution of rest pain, or cure of infection before thrombosing, leaving a viable limb. On the other hand a graft might remain patent, but because of a severely diseased distal vascular bed, the limb remains threatened and may never recover, and an amputation in the presence of a patent graft becomes necessary. In all published series, patency rates are inferior to limb salvage rates.[13,14]

Limb salvage rates vary from series to series. Most reports agree however, on the high early salvage rate. Collins and associates[15] reported an 86% early limb salvage rate after a variety of surgical procedures for severe lower limb ischemia. Yogasundaram[16] showed that arterial reconstruction was possible in 50% of his patients with threatened limbs, and the limb salvage rate was 76%. In a report on arterial reconstructions and limb salvage, Maini and Mannick[5] found the early limb salvage rate to be 96% at the end of the first month after surgery, 84% at 1 year, and 80% at 5 years. In addition, he found that patients were at greater risk of limb loss during the first year following vascular reconstruction.

In our series, the overall foot salvage rates for femoropopliteal bypasses performed for that indication were 70% at 5 years and 66% at 8 years. There was no

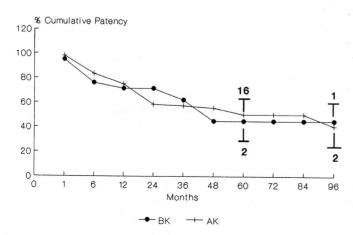

Figure 17–5. Primary patency rate for above-the-knee or below-the-knee femoropopliteal bypasses performed for critical ischemia.

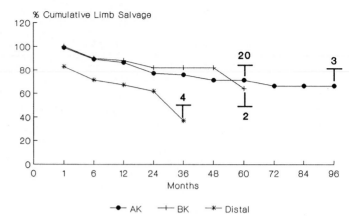

Figure 17–6. Limb salvage for grafts done for critical ischemia according to location of the distal anastomosis.

statistical difference in foot salvage rate between above-the-knee or below-the-knee anastomosis (Fig. 17–6).

For femoroinfrapopliteal grafts, however, the foot salvage rate was 37% at 5 years. When one considers the 22% patency rate for such grafts at that interval, the dependency of these limbs on graft patency is underscored.

GRAFT FAILURE

Graft failure is usually due to either *inflow failure* secondary to progression or development of new atherosclerotic lesions proximal to the graft or thrombosis of a proximal reconstruction. *Outflow failure* occurs as a result of progression of atherosclerosis distally or the development of an intimal hyperplastic lesion at the distal anastomotic site. Other causes of failure are technical, usually occurring soon after surgery, graft infection, and other patient-related causes, such as hypercoagulable state.

We have previously studied and reported our 10-year experience with 111 failures of ePTFE in infrainguinal revascularization.[17] Of these, 10 occurred during the first 30 days following surgery. Sixty percent of all failures (66 grafts) occurred in the first 12 months. Eighty-two percent of all failures occurred in the first 2 years, with only 19.5% of failures occurring after the second year.

Of the 111 failures, 28 occurred in patients operated on for severe claudication, with 22 being above-the-knee bypasses and 6 below the knee. Eighty-three failures occurred in patients operated on for limb salvage: 34 in the above-the-knee position, 31 in below-the-knee anastomosis, and 18 in the distal infrapopliteal position.

Progression of distal disease accounted for 40% of failures. Half of these were associated with intimal hyperplasia in the area of the distal anastomosis. In 22%, the cause of failure was attributed to progression of proximal disease, and only in 8% was intimal hyperplasia the sole cause of graft failure. Poor patient selection (patients with severe distal disease) accounted for 15% of the failures. Graft infection caused 6 failures, five of which had had multiple previous attempts at revascularization. In nine cases (8%), the cause of failure could not be determined (Table 17–3).

Various management alternatives were employed for treating the failed grafts, including thrombectomy with or without patch angioplasty, and extension with vein or PTFE to a more distal site. These methods of secondary revascularization yielded similar results, with a 30-month patency rate between 32% and 55%. On the other

TABLE 17–3. ANALYSIS OF 111 FAILED PTFE GRAFTS IN 322 INFRAINGUINAL REVASCULARIZATIONS

Distal Anastomosis	Interval from Surgery	Causes of Failure
Above the knee 56% (N=219)	0–30 days: 10 (9%)	Progression of distal disease: 40%[a]
Below the knee 37% (N=75)	0–12 months: 61 (60%)	Progression of proximal disease: 22%
Infrapopliteal 18% (N=28)	0–24 months: 91 (82%)	Severity of distal disease: 15%
		Intimal hyperplasia: 8%
		Infection: 5%
		Undetermined: 8%

[a] Fify percent of these were associated with intimal hyperplasia at the distal anastomosis.

hand, patients that underwent secondary revascularization with a completely new graft using the spared saphenous vein had a 30-month patency rate of 88%, with limb salvage achieved in all patients in whom the spare saphenous vein was used at the first reoperation.

These results agree with the work of Ascer and colleagues,[18] who recommended revision with an entirely new autogenous vein graft for failed PTFE reconstruction. Whittemore and coworkers[19] also recommended the placement of a new autogenous vein graft for the revision of failed previous reconstruction, based on their review of 109 failures of femoropopliteal reconstructions.

SUMMARY

Our results suggest that the failure rate of ePTFE grafts beyond 5 years is low in the femoropopliteal position, and thus the performance of PTFE grafts beyond that interval continues to be acceptable.

The most common cause of failure was progression of proximal or distal disease, or severity of distal disease, occurring mostly within the first year. We did not use oral anticoagulants routinely and thus cannot reach a definite conclusion about its benefit. It has been our experience, however, that patients do better with chronic long-term anticoagulants after failure of a PTFE graft when no clear cause of failure is identified.

In treating graft failures, it is tempting to revise the graft with minimal intervention, such as with thrombectomy and or angioplasty. Our experience, however, underlines the superiority of placing a new graft using autogenous saphenous vein if available, especially when the cause of failure is progression of distal disease.

Finally, the preferred primary conduit for infrainguinal reconstruction remains controversial, especially when the distal anastomosis could be performed above the knee. Our results show an acceptable performance of ePTFE in femoropopliteal reconstruction, but their use in the infrapopliteal position should be reserved as an alternative to amputation in patients with severe limb ischemia. For this reason we continue to recommend the preferential use of ePTFE for femoropopliteal reconstruction and the preservation of the autogenous saphenous vein for later use.

REFERENCES

1. Veith FJ, Gupta SK, Ascer E, et al. Six-year prospective multicenter randomized comparison of autologous saphenous vein and expanded polytetrafluoroethylene grafts in infrainguinal arterial reconstructions. *J Vasc Surg.* 1986;3:104–114.

2. Quiñones-Baldrich WJ, Busuttil RW, Baker JD, et al. Is the preferential use of polytetrafluoroethylene grafts for femoropopliteal bypass justified? *J Vasc Surg.* 1988;8:219–228.

3. Sterpetti AV, Schultz RD, Feldhaus RJ, et al. Seven year experience with polytetrafluoroethylene as above knee femoropopliteal graft. Is it worthwhile to preserve the autologous saphenous vein? *J Vasc Surg.* 1985;2:907–912.

4. Reichle FA, Tyson RR. Comparison of long-term results of 364 femoropopliteal or femorotibial bypasses for revascularization of severely ischemic lower extremities. *Ann Surg.* 1975;182:449–454.

5. Maini BS, Mannick JA. Effect of arterial reconstruction on limb salvage. *Arch Surg.* 1978;113:1297–1304.

6. Prendiville EJ, Yeager A, O'Donnell TF, et al. Long-term result with the above-knee popliteal expanded polytetrafluoroethylene. *J Vasc Surg.* 1990;11:517–524.

7. Reichle FA, Rankin KP, Tyson R, et al. Long-term results of 474 arterial reconstructions for severely ischemic limbs: a fourteen year follow up. *Surgery.* 1979;85:93–100.

8. Stoney RJ, James DR, Wylie EJ. Surgery for femoropopliteal atherosclerosis. *Arch Surg.* 1971;103:548–553.

9. DeWeese JA, Rob CG. Autogenous venous grafts 10 years later. *Surgery.* 1977;82:775–785.

10. Hobson RW, O'Donnell JA, Zafar J, et al. Below knee bypass for limb salvage. *Arch Surg.* 1980;115:833–837.

11. McAuley CE, Steed DL, Webster MW. Seven-year follow-up of expanded polytetrafluoroethylene (PTFE) femoropopliteal grafts. *Ann Surg.* 1984;199:57–60.

12. Ascer E, Veith FJ, Gupta SK, et al. Six year experience with expanded polytetrafluoroethylene arterial grafts for limb salvage. *J Cardiovasc Surg.* 1985;26:468–472.

13. Szilagyi DE, Hageman JH, Smith RS, et al. Autogenous vein grafting in femoropopliteal atherosclerosis: the limits to its effectiveness. *Surgery.* 1979;36:836–851.

14. Darling RC, Linton RR. Durability of femoropopliteal reconstruction. *Am J Surg.* 1972;123:472–479.

15. Collins GJ, Rich NM, Andersen CA. Limb salvage procedure for lower extremity ischemia. *Am J Surg.* 1976;132:707–715.

16. Yogasundaram YN. Salvage of the lower limb. *Br J Surg.* 1976;63:371–376.

17. Quiñones-Baldrich WJ, Prego A, Ucelay-Gomez R, et al. Failure of PTFE infrainguinal revascularization: patterns, management alternatives, and outcome. *Ann Vasc Surg.* 1991;5:163–169.

18. Ascer E, Collier P, Gupta SK, et al. Reoperation for polytetrafluoroethylene bypass failure: the importance of distal outflow site and operative technique in determining outcome. *J Vasc Surg.* 1987;5:298–310.

19. Whittemore AD, Clowes AW, Couch NP, et al. Secondary femoropopliteal reconstruction. *Ann Surg.* 1981;193:35–42.

20. Sladen JG, Maxwell TM. Experience with 130 polytetrafluoroethylene grafts. *Am J Surg.* 1980;141:546–548.

21. Gupta SK, Veith FJ. Three year experience with expanded polytetrafluoroethylene arterial grafts for limb salvage. *Am J Surg.* 1980;140:214–217.

18

Changing Disease Patterns and Management Strategies in Lower Limb-Threatening Ischemia:

A Sixteen-Year Experience

Frank J. Veith, MD, Sushil K. Gupta, MD, and Kurt R. Wengerter, MD

From January 1, 1974, to December 31, 1989, we treated 2,829 patients with critical lower extremity ischemia. In the last 5 years, 13% of those patients had therapeutically significant stenoses or occlusions above *and* below the groin, whereas 35% had them at two or three levels below the inguinal ligament. Unobstructed arterial flow to the distal half of the thigh was present in 26% of patients, and 16% had unobstructed flow to the upper third of the leg with occlusions of all three leg arteries distal to this point and reconstitution of some patent named artery in the lower leg or foot. In the last 2 years, 99% of all patients with a threatened limb and without severe organic mental syndrome or midfoot gangrene were amenable to revascularization by percutaneous transluminal angioplasty (PTA), arterial bypass, or a combination of the two, although some distal arteries used for bypass insertion were heavily diseased or isolated segments were without an intact plantar arch. Limb salvage was achieved and maintained in more than 90% of recent patient cohorts, with a mean procedural mortality rate of 3.3%. Recent strategies that contributed to these results include

1. distal origin short vein grafts from the below-the-knee popliteal or tibial arteries to an ankle or foot artery (291 cases)
2. combined PTA and bypass (245 cases)
3. more distal PTA of popliteal and tibial artery stenoses (233 cases)
4. use of *in situ* or ectopic reversed autogenous vein for infrapopliteal bypasses even when vein diameter was 3 to 4 mm
5. composite-sequential femoropopliteal–distal (PTFE–vein) bypasses
6. reintervention when a procedure thrombosed (637 cases) or was threatened by a hemodynamically significant inflow, outflow, or graft lesion (failing graft, 252 cases)

7. frequent follow-up to detect threatening lesions before graft thrombosis occurred and to permit correction of lesions by PTA (58%) or simple reoperation
8. unusual approaches to all infrainguinal arteries to facilitate secondary operations despite scarring and infection

Primary major amputation rates fell from 41% to 5%, and total amputation rates fell
from 49% to 14%. Aggressive policies to save threatened limbs are thereby supported.

Enormous strides have been made in the treatment of arteriosclerotic lower
extremity ischemia in the last 35 years. Surgical techniques for bypassing or otherwise
overcoming stenotic or occlusive lesions above and below the inguinal ligament have
been developed and proven effective. However, when the arteriosclerotic disease
process was advanced enough to produce ischemia that threatened limb viability,
major amputation above or below the knee has often been deemed necessary. Over
the last two decades, we and a few others have aggressively attempted revascularization in most patients whose lower extremities were threatened because of ischemic
gangrene, ulceration, or rest pain and have shown that these efforts were
worthwhile.[1-5] Although this aggressive approach to limb salvage was first received
with skepticism, such surgery is now widely accepted and practiced in many health
centers.

Although atherosclerosis is a segmental disease and although ideal candidates for
surgical and other endovascular treatments have hemodynamically significant lesions
of large proximal arteries interspersed in an otherwise normal arterial tree, it has
become apparent that many patients with limb-threatening ischemia have a different
pattern of arterial disease characterized by diffuse and multilevel arterial involvement. Moreover, occlusive or stenotic lesions may be present entirely or predominantly below the lower half of the thigh or entirely below the knee. Such patients
comprise those who are still thought by many surgeons to have arteries that are
inoperable because their disease is "too distal" and involves arteries that are "too
small." The frequency of such disease patterns remains unknown.

In the present study we reviewed our last 16 years' experience with patients with
lower limb-threatening ischemia to accomplish seven objectives. The first was to
examine the therapeutically important patterns of arteriosclerotic lesions in these
patients and to determine how frequently lesions at multiple levels above and below
the inguinal ligament required treatment. The second was to determine how these
patterns of disease have *appeared* to change over the years. These changes were
apparent because it was the *perception* or recognition of disease patterns that changed
rather than the pattern of the disease itself. These apparent patterns were reflected in
the level of surgical or other interventional therapy that was performed. A third
objective was to determine the frequency and extent of arterial involvement that
occurred only distal to the midthigh or distal to the knee. A fourth was to evaluate the
effect of PTA on the treatment of this entire patient group. A fifth was to determine
the importance of reintervention for failed (thrombosed) or failing (threatened but not
thrombosed) primary arterial procedures. A sixth was to describe new therapeutic
strategies that facilitate management of the patterns of disease and the need for
reintervention that were encountered in many patients. A final purpose of this review
was to evaluate the overall efficacy of treatment in these patients.

METHODS

During the past 16 years (January 1, 1974, to December 31, 1989) 2,829 patients on
whom we had not performed a previous ipsilateral revascularization were admitted

to Montefiore Medical Center with one or both lower extremities threatened by ischemia due to arteriosclerosis (Table 18–1). In this analysis we have included only diabetic and nondiabetic patients who had progressive or nonhealing toe, heel, foot, or leg gangrene or ulceration or severe rest pain uncontrolled by conservative treatment.[6] Excluded from this study were patients with only intermittent claudication (who constituted 2% to 5% of our patients undergoing operation or PTA) and those whose limbs were threatened because of infection and/or gangrene in association with intact major arterial circulation as indicated by palpable foot pulses and normal forefoot pulse volume recordings. Also excluded were patients with popliteal or femoral aneurysms without occlusive disease and patients whose limbs were threatened but who were treated by thromboembolectomy alone.

Patients with severe organic mental syndrome or gangrene and/or infection involving the deeper tissues of the midtarsal region of the foot were subjected to primary major amputation above or below the knee. Except for such patients, who constituted 4% of all those admitted to our institution,[1] all patients underwent arteriographic examination by the transfemoral or translumbar route. Visualization of all patent arteries from the renals to the forefoot was possible in almost all patients. This visualization showed that more than 94% of earlier patient cohorts[1] and virtually all of more recent patient cohorts had some patent visualized arterial segment, albeit sometimes relatively isolated, which could be used in an attempted revascularization. The only exceptions were patients who had undergone operation before or who had suffered an acute arterial occlusion. Extensive forefoot and heel gangrene, recent congestive heart failure or myocardial infarction, an incomplete plantar arch, and heavy circumferential calcification were not considered contraindications to attempting limb salvage, and successful revascularization has often been achieved in each of these circumstances.[1,7,8]

Our medical and surgical policies for treating these patients until 1981 have been detailed previously.[1] Important recent modifications are detailed below.

Graft Material

Until 1976, woven Dacron grafts were used for all bypass procedures above the groin or extending to the groin, and autologous vein grafts were used for all infrainguinal bypass operations. If no vein was available for the latter procedures, knitted Dacron grafts were used. From 1976 to 1987, woven Dacron was used for some aortofemoral grafts and expanded polytetrafluoroethylene (PTFE) grafts were used for some aortofemoral bypasses, all iliofemoral, axillofemoral, and femorofemoral procedures, and (until 1982) infrainguinal bypass operations if autologous vein was unavailable in the ipsilateral lower extremity. Some sick elderly patients requiring femoropopliteal bypass and those with veins that did not dilate beyond 3.5 mm had the procedure performed with PTFE grafts even if they had a usable ipsilateral vein. From 1978 to 1982, all patients undergoing infrainguinal bypass procedures who has usable ipsilateral autologous vein were randomized to receive either a vein or a PTFE graft.[9] From 1982 onward all patients requiring a bypass to an infrapopliteal artery had it performed with autologous vein if this was present in any of the four extremities as a single or composite graft of undiseased vein. Patency of long (>40 cm) reversed vein grafts smaller than 3.5 mm and all vein grafts smaller than 3.0 mm in minimal distended diameter were inferior to those of larger diameter vein grafts.[10] From 1982 to 1985, randomization of femoropopliteal bypass grafts to PTFE or ipsilateral vein continued. Thereafter these grafts were performed preferentially with ipsilateral vein if it was present and had a minimal distended diameter of 3.5 mm or more, except in

TABLE 18–1. PROCEDURES PERFORMED IN 2,829 PATIENTS WITH FIRST-TIME THREATENED LIMBS OVER 16 YEARS[a]

Period	I						II					III					Total
Year	1974	1975	1976	1977	1978	1979	1980	1981	1982	1983	1984	1985	1986	1987	1988	1989	Total
Total patients with threatened limbs	126	115	101	137	129	151	217	203	205	208	222	190	206	226	211	182	2829
Aorta- or iliac-to-femoral bypass	5	3	5	4	4	4	12	10	14	13	19	20	27	35	18	16	209
Axillofemoral bypass	6	6	3	25	20	17	19	14	10	13	19	12	9	12	11	12	208
Femorofemoral crossover bypass	8	10	5	24	15	16	22	20	28	23	18	25	23	32	19	19	307
Iliac PTA	0	0	0	0	2	20	31	26	45	40	53	51	55	67	47	48	485
CFA/DFA/PSFA to PA bypass	22	24	44	65	63	62	77	73	91	76	92	93	92	91	78	79	1122
SFA PTA	0	0	0	0	0	5	21	14	10	21	23	28	42	31	17	29	241
PA PTA	0	0	0	0	0	4	16	26	4	16	16	10	20	21	11	12	156
CFA/DFA/PSFA to DA bypass	10	7	8	38	19	41	43	34	49	51	42	36	34	39	41	41	533
DSFA/AK PA to DA bypass	0	1	3	6	4	8	9	9	11	20	10	13	15	18	21	23	171
BK PA to DA bypass	0	0	1	2	2	1	15	9	12	24	28	29	34	32	18	30	237
DA to DA bypass	0	0	0	0	0	0	1	2	4	2	5	7	12	8	6	7	54
DA PTA	0	0	0	0	0	3	9	8	1	0	6	8	13	10	8	11	77
Vein graft PTA	0	0	0	0	0	0	2	4	3	3	2	5	12	4	5	10	50
Sympathectomy alone	31	29	7	0	2	1	0	1	1	1	1	0	0	1	0	0	75
Primary BK/AK amputation	52	48	34	26	29	23	45	42	36	32	41	18	36	32	10	11	515
Total Procedures	134	128	110	190	160	205	322	292	319	335	375	355	424	433	310	348	4440
Secondary BK/AK amputation	7	11	23	28	44	33	38	44	43	41	34	22	34	31	17	18	468

[a] PTA = percutaneous transluminal angioplasty; CFA = common femoral artery; DFA = deep femoral artery; PSFA = proximal half of superficial femoral artery; DSFA = distal half of superficial femoral artery; PA = popliteal artery; DA = distal (Infrapopliteal) artery; AK = above the knee; BK = below the knee.

228

patients whose life expectancy was judged to be less than 2 to 3 years. In most patients requiring a femoropopliteal-to-infrapopliteal sequential bypass, the proximal graft was PTFE and the distal graft autologous vein. From 1983 onward, axillofemoral bypasses were performed with ringed PTFE grafts, and PTFE femoropopliteal bypasses were randomized to ringed or nonringed grafts.[11] From 1987 onward, bypasses originating from the aorta were performed with albumin-coated knitted Dacron or PTFE grafts. From July 1985 onward, all patients who had a usable ipsilateral greater saphenous vein and who required a bypass from the proximal half of the thigh to an infrapopliteal artery were randomized to receive a reversed or *in situ* vein graft.[12]

Graft Origin and Length

Increasingly over the 16 years of this study we have tried to minimize the length of infrainguinal vein bypasses by using more distal sites of origin in patients with unobstructed proximal arteries.[1,7,13] Short vein bypasses originating from the superficial femoral, deep femoral, popliteal, and infrapopliteal arteries and extending to distal arteries have become increasingly common (see Table 18–1). If vein length was limited, we have even placed grafts below stenoses of 20% to 40% of luminal diameter provided no postbypass pressure gradient was present. If such a gradient was present, a prosthetic extension was performed to a site proximal to the stenosis. The practice of using these distal-origin short vein grafts has maximized vein use, avoided dissection in scarred or infected groins, and simplified surgical procedures. Although it is not a topic of this review, problems arising from progression of disease proximal to a distal-origin graft have occurred in less than 5% of cases. They have almost *never* caused graft thrombosis and have been managed successfully by proximal prosthetic graft extension.

Improved Arteriographic Technique

In addition to the adjuncts previously outlined,[1] arteriographic visualization of patent foot arteries has been improved in the last 8 years by using digital augmentation techniques when necessary (3% of cases). Another advance has been the routine performance of aortic arch arteriography via a translumbar approach in patients who are possible candidates for axillofemoral bypass. Twenty-five percent of such patients had important and unsuspected axillary or subclavian disease that could have hampered bypass inflow.[14] When this was found, alternative adequate inflow sites were used.

Ankle and Foot Arteries as Bypass Insertion Sites

With adequate arteriographic visualization, it has been possible to find inframalleolar arteries that could provide bypass outflow in patients who previously would have been deemed unreconstructible.[1,7,15,16] The dorsalis pedis, the posterior tibial artery in the foot, and their main branches; the lateral tarsal artery, the deep metatarsal arch, and the medial and lateral plantar arteries have all been used to provide successful bypass outflow even when there was no patent plantar arch and other major pedal arteries were occluded (Fig. 18–1).

Use of Percutaneous Transluminal Angioplasty

Since 1978, if the procedure was technically feasible, we have used PTA to treat all gradient-producing or potentially gradient-producing (after distal papaverine administration) iliac artery stenoses and all potentially flow-reducing, high-grade (>70%

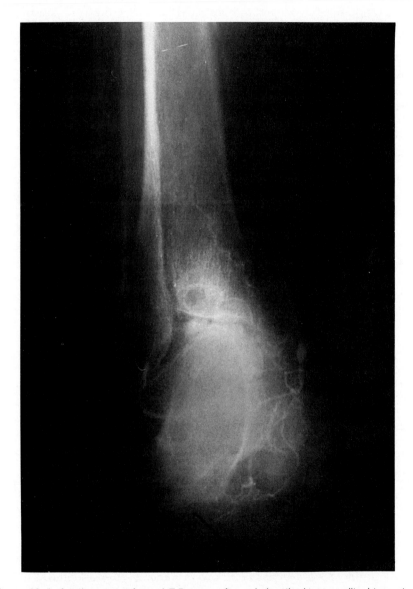

Figure 18–1. Arteriogram performed 7.5 years after a below-the-knee popliteal-to-posterio-tibial bypass. The outflow tract was limited and disadvantaged at operation and has remained so.

reduction of luminal diameter) stenoses in the femoral arteries (common, superficial, deep) and popliteal artery.[1] If a patient with a high-grade iliac stenosis with no measurable gradient across it was going to require an infrainguinal bypass of any sort (femorofemoral, femoropopliteal, or femoral to infrapopliteal), PTA of the iliac lesion was also performed.

In the last 8 years we have also extended the use of PTA with improved balloon catheters to treat stenotic lesions of the tibioperoneal trunk, the tibial or peroneal arteries at all levels in the leg, and even to the perimalleolar level.[17] Over the last 11 years, we have also used PTA to treat lesions that have developed proximal or distal to PTFE or vein grafts and to treat stenotic lesions developing within vein grafts.[18] However, intermediate (>1 yr) results with vein graft lesions over 2 cm in length have been so poor that PTA is no longer attempted for them, and vein patch angioplasty or bypass are employed instead. Angioplasty, if technically feasible, is still employed for short (≤2 cm) vein graft lesions.

Indications for Multilevel or Sequential Bypasses

These operations consisted of axillary artery or aorta-to-femoral-to-popliteal bypasses in patients with bilateral iliac disease that was not amenable to PTA and of femoral-to-popliteal-to-infrapopliteal artery bypasses. In the last 10 years, these operations were performed in one stage when extensive gangrene or infection was present in the foot and the more proximal insertion site artery ended blindly without direct luminal continuity to the lower leg or foot. In such circumstances, a simple bypass to the isolated segment would often remain patent but would not produce healing of foot lesions until a secondary distal sequential bypass was performed.[19,20] If patients had only one limb with extensive gangrene and required an axillary artery or aorta-to-femoral-to-popliteal bypass, we usually performed a unilateral procedure if the opposite limb was asymptomatic. This simplified a complicated operation, and if the opposite limb later became threatened, a simple crossover femorofemoral or femoropopliteal procedure from the unilateral prosthetic graft could easily be performed.

Postprocedural Patient Follow-up

Frequent patient observation to detect the development of flow-reducing lesions proximal to or distal to the arterial reconstruction before thrombosis occurs has been important to achieving the ultimate goal of limb salvage in these patients, except for those with only an aortofemoral bypass.[1,18,21–23] Failure from thrombosis of the arterial reconstruction or PTA site can occur from intimal hyperplasia involving vein grafts, anastomotic sites, or segments treated by PTA. Usually this process becomes apparent 2 to 24 months after the arterial manipulation.[22–25] Thereafter, disease progression is the most important threat to the arterial intervention. Fortunately these processes can often be detected before they cause thrombosis of an arterial reconstruction and corrective measures taken in the "failing" state. Improved extended patency and limb salvage can thereby be achieved.[18,25–27] Clinical observation with careful pulse examination by the operating surgeon every 1 to 2 months for the first postoperative year, every 3 months for the second year, and every 3 to 6 months thereafter has enabled us to detect 252 suspected failing arterial reconstructions in the last 10 years (Table 18–2). Urgent arteriography was usually performed, and patent arterial reconstructions that were threatened were confirmed and treated by PTA (145 cases) and/or by reoperation (107 cases).

In the last 4 years, frequent noninvasive, duplex examination of *in situ* vein grafts has been found helpful in detecting threatening lesions before they produce graft thrombosis (graft flow velocity <45 cm/s).[26] Simple and effective surgical intervention to improve graft patency is thereby facilitated. Accordingly, we have begun to supplement clinical follow-up with duplex examinations. However, this has not always been feasible with large numbers of patients, and cost factors remain a consideration. Moreover, some grafts to disadvantaged outflow tracts have had flows of less than 45 cm/s and remained patent for several years.

TABLE 18–2. SECONDARY PROCEDURES PERFORMED FOR OUR FAILED AND FAILING PRIMARY PROCEDURES OVER THE LAST 10 YEARS

Years	1980–1984	1985–1989	Total
Total number of patients with primarily threatened limb	1,055	1,015	2,070
Number of our patients requiring a secondary procedure (% of total patients)	286 (27%)	376 (37%)	662 (32%)
Number of secondary procedures on these patients[a]	394	495	889
Reoperations for failed procedures (% of secondary procedures)	295 (75%)	342 (69%)	637 (72%)
Suprainguinal	47	46	93
Infrainguinal	248	296	544
Reoperations for failing procedures			
Suprainguinal	8	8	16
Infrainguinal	24	67	91
PTAs for failing procedures			
Suprainguinal	25	15	34
Infrainguinal	42	63	111
Total reinterventions for failing procedures (% of secondary procedures)	99 (25%)	153 (31%)	252 (28%)

[a] Many patients had more than one secondary intervention.

Management of Failed (Thrombosed) Arterial Reconstructions

Throughout the 16-year period of this review, we have maintained an aggressive diagnostic and therapeutic attitude toward reintervening when a patient had a threatened limb because of failure from thrombosis of a previous arterial graft performed at our own or some other institution.[1,24] Such patients were subjected to arteriographic examination and correction of the problem that caused or contributed to the thrombosis. In the first 10 years of this review, reoperations tended to involve graft thrombectomy and salvage with patch grafting of hyperplastic outflow lesions and graft extension for progression of proximal or distal arteriosclerosis.[24] In the last 6 years, although we sometimes performed thrombectomies of prosthetic grafts terminating above the knee, we have tended to perform totally new bypasses to previously undissected arteries using vein grafts where possible and a variety of new or unusual approaches to gain access to the arteries via unscarred and uninfected tissue planes.[28,29] Failed PTA was generally treated with a bypass, except for occasional focal iliac artery lesions. Not every failure of a limb salvage procedure produced a renewed threat to a limb because the original toe or foot lesion may in part have been due to infection that never recurred. When a graft thrombosis did not threaten a limb, the patient was carefully observed and the noninterventional treatment was performed.[24,28] Although intra-arterial lytic agents have been used sporadically in the management of thrombosed reconstructions and although they may prove helpful in the future, they were rarely of value in our experience and not used routinely during the study period.

Management of Wound Hematoma, Necrosis, and Infection

Wound complications were frequent after infrainguinal operations in these patients, the majority (>60%) of whom were diabetic and who had lengthy operations with extensive vein harvest incisions. When these processes, which often occurred together, were extensive or involved more than the skin and superficial subcutaneous tissue, treatment usually involved surgical debridement, evacuation of blood and exudate, and excision of all necrotic tissue. With appropriate bedside care, healing by secondary intention usually occurred even when an autologous vein or prosthetic graft and its anastomosis to a native artery were exposed in the involved wound.[30] Skin grafts and muscle flaps were used only rarely but were helpful.

Data Maintenance and Analysis

Data for this study were culled from vascular service census sheets and logs of operations and PTAs. From 1976 onward, data on patients, their operations and PTAs, and their follow-up were entered prospectively into an IBM microcomputer database (Dataease International) that was specifically adapted to the monitoring of vascular patients.[31] Statistical evaluations of data were by the chi-squared test. The present review was performed by addressing specific queries to this database. Information on apparent disease patterns and their therapeutic significance was determined from the operations or other therapeutic interventions performed to treat the lesions that were deemed important. Amputation rates were derived from the number of amputations and the patients presenting primarily in the same period. Primary amputation rates minus 4% (for patients with severe organic mental syndrome and hopelessly extensive gangrene) were a reflection of untreatable arterial disease patterns. Secondary amputation rates were a reflection of early and late failures of arterial interventions that could not be salvaged by some form of secondary procedure. Although these failures and the resulting secondary amputations may have occurred remote to the arterial intervention, the overall rate calculations have validity because the number of patients treated annually remained relatively constant and because eventual failures, no matter how remote, would affect the secondary amputation rate of a subsequent year if it did not increase the rate for the same year.

RESULTS

Table 18–1 shows the number of patients presenting with a limb threatened from arteriosclerotic ischemia over the 16 years of the study and the therapeutic procedures performed on these patients. In the first 6 years of the study (period I) there was a sharp rise in the number of procedures extending to infrapopliteal arteries and a corresponding decrease in the number of sympathectomies and primary amputations. This is a reflection of our increasing recognition of the therapeutic significance of infrapopliteal lesions and our increasing ability to deal with them effectively. These trends continued and increased in the last 10 years of the study (periods II and III) and were associated with the introduction of iliac and femoral artery PTAs and increasing numbers of distal-origin bypass grafts and popliteal and infrapopliteal PTAs. These angioplasties were indicative of our increasing recognition that limb-threatening ischemia could be associated mainly with distal occlusive disease below the midthigh or knee, and that these patterns of disease often occurred without more proximal, therapeutically significant disease.

Another fact that can be derived from Table 18–1 was the increase in the number of procedures performed per patient, from 1.2 in period I, to 1.6 in period II, and to 1.8 in period III. This was due to our increasing inclination to deal with the multiple levels of disease these patients had and our willingness to reintervene when a primary procedure thrombosed or failed to save the limb.

Changing Patterns of Therapeutically Significant or Apparent Disease

Table 18–3 reflects the location and number of levels of therapeutically significant disease derived from the number of threatened limbs that received a particular

TABLE 18–3. LOCATIONS AND LEVEL OR LEVELS OF THERAPEUTICALLY SIGNIFICANT ARTERIOSCLEROTIC LESIONS IN ALL FIRST-TIME THREATENED LIMBS AS DETERMINED BY THE ARTERIAL PROCEDURES PERFORMED

Period	I							II				III					Total
Year	1974	1975	1976	1977	1978	1979	1980	1981	1982	1983	1984	1985	1986	1987	1988	1989	Total
Total limbs threatened for first time	132	124	117	163	147	191	255	244	247	264	290	240	262	281	220	188	3365
Primary major amputation	52	48	34	26	29	23	45	42	36	32	41	18	36	32	11	10	515
Sympathectomy alone	26	27	5	2	0	0	0	0	1	0	0	0	0	0	0	0	61
Arterial procedures	54	49	78	135	118	168	210	202	210	232	249	222	226	249	209	178	2789
Suprainguinal procedures alone[a] (%)	19 (35)	16 (33)	17 (22)	33 (24)	32 (27)	29 (17)	63 (30)	53 (26)	56 (27)	52 (22)	58 (23)	63 (28)	57 (25)	73 (29)	51 (24)	41 (25)	713 (26)
Infrainguinal procedures alone[a] (%)	32 (59)	32 (65)	56 (72)	85 (63)	75 (64)	113 (67)	118 (56)	131 (65)	132 (63)	159 (69)	169 (68)	132 (59)	141 (62)	145 (58)	131 (63)	111 (62)	1762 (63)
Multilevel supra- and infrainguinal procedures[a] (%)	3 (6)	1 (2)	5 (6)	17 (13)	11 (9)	26 (15)	29 (14)	18 (9)	22 (10)	21 (9)	22 (9)	27 (12)	28 (12)	31 (12)	27 (13)	26 (15)	314 (11)
Multilevel infrainguinal procedures[a] (%)	12 (22)	11 (22)	16 (21)	39 (29)	31 (26)	56 (33)	59 (28)	70 (35)	72 (34)	82 (35)	85 (34)	71 (32)	82 (36)	84 (34)	80 (38)	62 (35)	912 (33)
Total multilevel procedures	15	12	21	56	42	82	88	88	94	103	107	98	110	115	107	88	1226
Percentage of total multilevel procedures[a]	28	24	27	41	36	49	42	44	45	44	43	44	49	46	51	49	44

[a] Percentages represent fraction of total arterial procedures in that year receiving that treatment.

234

treatment or had an operation or PTA to overcome a significant arterial lesion. Of the patients undergoing therapeutic arterial procedures, the proportions with therapeutically significant disease above and below the inguinal ligament did not change significantly over the 16 years of the study. However, the proportion of patients undergoing treatment at multiple levels, either above and below or all below the groin, increased from 28% to 49%. Even the high proportions of multilevel procedures in the last 5 years of the study (44% to 51%) are misleadingly low since many patients with multilevel disease could often be adequately treated by overcoming only one of several lesions in a series.

From 56% to 72% (mean 63%) of threatened limbs were associated only with therapeutically significant disease below the inguinal ligament, almost always occurring at two or more levels although only 21% to 38% (mean 33%) required a therapeutic procedure for at least two of these infrainguinal levels of disease. An additional 2% to 15% (mean 11%) of threatened limbs were associated with suprainguinal and infrainguinal lesions that both required interventional treatment.

Table 18–4 summarizes data for the three time periods on numbers and percentages of patients who had sympathectomy, primary amputation, or initial therapeutic interventions at various levels of the arterial tree. The groups treated by arterial procedures reflect the predominant patterns of therapeutically significant arteriosclerotic lesions although these data do not stratify for single-level and multilevel lesions requiring treatment. The most striking change in the therapeutically significant disease patterns in these patients was the increase in the proportion receiving treatment of infrapopliteal arterial lesions. This increased from 13% in the first period to 32% in the last period ($P<.001$). Since there was a concomitant decrease in the proportion of patients treated by primary amputation and sympathectomy, it is probable that many of these latter patients in the earlier periods could have been better treated by an intervention extending to the infrapopliteal arteries. However, the significance of their distal disease was unrecognized, and often techniques and strategies for dealing with it had not yet been developed.

Table 18–5 summarizes for the three time periods the increasing frequency of

TABLE 18–4. THERAPEUTICALLY SIGNIFICANT PATTERNS OF ARTERIOSCLEROTIC LESIONS IN 2,829 PATIENTS WITH A FIRST-TIME THREATENED LIMB[a]

	Period I	Period II	Period III
Years	1974–1979	1980–1984	1985–1989
Total number of patients	759	1,055	1,015
Number treated sympathectomy alone (%)	65(9)	4(0.4)	0(0)
Number treated by primary major amputation (%)	212(28)	196(19)	107(11)
Number treated by operation or PTA of aortoiliac lesion (%)	146(19)	252(24)	252(25)
Number treated by operation or PTA of superficial femoral and popliteal artery lesions (%)	238(31)	374(35)	336(33)
Number treated by operation or PTA of infrapopliteal artery lesions (%)	98(13)	229(22)	320(32)

[a] When patients treated by sympathectomy and primary amputation were excluded, the initial arterial intervention indicated the pattern of arteriosclerotic lesions. Arterial interventions were classified on the basis of the most proximal lesion treated, except for the group undergoing treatment of infrapopliteal artery lesions. Many of these latter patients also had treatment for lesions of the superficial femoral and proximal popliteal arteries. PTA = percutaneous transluminal angioplasty.

TABLE 18–5. NUMBERS AND PERCENTAGE OF PATIENTS WITH FIRST-TIME THREATENED LIMBS[a]

Years	Period I 1974–1979	Period II 1980–1984	Period III 1985–1989
Total number of patients	759	1,055	1,015
Number treated with operation or PTA only distal to midthigh (%)	8(1.1)	182(17)	262(26)
Number treated with operation or PTA only distal to knee joint (%)	6(0.8)	107(10)	160(16)

[a] These patients had therapeutically significant disease only distal to the midthigh or the knee joint as indicated by the performance of therapeutic procedures only distal to these levels. PTA = percutaneous transluminal angioplasty.

recognized, therapeutically significant disease restricted to the arterial tree distal to the midthigh and distal to the knee joint. Over one-quarter of our patients in the last 5 years were recognized to have these distal disease patterns. Undoubtedly, many other patients in the earlier periods of the study had similar patterns of disease although they were not recognized. Many of these patients were probably treated less effectively by sympathectomy and amputation.

Effect of Percutaneous Transluminal Angioplasty

Table 18–6 shows that 34% of all 2,221 patients presenting for the first time with a threatened limb in the last 11 years were treated by PTA. However, only 426, or 19%, had PTA alone. The remaining 331 patients, or 15%, of the total had a PTA and an operation. Usually this was for another lesion proximal or distal to the one treated by

TABLE 18–6. ROLE OF PTA IN TREATING PATIENTS PRESENTING FOR THE FIRST TIME WITH A THREATENED LIMB FROM JANUARY 1, 1979 TO DECEMBER 31, 1989[a]

	Number	Percentage of All Patients	Percentage of PTA-Treated Patients
Total patients	2,221	100	0
Total patients treated by PTA	757	34	100
Total patients treated by PTA alone	426	19	56
Iliac arteries	347		
SFA/PA	342		
DA	72		
Deaths (%)	40.9		
Total patients treated by PTA and operation	331	15	44
Proximal to bypass	184	8	24
Iliac arteries	136		
SFA/PA	48		
In or distal to bypass	61	3	8
SFA/PA/DA	11		
Vein graft	50		
For PTA complication or failure	86	4	11
Iliac arteries	36		
SFA/PA	36		
DA	14		

[a] PTA = Percutaneous transluminal angioplasty. SFA = superficial femoral artery. PA = popliteal artery. DA = infrapopliteal artery. Patients having PTA alone often had lesions treated at several levels.

PTA. However, in 86, or 11%, of patients treated with PTA, the operation was because the PTA had a complication or failed.

Secondary Procedures

Secondary interventions performed for failed or failing previous procedures in the latter two 5-year periods are recorded in Table 18–2. Of all patients treated in those 10 years, 32% required some secondary procedure. Reoperations for *failed* or thrombosed procedures constituted 72% of the secondary procedures, whereas 28% of the secondary procedures (either reoperations or PTA) were performed for *failing* or threatened but unthrombosed previous interventions. The total number of secondary procedures and the proportion for failing interventions increased significantly ($P<.001$) in the most recent 5-year period.

Mortality, Failures, and Amputations

Table 18–7 lists the proportion of prosthetic grafts and the 30-day mortality, failure (thrombosis), and major amputation rates for the various surgical procedures over the last 5 years. The overall 30-day mortality rate was 3.3%, the failure rate 4.1%, and the major amputation rate 2.4%. The procedural mortality rate for PTA alone over an 11-year period was 0.9% (see Table 18–6).

Major Amputation Rates

Overall major *primary, secondary,* and *total* amputation rates for the entire 16 years of the study are shown in Figure 18–2. The gradual decrease in total amputation rates from 49% to 14% is highly significant ($P<.001$) and reflects overall improvement in the treatment of this disease process. The gradual decrease in the primary amputation rate from 41% to 5% is also highly significant ($P<.001$) and approaches the 4% of our patients who are subjected to primary amputation because of extensive midfoot infection, necrosis, or severe organic mental syndrome. This means that few recent

TABLE 18–7. SURGICAL PROCEDURES INITIALLY PERFORMED FOR THREATENED LIMBS IN THE LAST 5 YEARS (JANUARY 1, 1985–DECEMBER 31, 1989) AND 30-DAY MORTALITY, FAILURE, AND AMPUTATION RATES[a]

Operation	Number Performed	Percentage Prosthetic Grafts	30-Day Mortality Rate (%)	30-Day Failure Rate (%)	30-Day Major Amputation Rate (%)
Aorta- or iliac-to-femoral bypass	116	100	2	2	1
Axillofemoral bypass	56	100	6	4	2
Femorofemoral bypass	118	100	2	3	1
Femoropopliteal bypass	433	42	3	4	2
Femorotibial–peroneal bypass	191	16	4	5	4
Popliteal- or tibial-to-tibial–peroneal bypass	233	4	3	4	4
Total	1,147	44	3.3	4.1	2.4

[a] When multilevel lesions were treated, the operation performed for the most proximal lesion was the one included in this table.

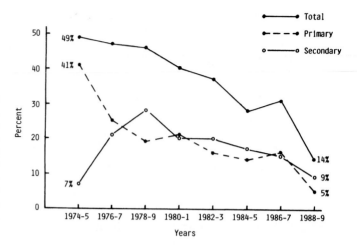

Figure 18–2. Amputation rates in all patients with threatened limbs. Primary amputations were those at the above-the-knee or below-the-knee levels without previous vascular interventions. Secondary amputations were major amputations performed at any time after an arterial intervention. Total amputations included all major amputations.

patients (<1%) were undergoing primary amputation because of arterial disease that was deemed impossible to treat. The decrease in the secondary amputation rate after 1978 from 28% to 9% was also significant ($P<.001$), because it means that more aggressive arterial interventions and increasing operability were providing durable limb salvage and not merely delaying amputation by converting primary major amputations to secondary ones.

DISCUSSION

This review of 16 years' experience with patients who have lower limb-threatening ischemia from infrarenal arteriosclerosis establishes several facts and raises several questions. Patients who present with this problem generally have diffuse, multilevel disease that often requires treatment by PTA or bypass procedures above and below the inguinal ligament or at multiple levels below the groin to save the limb. Furthermore, the occlusive or stenotic disease process involves infrapopliteal arteries in at least one-third of these patients, and in about one-quarter it involves the arterial tree predominantly below the midthigh or knee. Although patterns of arteriosclerotic disease in the lower extremity have been studied for many years and the frequency of distal popliteal and infrapopliteal disease appreciated,[32] only recently has the therapeutic significance of this distal disease been realized and methods developed for visualizing it arteriographically and for treating it with a high degree of success. Recognition of the importance of distal disease and development of effective techniques for overcoming it have contributed importantly to recent improved operability rates and declining primary amputation rates. In the last few years less than 1% of patients who had threatened limbs and had not been invasively treated before had patterns of arterial disease that were unsuitable for some attempt at revascularization. Although our data document a progressive increase in the proportion of therapeutic procedures to overcome multilevel and distal arteriosclerotic lesions (see Tables 18–1 and 18–3), these changes in treatment do not indicate that the actual pattern of the disease is changing, but rather that our perception or recognition of its therapeutic significance is changing.

Opinions diverge over the frequency of predominantly infrainguinal disease and that mainly or only below the midthigh and knee. Although our review suggests that these therapeutically significant patterns of disease are common (see Tables 18–3, 18–4, and 18–5), it is possible that we are seeing a selected population of patients with a misleadingly high incidence of predominantly infrainguinal and distal disease. This can only be determined when data from other health centers becomes available. Similar confirmation of the high incidence of multilevel disease in limb salvage patients should also be sought. However, our therapeutically derived data (see Table 18–3) tends to underestimate the frequency of multilevel disease since many hemodynamically significant lesions were present in our patients but did not require treatment to save the involved limb.

Our review underscores the importance of careful follow-up of limb salvage patients with reintervention if an initial procedure thromboses and fails and the limb is rethreatened. Such secondary procedures are worthwhile in terms of enhanced limb salvage rates.[1,24,25,27] Even more important is reintervention for a failing graft that is not yet thrombosed but is threatened because of intimal hyperplasia or progressive disease in its inflow or outflow tract or in the graft itself.[18,21–27] Even though the need for some secondary procedures may be reduced due to improving surgical management, the number remains high (see Table 18–2). This indicates that secondary treatment of disease progression and other problems and failures of primary procedures remain an important part of the treatment of these patients and one that must be pursued diligently if the optimum limb salvage results are to be achieved.

In situ vein graft techniques have been credited with much of the improvement that has occurred in the treatment of patients with threatened lower limbs.[33] We believe that this is true but not because *in situ* vein grafts have been proven to have better patency than reversed vein grafts.[34] As *in situ* techniques have been popularized, they have led to more widespread use of careful microtechniques using special instruments, headlight illumination, and, sometimes, loupe magnification, all methods that we have used and advocated for many years.[1,35] When such methods are used with reversed vein grafts, excellent results can also be obtained even in disadvantaged circumstances.[7,34] Moreover, *in situ* techniques are not feasible in many patients requiring a secondary operation, but use of an ectopic reversed vein graft is. It is, therefore, important that vascular surgeons not restrict themselves to *in situ* techniques.

Another technical modification that facilitates use of autologous vein grafts, particularly in the increasingly common group of patients requiring a secondary operation, is use of short distal-origin grafts. Our data suggests that such grafts work well and have other advantages besides increasing vein use.[7,13] However, proximal disease progression is a consideration, although it rarely causes graft thrombosis in our experience.

The present review demonstrates that PTA, when it was feasible in limb salvage patients, was usually a simpler, safer, often complimentary mode of therapy. In the last 10 years, 34% of our limb salvage patients were treated by PTA (see Table 18–6). However, 44% of these patients required an operation as well. Usually the operation was needed for a second lesion that could not be treated by PTA. Overall treatment was thereby simplified as has been found by others.[36] On other occasions PTA of a lesion in, proximal to, or distal to a bypass graft improved graft flow and relieved ischemia or prevented graft thrombosis. In only 11% of patients treated by PTA was an operation needed because a PTA failed or had a complication. Usually these latter operations, although more urgent, were the same or only slightly more complex than the operation that would have been required had the PTA not been attempted.[37] Moreover, when PTAs failed early or late, reintervention (usually by operation) was almost always possible. We, therefore, remain enthusiastic about PTA, when it is feasible in this group of patients. It is more an adjunct and aid to the surgical treatment than a competing mode of therapy. This may not be true with other forms of endovascular treatment by lasers, stents, and atherectmoy devices, but that remains to be determined. It certainly is not true in the treatment of patients with intermittent claudication, who generally have easier lesions to treat within a less diseased arterial tree. If treatment is warranted in such patients, it may be accomplished more safely by endovascular means alone than by open operation. However, this remains to be proven, and the long-term risks and benefits of these treatments have yet to be determined. Until they are, we believe that patients with arterial lesions that are easy to treat generally do not need treatment. In contrast, the limb salvage patients, who clearly need improved circulation but are difficult to treat by any interventional method, should be treated by whatever method proves safest and most effective. Because of the complexity and extensive nature of their disease, some form of surgical bypass treatment was required in 81% of recent limb salvage patients although it was often simplified or facilitated by PTA. In the future, other newer endovascular methods may provide additional improvements in the treatment of these patients.

Our previous work showed that aggressive efforts by surgeons and other medical specialists to save limbs were effective. Despite the fact that 90% of patients had attempts at limb salvage, procedural mortality rates averaged 3%, and over 85% of patients retained a functional limb until they died.[1] The present review provides further documentation of the effectiveness of this aggressive approach. The *primary major amputation* rate of 5% in the last 2 years approaches the irreducible minimum proportion of patients (4%) who have severe organic mental syndrome and extensive midfoot gangrene or infection. Moreover, the proportion of patients subjected to *secondary major amputation* ranged between 9% and 15% over the last 5 years. These secondary amputations resulted from final, uncorrectible early or late failure of limb salvage procedures. If our extension of limb salvage efforts to additional patients with more difficult distal patterns of disease had not been successful, it would have been reflected in an increasing number and proportion of secondary amputations.

We therefore conclude that limb salvage efforts are worthwhile and that they should be extended to mentally functional patients with all apparent patterns of arteriosclerotic disease, provided extensive gangrene or infection does not involve the midtarsal region of the foot. Although the surgical and radiographic procedures required to treat many of these patients are often difficult and require skill and commitment, they are rewarded with success in most instances. The resulting outcome is beneficial both to the patient and to society.

Acknowledgments
Portions of this chapter were taken from an article published in Ann Surg. *1990;212:402–414. Veith FJ, Gupta SK, Wengerter KR, et al. Changing arteriosclerotic disease patterns and management strategies in lower limb threatening ischemia.*

REFERENCES

1. Veith FJ, Gupta SK, Samson RH, et al. Progress in limb salvage by reconstructive arterial surgery combined with new or improved adjunctive procedures. *Ann Surg.* 1981;194: 386–401.
2. Reichle FA, Tyson R. Comparison of long-term results of 364 femoropopliteal or femorotibial bypasses for revascularization of severely ischemic lower extremities. *Ann Surg.* 1975;182:449–455.
3. Maini BS, Mannick JA. Effect of arterial reconstruction on limb salvage: a ten-year appraisal. *Arch Surg.* 1978;113:1297–1304.
4. Perdue GD, Smith RB, Veazey CR, et al. Revascularization for severe limb ischemia. *Arch Surg.* 1980;115:168–171.
5. Bartlett ST, Olinde AJ, Flinn WR, et al. The reoperative potential of infrainguinal bypass: long-term limb and patient survival. *J Vasc Surg.* 1987;5:170–179.

venipuncture even in patients who have been chronically ill or who have undergone multiple operations; it is often the only vein available. By virtue of its far posteriomedial location, the forearm basilic is also surprisingly undamaged and usable (Fig. 20–1). Tattoos of the overlying skin do not seem to damage the arm veins. Moreover, most venipuncturists are hesitant to perform venipunctures through tattoos.

Recanalization of thrombosed arm veins results in diameter narrowing, perivenous fibrosis formation, and a coarse network of internal synechial webs. The vein may become a fibrous cord without a lumen. Short or skip areas of intraluminal fibrous trabeculation may occur with minimal external evidence of the internal scarring. Usually, after the vein is excised, thickness may be palpated or visualized, and the vein fails to distend normally. In the areas of minimal scarring, the vein may appear normal but has lost its distensibility and compliance. It is likely that these scarred segments, developed while the vein is in the venous circulation, become the nidus of fibrous stricturing once the vein has been translocated to the arterial system.

Diseased segments are found most often in the median antecubital vein, followed in frequency by the forearm cephalic vein and the upper arm cephalic vein. Arm veins harvested from diabetics and patients with end-stage renal failure on hemodialysis are usable but are often subject to vein damage or *de novo* calcification.

Imaging Strategies

Steps must be taken to ascertain the availability of nonsaphenous autogenous conduit if the patient has varicose veins, previous deep or superficial thrombophlebitis, or if the saphenous vein has been previously harvested or stripped. When potential need exists, we visualize the lesser saphenous veins, the contralateral saphenous vein, and all arm veins bilaterally to estimate the length of vein available for harvesting either as a single length or as segments for an autogenous composite conduit. Except in muscular or slim patients whose arm veins are readily seen, we image both the cephalic and basilic segments. Venous flow, caliber, compressibility, distensibility, and continuity are assessed. The veins are examined in a warm room with tourni-

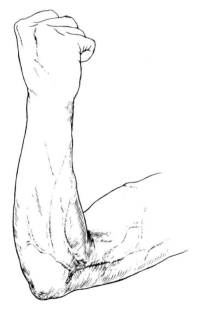

Figure 20–1. The forearm basilic vein lies posteromedially and is dissected with the forearm flexed. (*Reproduced with permission from Andros et al. In: Bergan JJ, Yao ST, eds.* Arterial Surgery: New Diagnostic and Operative Techniques. *Orlando FL: Grune & Stratton, Inc; 1988:528.*)

quets. An arm diagram designates usable veins in green, questionable veins in grey, and unusable veins in red, showing continuity and indicating diameters every 2 to 3 in. This map is available to the surgeon in the operating room. We have not felt the need to employ pre-bypass arterialization of the vein with construction of a Cimino fistula, nor have we found preoperative phlebography necessary.

SURGICAL PREPARATION

Patients arrive at the operating room with a detailed arteriogram. Although regional anesthesia is possible for the femorodistal reconstruction, we have not adopted its use for harvesting of the arm vein, either by axillary block or with local anesthesia. If, however, short segments of vein are obtainable distal to the middle upper arm, regional anesthesia may be considered. Intravenous infusion is achieved by internal jugular placement of a triple-lumen catheter; blood pressure is monitored via radial artery canalization (Fig. 20–2). By using two surgical teams, arm vein bypass often requires less time than saphenous vein bypass. Rarely, it is necessary to harvest vein from both arms.

SURGICAL TECHNIQUES

Intra-operative Assessment and Excision Strategies

With many conduit options available among the arm veins and their interconnections, the selection of a specific arm vein bypass may be bewildering. Our order of

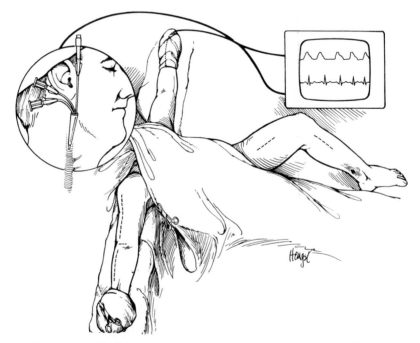

Figure 20–2. The radial artery site is sterily prepped and draped to allow complete harvesting of the cephalic and/or basilic veins. Extremities not actively being dissected are covered to minimize heat loss. A triple-lumen catheter is inserted via the internal jugular vein.

preference of autogenous veins is listed in Table 20–1. The cephalic vein is excised from the anatomic snuff-box to its confluence with the axillary subclavian vein in the deltopectoral groove. The cephalic vein is normally thickest at the wrist and may be gossamer thin at the shoulder; it is uniform in diameter and is implanted in the reversed configuration. Despite being the least commonly used vein, the complete basilic vein, from the axilla to the ulnar styloid process, is desirable because of its natural taper; it is of course used nonreversed and valve-incised. Even when arms appear devoid of usable veins, the basilic veins are nearly always available for harvesting. The left and right basilic veins as a composite graft yield a conduit to span from the common femoral artery to the knee.

If the cephalic vein is clearly visible at the wrist, excision is begun at this point. After duplex ultrasonic evaluation, if the forearm cephalic vein is deemed unusable and the upper arm segment is satisfactory, unroofing is begun lateral to the biceps just above the antecubital fossa. Dissection is carried toward the clavicle, incising the skin directly over the vein with scissors. Unroofing is carried distally by making a separate forearm incision leaving a skin bridge of 1 to 2 cm at the antecubital fossa. The cephalic vein is traced distally until it is obviously unusable. If the forearm cephalic vein is abandoned and a transverse antecubital fossa incision has been made, the median antecubital vein is dissected from the cephalic to the basilic juncture. Should this segment be disease-free, a new incision is made on the medial upper arm, and the basilic vein is unroofed. The forearm basilic vein, as it passes anterior to the median epicondyle is dissected but not divided until all veins have been assessed.

Intraoperative assessment of the arm veins either by *in situ* distension or angioscopy is undertaken prior to excision. All large tributaries are divided. A soft irrigating catheter is inserted distally, and, using either finger compression or bulldog clamps, the vein is distended to determine its diameter. Ease of irrigation is noted. Distensibility of the median antecubital and basilic veins can be determined by passing a No. 5 or 8 pediatric feeding tube; this maneuver permits selective venous distension and helps to confirm a patent lumen.

Angioscopy has confirmed the clinical observations made with *in situ* distension. Although Stonebridge and colleagues recommend routine angioscopic inspection of veins,[19] our experience is that this procedure has not added to preoperative and intraoperative assessment of veins.

TABLE 20–1. ORDER OF PREFERENCE IN THE USE OF AUTOGENOUS VEINS

1.	Ipsilateral greater saphenous vein
	    In situ or reversed
	    Translocated or nonreversed

2.	Contralateral greater saphenous vein Reversed or nonreversed
3.	Forearm-to-upper arm cephalic vein Reversed
4.	Forearm cephalic-to-median antecubital-to-upper arm basilic vein Reversed or nonreversed
5.	Upper arm basilic-to-median antecubital-to-upper arm cephalic Nonreversed basilic
6.	Forearm basilic-to-upper arm basilic Nonreversed valve-incised
7	Composite autogenous grafts
8.	Lesser saphenous Short or composite grafts

After unroofing but before excision, the length of the intended bypass is deter-mined with a measuring catheter; the arm vein or veins available are measured to correspond to the length necessary for the bypass. Five or 6 extra cm of vein are harvested for the anastomoses. The vein is then excised and irrigated with heparin-ized saline. Hemostasis is achieved in the arm incisions, and they are closed in two layers. All bony prominences are generously padded, and before the patient receives heparin, the arm is wrapped with a compression dressing from the base of the fingers to the axilla.

Composite Grafting and Implantation

Arm veins as part of composite grafts with other autogenous segments to produce a long autogenous graft have been described elsewhere.[8,14] In some series the number of composite grafts approximates the number of single-length grafts.[24,25]

Composite grafts are subject to anastomotic myointimal hyperplasia (AMH) at each suture line: the greater the number of segments joined in series, the greater the risk of secondary vein graft stenosis. Anastomotic hyperplasia has occurred at the venous and arterial ends of arm vein bypass grafts as well as in the body of the graft at venovenous anastomoses.

Arm vein bypasses originating from Dacron bypass grafts are also susceptible to AMH (Fig. 20–3). Consequently, autogenous inflow sites are preferred. Alternative

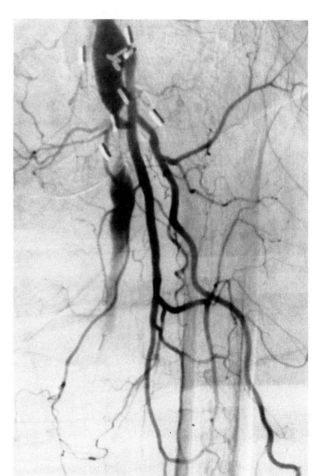

Figure 20–3. Anastomotic myointimal hyperplasia in a nonreversed basilic vein just distal to its origin from an aortofem-oral bypass graft.

strategies include anastomosing the autogenous graft to the deep femoral or superficial femoral artery. Superficial femoral endarterectomy for 3 to 4 cm distal to the Dacron graft to originate the bypass is a less desirable option.

The sequence of arm vein segments places the largest segments proximally. The basilic vein in the nonreversed, valve-incised configuration is usually placed proximally. The brachial vein tends to be smaller than the basilic vein and can be placed more distal in the sequence. After the basilic vein, we insert reversed cephalic vein segment(s), and finally forearm basilic vein. Further in the sequence come saphenous veins from the leg. The reversed short saphenous vein is placed most distally because, on average, it is the smallest of the available autogenous veins.

Orthotopic tunnels adjacent to the native artery are preferred for femorodistal arm vein bypasses. However, subcutaneously tunneled grafts have demonstrated long-term patency both in the single length and the composite configuration. Long-term durability has also been obtained with infrapopliteal and paramalleolar grafts in extra-anatomic tunnels extending from the groin laterally over the thigh and the knee.

Composite grafts are sutured and tunnelled, segment by segment. The proximal anastomosis is sutured, inspected for unsecured side branches and adventitial bands, and the graft is flushed. The graft segment is then tunnelled to the next skin incision. The venovenous anastomosis is constructed at that site, and the bypass graft is again evaluated. The next segment is then tunnelled either to the distal anastomotic site or to the next intermediate incision. In this way, no anastomosis is pulled through a tunnel. This technique prolongs the period of heparinization but avoids disrupting venovenous anastomoses. Alternatively, the completed composite graft can be passsed in one maneuver through a rigid hollow tunneller. Composite anastomoses, about 2 cm in length, are sutured over a No. 8 feeding tube, which serves both as a stent and as a calibrator of the diameter of the venous segment. The assistant maintains traction on the anastomosis after the toe-and-heel sutures have been placed. Additionally, two lateral sutures minimize the risk of "purse stringing" the anastomosis.

COMPLICATIONS AND THEIR MANAGEMENT

Bleeding

The most common cause of immediate postoperative bleeding is a ligature slipping off a side branch; the basilic vein is most susceptible, with bleeding occurring within a few minutes to hours after surgery. We have observed this slippage of a tie on three occasions, all requiring immediate reoperation to treat life-threatening hemorrhage. We now doubly ligate all large branches, particularly those of the basilic and median antecubital veins. If the stump of the vein does not accommodate two ties, the tributary is tied and oversown. On two occasions we have encountered particularly fragile veins with multiple side branches and areas of nonstenosing transmural fibrosis. In both instances the implanted vein developed multiple holes and longitudinal splits. Control with sutures was impossible, and the vein was removed. We seldom use arm veins for arterial patching, but when doing so we prefer forearm cephalic, median antecubital, or distal upper arm basilic veins. Delayed hemorrhage associated with sepsis as reported with saphenous veins[26] has not been observed.

Thrombosis and Occlusion

Occlusion of arm vein bypasses occurs most often in the early postoperative period (within the first 48 hours after surgery). Most grafts thrombose because of technical problems or inadequate vein. When early thrombosis occurs, the proximal and distal anastomoses are investigated. The vein graft is removed completely from its tunnel, stripped of all clot, copiously irrigated with heparinized saline and reimplanted. Inadequate inflow and outflow sites may require vein patch angioplasty. Efforts are made to avoid passage of embolectomy catheters through the vein. Additionally, by transilluminating the vein against a bright light, one can be assured that all clot has been removed. Angioscopy is a useful adjunct if available on an emergency basis. We attribute the lower incidence of acute vein thrombosis with arm veins to their diameters, which are 1 to 2 mm larger than saphenous veins.[2] After salvage of the acutely occluded graft, we administer heparin and dextran and investigate the patient for hematologic conditions predisposing to thrombosis.[27] Prior to discharge, this group of patients undergoes complete arteriography and noninvasive evaluation.

Between 2 and 20 months, AMH results in stenotic lesions at suture lines and in the body of the graft. In veins of uniform diameter, such as the cephalic, this anastomotic stenosis normally occurs proximally, whereas in the tapered, nonreversed, valve-incised basilic vein, the stenosis appears distally. By the time such anastomotic stenoses develop, arm veins have become well arterialized and are difficult to differentiate from saphenous veins. As with saphenous veins, AMH can be repaired by vein patch angioplasty, although inflow jump grafting, transposition angioplasty,[28] and balloon angioplasty have all been successful. We have observed areas of fibrostenosis in the body of an otherwise normal-looking vein graft. They are not associated with vein valves, and we have speculated that preexisting venous lesions induced by venipuncture predispose the arterialized arm vein to myointimal hyperplasia.

Late occlusions result mainly from progressive inflow and outflow occlusive disease. Arm veins, like saphenous veins, tolerate low flow remarkably well. Concern over the occurrence of graft aneurysmosis appears to have been unfounded. The only examples we have seen occurred in two young patients in their 40s, who were operated on for thrombosed popliteal aneurysms. Large-diameter basilic veins should not be mistaken for aneurysms because these veins may be 9 to 11 mm in diameter at the time of implantation. Mild dilatation and elongation have been observed.

Complications with donor arms have been remarkably infrequent. We have harvested both the cephalic and basilic veins as well as the median antecubital vein in more than 40 arms and have observed only 2 instances of persisting edema, both of which subsided after 12 months.

APPLICATIONS

Arm veins have been successfully used in nearly every clinical setting amenable to saphenous vein grafting in the lower extremity. In brachiocephalic reconstructions both basilic and cephalic veins have been used for carotid-to-brachial bypass. We have not used arm vein in the carotid–subclavian position. Axillobrachial and brachiobrachial bypasses are possible using either translocated veins[29] or the *in situ* technique.[17,18] The latter method may result in a bypass longer than might be dictated by the actual length of the occlusion.

Miscellaneous applications include hepatorenal bypass, vein patch angioplasty, and aortocoronary bypass.[30] These cardiac grafts appeared to be particularly susceptible to late stenosis leading to occlusion.

RESULTS

Our experience with arm vein bypasses began in 1969 with single-length cephalic conduits and now comprises more than 300 arterial reconstructions. Arm vein bypass grafts can last for decades (Fig. 20–4). The results obtained with the various autogenous veins, including arm veins, used in our practice parallel published results obtained with saphenous and arm vein bypass grafts. These results are a function of several factors, such as primary versus secondary revascularization, claudication versus limb salvage as indications for surgery, popliteal versus infrapopliteal arteries as distal anastomotic sites, single-length versus composite grafts, and, possibly, initial experience versus present experience.[7–9,11,14,22–25,31–39] Table 20–2 summarizes our published data on 1-year secondary patency rates for various grafts. The observation of Whittemore and colleagues[7] that both arm veins and saphenous veins have a lower

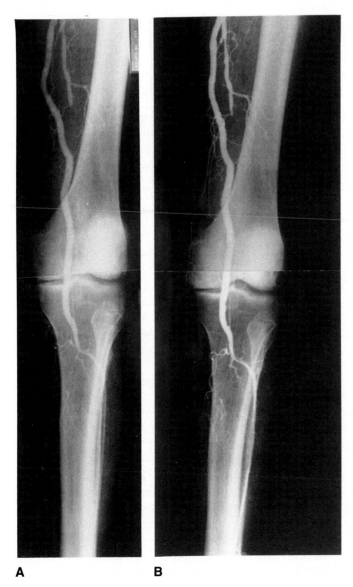

A   **B**

Figure 20–4. Cephalic vein bypass graft from the superficial femoral to the infrageniculate popliteal artery. Arteriography revealed no change in the appearance of the graft between (**A**) 15 years and (**B**) 17 years after implantation.

TABLE 20–2. A COMPARISON OF ONE-YEAR SECONDARY PATENCY RATES FOR INFRAGENICULAR AUTOGENOUS VEIN BYPASS GRAFTS[a]

Graft	Method	Patency Rate (%)
Popliteoparamalleolar	*In situ*	100
Popliteoparamalleolar	Autogenous non *in situ*	96
Claudication	*In situ* (initial experience)	96
Femoropopliteal	*In situ* (initial experience)	92
Femoroperamalleolar	*In situ*	92
Femoropopliteal	Arm vein single length	90
Femoroinfrageniculate	Arm vein (first graft)	87
Limb salvage	*In situ* (initial experience)	87
Femoroinfrapopliteal	*In situ* (initial experience)	86
Femoroparamalleolar	Autogenous non *in situ* single length	82
Femoroinfrapopliteal	Arm vein single length	80
Femoroinfrapopliteal	Composite autogenous	74
Femoroparamalleolar	Composite autogenous	73
Femoroinfrageniculate	Arm vein secondary reconstruction	70

[a] From our experience, Andros et al,[11] Harris et al,[14] Andros et al,[22] and Harris et al.[31]

long-term patency for repeat bypasses than for primary procedures has been confirmed in our own series.[11] The reasons for this reduced patency despite the implantation of an entirely new conduit are unexplained but may be the result of progressive arteriosclerosis or a group of patients predisposed to graft failure because of anastomotic hyperplasia. Established arm vein bypasses have been successfully thrombolysed with urokinase as late as 4 weeks following acute occlusion.[20]

COMMENTS

The growing numbers of reports on the use of arm veins are testimony to their versatility. The indications of when and where to use arm veins coupled with improved familiarity with the technical features of their implantation have enhanced their popularity. This heightened awareness of the applicability of arm veins has contributed to the growth of the "all autogenous" approach to infrainguinal revascularization fostered by several groups.[14,23,36] This strategy has developed in the wake of the observations that autogenous reconstructions are more durable and less prone to complication than reconstructions using prosthetic materials.[38]

In contrast to procedures using saphenous veins, particularly those implanted using the *in situ* technique, comprehensive postoperative graft surveillance programs using ultrasonic imaging have not been specifically reported.[40,41] Frequent postoperative clinical evaluation is highly desirable because these bypasses are subject to the same defects that develop in saphenous vein bypass grafts. Cost constraints may restrict serial noninvasive examination, but it should be pointed out that careful surveillance detects failing grafts and permits repair of focal lesions prior to graft thrombosis. Many of these patients already have failed grafts, and their options for further autogenous revascularization are already diminished.

As experience with arm-vein-based revascularization accumulates, accurate reporting methods must be sedulously applied. Grafts should be categorized into cephalic, basilic, composite, and inflow or outflow jump grafts. Stratification and analysis of subgroups may yield new information despite the creation of smaller sample sizes. This new information will refine the appropriate applications of arm veins for arterial revascularization.

REFERENCES

1. Kakkar VV, Tsapogas MJ. The use of the cephalic vein as a peripheral vascular graft. *Br J Surg.* 1968;55:384.
2. Kakkar VV. The cephalic vein as a peripheral vascular graft. *Surg Gynecol Obstet.* 1969;128:551–556.
3. Andros G, Harris RW, Salles-Cunha SX. Arm veins as arterial autografts. In: Rutherford RB, ed. *Vascular Surgery.* 3rd ed. Philadelphia: WB Saunders Co.; 1989:434–449.
4. Vellar IDA, Doyle JC. The use of cephalic and basilic veins as peripheral vascular grafts. *Aust N Z J Surg.* 1970;40:52–57.
5. Stipa S. The cephalic and basilic veins in peripheral arterial reconstructive surgery. *Ann Surg.* 1972;175:581–587.
6. Bernhard VM, Ashmore CS, Evans WE, et al. Bypass grafting to distal arteries for limb salvage. *Surg Gynecol Obstet.* 1972;135:219–224.
7. Whittemore AD, Clowes AW, Couch NP, et al. Secondary femoropopliteal reconstruction. *Ann Surg.* 1981;193:35–42.
8. Graham JW, Lusby RJ. Infrapopliteal bypass grafting: use of upper limb vein alone and in autogenous composite grafts. *Surgery.* 1982;91:646–649.
9. Harris RW, Andros G, Dulawa LB, et al. Successful long-term limb salvage using cephalic vein bypass grafts. *Ann Surg.* 1984;200:785–792.
10. Schulman ML, Badrey MR. Late results and angiographic evaluation of arm veins as long bypass grafts. *Surgery.* 1982;92:1032–1041.
11. Andros G, Harris RW, Salles-Cunha SX, et al. Arm veins for arterial revascularization of the leg: arteriographic and clinical observations. *J Vasc Surg.* 1986;4:416–427.
12. Andros G, Harris RW, Dulawa LB, et al. The use of cephalic vein as a conduit. In: Greenhalgh RM, ed. *Vascular Surgical Techniques.* London: Butherworth Publ; 1984:169–176.
13. Salles-Cunha SX, Andros G, Harris RW, et al. Preoperative noninvasive assessment of arm veins to be used as bypass grafts in the lower extremities. *J Vasc Surg.* 1986;3:813–816.
14. Harris RW, Andros G, Salles-Cunha SX, et al. Totally autogenous venovenous composite bypass grafts. *Arch Surg.* 1986;121:1128–1132.
15. Logerfo FW, Paniszyn CW, Menzoian J. A new arm vein graft for distal bypass. *J Vasc Surg.* 1987;5:889–891.
16. Grigg MJ, Wolfe JHN. Combination reversed and non-reversed upper arm vein for femoro-distal grafting. *Eur J Vasc Surg.* 1988;2:49–52.
17. Cohen ES, Holtzman RB, Johnson GW. Axillobrachial artery bypass grafting with in situ cephalic vein for axillary artery occlusion: a case report. *J Vasc Surg.* 1989;10:683–687.
18. Kniemeyer HW, Sandman W. In situ and composite in situ vein bypass for upper extremity ischaemia. *Eur J Vasc Surg.* 1992;6:41–46.
19. Stonebridge PA, Miller A, Tsoukas A, et al. Angioscopy of arm vein infrainguinal bypass grafts. *Ann Vasc Surg.* 1991;5:170–175.
20. Andros G, Salles-Cunha SX, Harris RW. Arm veins for arterial reconstruction. In: Ernst CB and Stanley JC, eds. *Current Therapy in Vascular Surgery.* 2nd ed. Philadelphia: BC Decker Inc; 1991:505–512.
21. Veith FJ, Gupta SK, Samson RH, et al. Superficial femoral and popliteal arteries as inflow sites for distal bypasses. *Surgery.* 1981;90:980–990.
22. Andros G, Harris RW, Salles-Cunha SX, et al. Bypass grafts to the ankle and foot. *J Vasc Surg.* 1988;7:785–794.
23. Kent RC, Whittemore AD, Mannick JA. Short-term and midterm results of an all-autogenous tissue policy for infrainguinal reconstruction. *J Vasc Surg.* 1989;9:107–114.

24. Sesto ME, Sullivan TM, Hertzer MR, et al. Cephalic vein grafts for lower extremity revascularization. *J Vasc Surg.* 1992;15:543–549.
25. Coe D, Harward TRS, Flynn TC, et al. Use of arm vein conduits for arterial bypass. *J Vasc Surg.* 1992;15:250. Abstract.
26. Craver JM, Ottinger LW, Darling RC, et al. Hemorrhage and thrombosis as early complications of femoropopliteal bypass grafts: causes, treatment, and prognostic implications. *Surgery.* 1973;74:839–845.
27. Donaldson MC, Weinberg DS, Belkin M, et al. Screening for hypercoagulable states in vascular surgical practice: a preliminary study. *J Vasc Surg.* 1990;11:825–831.
28. Andros G, Harris RW, Dulawa LB, et al. Transposition angioplasty: a technique for the correction of proximal anastomotic neointimal hyperplasia in femorodistal bypasses. *Surgery.* 1988;103:698–700.
29. Harris RW, Andros G, Dulawa LB, et al. Large-vessel arterial occlusive disease in symptomatic upper extremity. *Arch Surg.* 1984;119:1277–1282.
30. Prieto I, Basile F, Abdulnour E. Upper extremity vein graft for aortocoronary bypass. *Ann Thorac Surg.* 1984;37:218.
31. Harris RW, Andros G, Dulawa LB, et al. The transition to "in situ" vein bypass grafts. *Surgery.* 1986;163:21–28.
32. Clayson KR, Edwards WH, Allen TR, et al. Arm veins for peripheral arterial reconstruction. *Arch Surg.* 1976;111:1276–1280.
33. Campbell DR, Hoar CS Jr, Gibbons GW. The use of arm veins in femoral-popliteal bypass grafts. *Ann Surg.* 1979;190:740–774.
34. Balshi JD, Cantelmo NL, Menzoian JO, et al. The use of arm veins for infrainguinal bypass in end-stage peripheral vascular disease. *Arch Surg.* 1989;124:1078–1081.
35. Bergamini TM, Towne JB, Bandyk DF, et al. Experience with in situ saphenous vein bypasses during 1981 to 1989: determinant factors of long-term patency. *J Vasc Surg.* 1991;13:137–149.
36. Taylor LM Jr, Edwards JM, Phinney ES, et al. Reversed vein bypass to infrapopliteal arteries. *Ann Surg.* 1987;205:90–97.
37. Leather RP, Shah DM, Change BD, et al. Resurrection of the in situ saphenous vein bypass: 1000 cases later. *Ann Surg.* 1988;208:435–442.
38. Veith FJ, Gupta SK, Ascer E, et al. Six-year prospective multicenter randomized comparison of autologous saphenous vein and expanded polytetrafluoroethylene grafts in infrainguinal arterial reconstructions. *J Vasc Surg.* 1986;3:104.
39. Weaver FA, Barlow CB, Edwards WH, et al. The lesser saphenous vein: autogenous tissue for lower extremity revascularization. *J Vasc Surg.* 1987;5:687–692.
40. Bandyk DF. Postoperative surveillance of infrainguinal bypass. In: Pearce WH, Yao JS, eds. *The Surgical Clinics of North America Noninvasive Diagnosis of Vascular Diseases.* Philadelphia: WB Saunders Co; 1990:71–85.
41. Mofford R, Salles-Cunha SX, Andros G. Duplex imaging of femorodistal bypass grafts. *Bruit.* 1986;10:213–217.

21

Long-Term Results of *In Situ* Saphenous Vein Arterial Bypass

Robert P. Leather, MD, and Benjamin B. Chang, MD

The surgical treatment of infrainguinal occlusive disease is most effectively performed with autogenous vein bypass. This is generally accepted; however, the ideal method of vein preparation has been a matter of controversy in the surgical literature for over a decade. The relative advantages of *in situ* bypass (ISB) versus reversed vein graft in the modern setting continues to be argued.[1–3]

In spite of this continuing debate, it is evident that ISB performs at least as well or better than reversed vein graft in almost all reported series. Thus, ISB has been established as an effective technique that should be within the capabilities of all committed vascular surgeons.

The general concept of using the saphenous vein *in situ* dates back at least to the work of Hall and Rob in the early 1960s. Although the technique used in these cases recognized the need for rendering the valves nonfunctional—the hallmark of *in situ* techniques in general—it did not recognize the importance of preserving the microstructure of the vein itself and, in particular, the endothelial monolayer. Use of a blunt instrument passed proximally to distally to disrupt the venous valves sufficiently traumatized the lumen to result in poor long-term patency. Recognition of the poor results of this specific methodology led to the abandonment of *in situ* techniques in the late 1960s.[4]

In spite of this report, Hall continued to develop his own *in situ* technique independently. Instead of using an intraluminal device to produce valvular incompetence, he excised valve leaflets sharply through the use of separate venotomies in sequence following arterialization of the great saphenous vein. Although largely ignored by the majority of the surgical community, this refinement in technique produced significantly improved results, undoubtedly because of decreased trauma to the endothelium.[5,6]

In 1974, during an *in situ* procedure using Hall's improved technique, it was serendipitously noted that bisection of the valve leaflets along their long axes was sufficient to produce valve incompetence. This technique—termed *valve incision*—has formed the basis for the development of a series of instruments for the *in situ* technique. This concept has been used more extensively than any other method of *in situ* vein bypass preparation and has produced most of the favorable results.

Several alternative instruments have been developed for performing *in situ* bypasses. However, they generally employ a blunt edge that avulses the valve (Hall & Cartier) or a circular blade that attempts to partially excise the valve leaflet (Le-Maitre). These instruments carry with them two basic limitations that translate into the potential for intraluminal trauma during valve lysis. The first limitation is the mechanism by which valvular incompetence is produced. The second, and far more significant, is that the instruments must be introduced and withdrawn through the distal divided end of the vein, which is not only invariably that portion of the vein smallest in diameter, but, prior to arterialization, it has little if any distending (venous) pressure. In addition, such small-diameter veins are more prone to be further narrowed by spasm when manipulated by exposure and by the intraluminal passage of such devices. These factors all conspire to potentially produce the maximum endothelial injury, or circumferential denudation. This has been demonstrated by scanning electron microscopy of prepared vein segments, which show a higher frequency and extent of endothelial damage using these alternative methods of valve lysis.

Although the effects of this type of injury may be compensated for by high flow rates (as evidenced by reasonable patency rates in bypasses performed for claudication or limb salvage to the popliteal arteries with good runoff), when longer low-flow bypasses to the crural arteries performed for limb salvage are analyzed, the results are the same or worse than those historically obtained with reversed vein bypass grafts.[7–9]

In spite of the apparent simplicity of such variants of the *in situ* technique, it is evident that consistently successful *in situ* vein preparation is technically exacting and a major determinant of bypass function. Therefore, assiduous attention to the technical minutiae of the *in situ* vein arterial bypass is critically important in achieving the best results. This chapter seeks to identify many of the important details that may be used by the surgeon to critically examine his or her particular technique.

PATIENT SELECTION AND VEIN IMAGING PRIOR TO BYPASS SURGERY

In general, the majority of patients undergoing an *in situ* bypass have had critical ischemia. Use of this technique to alleviate claudication, as with all reconstructive methods at the infrainguinal level, should be applied conservatively, as evidenced in our series where less than 5% of these bypasses have been performed for this indication.

For appropriate *in situ* bypass candidates, detailed angiography is necessary. Imaging of the tibial arteries is particularly important and may well require modification of the angiographer's technique. Biplanar views of the infrageniculate arteries are critical in distinguishing the peroneal from the anterior tibial artery.

Prebypass imaging of the greater saphenous vein is as important as detailed angiography. Conventional or intraoperative prebypass contrast venography may be performed with good results; however, B-mode ultrasonography provides the same information noninvasively.[10] It should be noted, however, that neither of these methods accurately assesses the eventual diameter of the vein under arterial pressure, in part because they delineate the internal diameter under venous pressure, whereas surgeons historically have considered the outside diameter under arterial pressure as being a critical factor in vein bypass patency. Thus, patients should not be denied *in situ* bypass on the basis of a small vein diameter measured preoperatively; all continuous patent veins should be assessed by direct inspection with distention before decisions based on the ultimate vein diameter are made.

Use of ultrasonography allows the imager to map the course of the vein upon the skin as well as to determine its depth. Preoperative knowledge of this type is important, especially because the frequency of anatomic variants in the greater saphenous vein is as high as 30%. A cutaneous map of the vein may be used by the surgeon to minimize necessary dissection and thereby expedite the completion of the bypass and minimize postoperative wound complications.

Recent reports have discussed the use of angioscopy to identify other forms of vein pathology not apparent by conventional methods and to allow valve incision using the Mills valvulotome under direct vision. Whether the information gained compensates for the extra time, expense, and intraluminal trauma produced by the angioscope remains to be seen. Furthermore, safe, consistent valve lysis can be accomplished without such intraluminal visualization, and the frequency of such pathology is extremely low. When disease is present, it can be detected on completion angiography and corrected if necessary.

VESSEL SELECTION

With the preoperative studies completed, careful and deliberate planning will maximize bypass patency. Obviously, selection of the appropriate inflow and outflow vessels is necessary. The common femoral, superficial femoral, or profunda femoris arteries may be used as inflow vessels with equal expectations of success. There has been no long-term difference in patency using any of these arteries. As the greater saphenous vein generally terminates at the level of the femoral artery bifurcation, use of either of the two more distal arteries is technically easier, requiring less mobilization of the saphenofemoral junction and, in general, expediting the procedure. Furthermore, use of alternatives to the common femoral arteries allows the surgeon to avoid previous scar tissue when present and to ''debride'' the proximal manipulated vein.

Given a continuous greater saphenous vein, the site of the distal anastomosis is selected so as to bypass all significant occlusive disease and thereby directly to perfuse the most affected tissue (usually the foot). This policy emphasizes the use of tibial arteries while minimizing the use of the more proximal isolated popliteal artery as an outflow site.

Among the three tibial arteries, the peroneal is the most likely to remain patent and relatively free of atherosclerotic changes.[11] Therefore, this is the most common site for the distal anastomosis in this series; fully 45% of all infrapopliteal bypasses use this artery. The *in situ* bypass performs equally well with any of the four infrageniculate arteries; in addition, bypasses to the foot and ankle have patencies comparable to bypasses to more proximal sites.[12]

The above-the-knee popliteal artery is rarely used for distal anastomosis of an *in situ* bypass because there is relatively little of the vein actually not mobilized in this case and it is rarely a viable option in patients with critical ischemia. Therefore, there is little choice between reversed and *in situ* techniques in such cases. In general, ISB is especially to be preferred in long infrageniculate bypasses performed for limb salvage.

VEIN PREPARATION

During the conduct of the procedure, loupe magnification (preferably at least 3.5 ×) and coaxial fiberoptic lighting is essential to adequately visualize the field, especially of the vein preparation and distal anastomosis. Although many surgeons resist this suggestion, we feel that this detail is a critical feature of consistent *in situ* bypass success.

After the inflow and outflow arteries are exposed, the vein is prepared. Several instruments have been developed for use in the valve incision technique, for example, scissors, Mills' valvulotome, and the valve cutter; it should be noted that these instruments are all capable of producing excellent long-term results and differ largely in the ease with which vein preparation may be completed.[3] In our current method of vein preparation, which has remained unchanged for over 10 years, we use scissors and the intraluminal valve cutter for the proximal vein (thigh portion) and the modified Mills' valvulotome for the infrageniculate portion of the vein.

This approach transects the saphenous vein at or near its junction with the common femoral vein. It is critically important to try to obtain slightly more vein than is necessary for the completion of the proximal anastomosis because there is inevitably some trauma produced to the endothelium in the most proximal centimeter of vein during manipulation to achieve valve lysis. Having a little extra vein allows the surgeon to amputate (debride) the proximal damaged centimeter or at least position this area in the widest (patch) portion of the proximal anastomosis. This maneuver reduces both early failures and the formation of late proximal perianastomotic strictures.

VALVE INCISION METHOD

The specifics of the valve incision method as we perform it have been presented elsewhere and should be referred to for the technical details.[13] There are, however, some aspects that should be emphasized here. Most importantly, the surgeon should be constantly aware that the use of instruments within the lumen of the vein is potentially very damaging if done improperly and that every effort should be taken to minimize this possibility. To this end, instruments should never be inserted into the vein without prior distention under pressure. Although heparinized blood can and has been used, we employ a mixture of dextran 70, heparin, and papaverine pressurized to between 200 and 300 mm Hg. Intraluminal instrumentation without previous distention will almost always result in significant vein damage, leading to short- or long-term failure.

The intraluminal valve cutter is designed to incise venous valves without trauma because it "floats" within the lumen of the vein. When using the valve cutter it is necessary to use a following catheter to distend the vein and necessary to place the valve leaflets in the functionally closed position as the cutter is drawn down the vein. In general, the cutter is not used beyond the knee because the vein is usually smaller below this point and the many interconnections with the deep venous system may make it difficult to ensure that the cutter will float properly. Use of the cutter in the proximal segment obviates the need for an incision along the entire length of the vein and expedites the procedure considerably without any sacrifice in immediate or long-term patency.

After the proximal segment of vein has been thus prepared, the vein is arterialized. The proximal clamps are then removed to permit arterialized (oxygenated) blood to perfuse the vein. This procedure minimizes the ischemic insult produced by mobilizing the vein and transecting its vasa vasorum, which normally helps oxygenate the vein wall. Expedient perfusion of the vein greatly increases the possibility of endothelial preservation.

The infrageniculate portion of the vein is then prepared. The modified Mills' valvulotome is most commonly employed at this time. This instrument is the least trauma-producing means of incising venous valves. As detailed above the same effort should be taken to distend the vein prior to insertion of the instrument. Arterialized blood is thereby allowed to preserve the vein wall. Ideally, an additional 2 to 4 cm of vein is prepared, allowing the surgeon to amputate the most distal segment, which is the most vulnerable portion of the bypass.

To better understand the problems encountered with valve lysis, it is important to have a clear concept of venous valve function. The normal closing mechanism in a symmetrical venous valve is triggered by expansion of the valve sinus in response to increased intraluminal pressure. The valve expansion creates tension along the leading edge of the valve, which brings the cusps toward the center of the lumen. Reverse flow then forces the cusps into a closed and competent position. In a segment of vein where a valve has been mechanically opened from below by passage of an instrument in the proximal direction (e.g., valvulotome, balloon catheter, or, especially, cylindrical valve disruptors), a valve leaflet may temporarily adhere to the wall of the valve sinus in the open position. This phenomenon is most likely to occur in asymmetrical valves because the normal closing mechanism may not be functioning. Subsequent closure of such an artificially opened valve leaflet results in partial or complete obstruction to prograde arterial flow. In these circumstances, an incompletely lysed leaflet can close during extraluminal manipulation of the vein (e.g., during attempts to palpate a pulse). Therefore, before the operation is completed, deliberate attempts should be made to precipitate closure of any incompletely lysed valves by the following maneuver: with the distal vein open and free flow observed, a sponge is rolled along the *in situ* conduit from top to bottom. The most reliable test of the absence of a flow-limiting stenosis in the bypass conduit before construction of the distal anastomosis is to observe free flow through the distal divided end of the arterialized *in situ* vein. Strong, persistent pulsatile flow (for more than 5 to 10 seconds) is absolute evidence that no proximal hemodynamically significant stenotic lesion exists. If, however, there is initial strong flow (one to two pulses) followed by diminished flow, one should palpate along the conduit until a strong pulse is palpable. This is the site of obstruction or stenosis. If no valve leaflet is encountered by reintroduction of the valvulotome then spasm or a platelet plug is the cause.

ANASTOMOSIS

With the vein completely prepared, distal anastomosis is made. The artery is best controlled with Yasargil's neurosurgic aneurysm clips. Use of heavy, Cooley-type clamps often leads to permanent damage and possible stricturing of the artery. Intraluminal occluders or balloon catheters carry with them the potential for endothelial injury and should be avoided. If necessary, an orthopedic tourniquet can be used to obtain arterial control, especially with calcified arteries.[14]

As the anastomosis is made, no instruments should be inserted within the luminal surface of the vein. Injury to the vein at this point leads to platelet deposition and subsequent occlusion. There is no need to create an overly long anastomosis; usually 1.5 to 2 times the diameter of the vein is sufficient.

With completion of the second anastomosis, flow is instituted in the bypass. Sterile intraoperative Doppler ultrasonography assesses flow, and intraoperative arteriography identifies fistulas and technical problems along the bypass. Fistulas that connect the greater saphenous vein with the deep system should be ligated. Most

TABLE 21–1. TOTAL *IN SITU* BYPASSES—SECONDARY PATENCY

Interval	Number Entering Interval	Occlusions	Interval Patency	Cumulative Patency
0–1	1,473	56	0.960	0.960
2–12	1,244	51	0.951	0.912
13–24	766	24	0.963	0.879
25–36	524	10	0.977	0.859
37–48	351	11	0.963	0.827
49–60	235	4	0.980	0.810
61–72	152	4	0.968	0.784
73–84	92	2	0.974	0.764
85–96	58	0	1.000	0.764
97–108	39	4	0.879	0.671
109–120	23	1	0.947	0.636

other fistulas will spontaneously occlude during the first postoperative year. In any case, there is no need to ligate every branch of the vein because patent fistulas will not cause thrombosis in a properly constructed ISB, contrary to the beliefs of some surgeons.

All identified intraluminal defects should be repaired or replaced. In general, segmental replacement is favored over patching.

In practice, every effort should be made to prevent intimal injury and its resulting platelet aggregation. Instruments should be passed only when the vein is fully distended, preferably by arterialized blood and pressure, so that contact with the endothelium is minimized. Particularly devastating is circumferential shear, especially in the distal mobilized segment, which is smallest in diameter and where the protective effect of flowing blood through a coincident fistula before completion of the distal anastomosis is absent. Fortunately, with proper care of this critical segment by strictly preventing instruments, such as catheters, sounds, dilators, and cylindrical valve cutters or disruptors, from making circumferential contact, this problem is infrequent.

TABLE 21–2. POPLITEAL *IN SITU* BYPASSES—SECONDARY PATENCY

Interval	Number Entering Interval	Occlusions	Interval Patency	Cumulative Patency
0–1	475	20	0.956	0.956
2–12	412	14	0.960	0.917
13–24	271	9	0.963	0.884
25–36	207	1	0.994	0.879
37–48	142	6	0.951	0.835
49–60	95	1	0.987	0.824
61–72	58	3	0.936	0.772
73–84	33	0	1.000	0.772
85–96	28	0	1.000	0.772
97–108	21	3	0.842	0.650
109–120	14	0	1.000	0.650

TABLE 21–3. TIBIAL *IN SITU* BYPASSES—SECONDARY PATENCY

Interval	Number Entering Interval	Occlusions	Interval Patency	Cumulative Patency
0–1	998	36	0.961	0.961
2–12	832	37	0.946	0.909
13–24	495	15	0.964	0.876
25–36	317	9	0.966	0.847
37–48	209	5	0.972	0.823
49–60	140	3	0.975	0.802
61–72	94	1	0.987	0.792
73–84	59	2	0.956	0.757
85–96	30	0	1.000	0.757
97–108	18	1	0.929	0.703

POSTOPERATIVE SURVEILLANCE AND LONG-TERM RESULTS

After surgery, pulse volume recordings and duplex scans of each ISB are performed serially. Although the criteria used to identify preocclusive stenoses vary from one health center to another, use of some form of strict postoperative surveillance will identify these problems prior to bypass failure in many cases.[15] Correction of these lesions, which probably result from vein injury at the time of the original procedure, is again best performed with segmental replacement. We have had disappointing results with balloon dilatation. Serial follow-up and revision generate an approximately 15% improvement in patency (secondary patency) by Life Table methods.

Overall long-term results of ISB performed by the valve incision technique are presented in Tables 21–1 through 21–3. There are points in these data that should be emphasized. As discussed previously, bypass patency is independent of the inflow or outflow artery used, the length of the bypass, and the size of the vein. It is also notable that these results have remained stable despite the evolution in the instruments used for valve incision (i.e., from scissors to Mills' valvulotome to valve cutter). That the ISB is so insensitive to factors that are often felt to determine the patency of reversed saphenous vein bypasses bespeaks the inherent soundness of this method of valve lysis.

Conversely, the careful surgeon will realize that there is much that differs between the method of vein preparation used in this series and other techniques. Therefore, any critical analysis of ISB patency should take into account these differences.

REFERENCES

1. Taylor LM, Edwards JM, Phinney ES, et al. Reversed vein bypass to infrapopliteal arteries: modern results are superior to or equivalent to in situ bypass for patency and for vein utilization. *Ann Surg.* 1987;205:90–97.
2. Fogle MA, Whittemore AD, Couch N, et al. A comparison of in situ and reversed saphenous vein grafts for infra-inguinal reconstruction. *J Vasc Surg.* 1987;5:46–52.
3. Leather RP, Shah DM, Chang BB, et al. Resurrection of the in situ saphenous vein bypass: 1000 cases later. *Ann of Surg.* 1988;208:435–442.
4. Barner HB, Judd DR, Kaiser GC, et al. Late failure of arteriologic "in situ" saphenous vein. *Arch Surg.* 1969;99:781.

5. Hall KV. The great saphenous vein used *in situ* as an arterial shunt after extirpation of the vein valves: a preliminary report. *Surgery.* 1962;51:492.

6. Hall KV. The great saphenous vein used *in situ* as an arterial shunt after vein valve extirpation. *Acta Chir Scand.* 1964;128:365.

7. Gruss JD, Bartels D, Vargas H. Arterial reconstruction for distal disease of the lower extremities by the in situ vein graft technique. *J Cardiovasc Surg.* 1982;23:231–234.

8. Fietze-Fischer B, Gruss JD, Bartels D, et al. Prostaglandin E_1 as an adjuvant therapy in the event of femoropopliteal and crural great saphenous vein in situ bypass surgery. *Vasa.* 1987;(suppl)17:23–25.

9. Denton MJ, Hill D, Fairgrieve J. In situ femoropopliteal and distal vein bypass for limb salvage: experience of 50 cases. *Br J Surg.* 1983;70:358–361.

10. Kupinski AM, Leather RP, Chang BB, et al. Pre-operative mapping of the saphenous vein. In: Bernstein EF, ed. *Vascular Diagnosis.* St Louis: CV Mosby; In press.

11. Dible JH. *The Pathology of Limb Ischemia.* Edinburgh: Oliver & Boyd; 1966:39–71.

12. Shah DM, Darling RC III, Chang BB, et al. Is long vein bypass from groin to ankle a durable procedure? An analysis of a ten year experience. *J Vasc Surg.* 1992;15:402–408.

13. Leather RP, Shah DM. In situ saphenous vein bypass. In: Rutherford RB, ed. *Vascular Surgery.* Denver: WB Saunders; Philadelphia. 1989:414–425.

14. Bernhard V, Boren C, Towne J. Pneumatic tourniquet as a substitute for vascular clamps in distal bypass surgery. *Surgery.* 1980;87:709.

15. Bandyk DF, Cato RF, Towne JB. A low flow velocity predicts failure of femoropopliteal and femorotibial bypass grafts. *Surgery.* 1985;98:799–809.

22

Patency Potential of Composite Sequential Femoral Bypass

Walter J. McCarthy, MD, William H. Pearce, MD,
William R. Flinn, MD, Roger Wang, BS, and
James S. T. Yao, MD, PhD

Most surgeons would agree that the surgical management of femoral tibial occlusive disease requiring bypass to the tibial level is most successfully managed using autogenous vein. This may be accomplished using reversed greater saphenous vein or *in situ* techniques or by combining segments of vein from different locations to afford a complete conduit. The exact technique of bypass construction is still open for debate, but none among us would argue for routinely using prosthetic graft to the tibial level if vein is available. Despite this preference, patients are occasionally seen who have arterial occlusive disease with limb-threatening ischemia and insufficient vein for complete arterial bypass. The management of these individuals requires more ingenuity than the usual case. All-prosthetic bypasses often will establish excellent foot perfusion but are subject to early occlusion from distal anastomotic intimal hyperplasia.[1] Thus, several alternatives have been devised to use even short segments of autogenous venous conduit. These include composite grafts where the distal portion is autogenous vein anastomosed end-to-end to a more proximal prosthesis. A variation of this is the composite sequential graft, defined as having an intermediate arterial anastomosis (Fig. 22–1). The focus of this chapter is on composite sequential bypassing, which has attained a more encouraging patency record than strictly composite grafting (Table 22–1).

BACKGROUND

DeLaurentis and Friedmann[2] were the first to describe the composite sequential configuration as currently practiced. They reviewed work performed in Springfield, Massachusetts, over 4 years beginning in 1966 for the New England Surgical Society and subsequently published their experience with 74 femoral bypasses in 1971. DeLaurentis was familiar with simple, end-to-end, composite bypass grafts and said that the technique had been "mostly abandoned," quoting work by Dale et al,[3] publishing a high failure rate in 1962. One may wonder what advantage composite

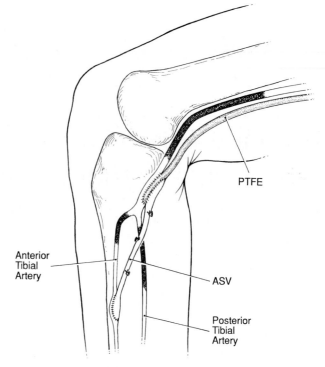

Figure 22–1. Composite sequential bypassing is defined for this presentation as prosthetic material (PTFE) anastomosed either above the knee or below the knee to the popliteal artery. Following this anastomosis, autogenous vein is brought to a patent tibial vessel. Both greater saphenous and lesser saphenous vein have been used with success. (*Reprinted with permission* from: McCarthy WJ, Pearce WH, Flinn WR, et al. Long-term evaluation of composite sequential bypass for limb-threatening ischemia. *J Vasc Surg.* 1992;15:765.)

sequential grafting with its intermediate anastomosis has. DeLaurentis and Friedmann in this early paper suggested three inherent superiorities, probably still pertinent today: (a) There is less likely to be any kinking effect at the vein graft junction; (b) the prosthetic material can be of large diameter, and (c) good quality autogenous vein can be used and, it is hoped, can be used to traverse the knee joint. To these three we might add that a vein graft to tibial artery anastomosis is superior to one involving prosthetic material. Finally, the distal venous graft affords greater blood flow through the proximal prosthetic section, making it less likely to thrombose from a low flow state. In their review of these 74 bypasses above and below the knee, three patients

TABLE 22–1. SELECTED REPORTS OF COMPOSITE SEQUENTIAL BYPASS PATENCY

Reference	Date	Location	Journal	Number of Grafts	Follow-up	Patency
Delaurentis and Friedmann[2]	1971	Springfield, MA	*Am J Surg*	3	To 6 mo	100%, 6 mo
Bliss and Fonseka[4]	1976	London	*Br J Surg*	16	2–14 mo	11/16 at 2–14 mo
Rosenfeld et al[8]	1981	Philadelphia	*Arch Surg*	22	1–72 mo	59%, 24 mo 42%, 48 mo
Verta[6]	1984	Chicago	*J Vasc Surg*	54	26 mo mean	81%, 24 mo 72%, 48 mo
Flinn et al[7]	1984	Chicago	*J Vasc Surg*	30	1–27 mo	93%, 12 mo 80%, 24 mo
McCarthy et al[9]	1992	Chicago	*J Vasc Surg*	67	33 mo mean (1–91 mo)	72%, 12 mo 64%, 24 mo 48%, 36 mo 40%, 48 mo

were reconstructed using what DeLaurentis called a "double bypass." These three constitute the first published cases using composite segmental technique. Eight-millimeter Dacron graft was used between the common femoral artery and a patent or "endarterectomized" popliteal vessel. Next, a short segment of saphenous vein was anastomosed adjacent to this Dacron graft onto the popliteal segment and taken to a patent distal vessel. With only 6 months follow-up, the authors were only cautiously enthusiastic but reported that all grafts were functioning well. The double bypass caught the attention of Bliss and Fonseka,[4] working at the Charing Cross Hospital, London. By August 1975, they had completed 16 such procedures for patients without adequate saphenous vein for a complete tibial bypass. Their bypass called a "hitch-hike" graft, had seen only four failures of 16 grafts with follow-up at 2 to 14 months after operation. The technique used was with Dacron as a proximal graft limb with the distal Dacron anastomosis abutting the proximal venous hood on a patent popliteal segment.

By the late 1970s, these principles were well known in Chicago and frequently used at both the University of Illinois and Northwestern University. Flinn et al[5] presented the combined experience of these two university centers to the Central Surgical Association in 1980 with an evaluation of 40 bypasses. All 40 grafts originated with the femoral artery and had a distal anastomosis made to one of the tibial vessels. Thirty of these grafts were performed with an intermediate side-to-side anastomosis termed "kiss-and-run" and thus were sequential, not composite sequential bypasses. Of those, 28 were completely polytetrafluoroethylene (PTFE) and the remaining two with all-autogenous vein. However, from this presentation, nine grafts stand out as truly composite sequential bypasses with PTFE material to the popliteal position and autogenous vein brought to a patent distal tibial vessel. From this series, with follow-up ranging from 3 to 18 months, limb salvage was 76%.

The compilation of this information made several things apparent. The kiss-and-run intermediate side-to-side anastomosis seemed to offer little or no advantage. For all-venous bypass, it is not necessary to enhance flow through the proximal segment. If all-prosthetic grafting is used, the side-to-side configuration will actually decrease flow through the distal portion and possibly hinder patency. Thus, the intermediate anastomosis was abandoned in future years. The nine patients with venous extensions of their graft did, however, maintain reasonable patency and that configuration has remained predominant. The next publication related to this work was by Verta,[6] a co-author of Flinn's paper. His analysis of 54 patients emphasized distal vein graft placement to the foot or distal tibial vessels and contained follow-up to 48 months, with a mean of 26.4 months. Cumulative Life Table patency rates of 81% at 2 years and 72% at 4 years were presented.

In an attempt to better understand composite sequential as compared with sequential bypasses, Flinn et al[7] then analyzed a 5-year experience with such grafts at Northwestern. This work, which was presented to the Midwest Vascular Surgical Society in 1983, reviewed 12 sequential grafts performed with saphenous vein alone, 22 with PTFE alone, and 30 in the composite sequential configuration. The sequential grafts each had an intermediate side-to-side popliteal anastomosis performed. Cumulative Life Table patency rates were compared and were illuminating. The composite sequential bypasses showed a 1-year 93% patency and 2-year 80% rate. Sequential grafts performed entirely with reversed saphenous vein had 90% patency at 1 and 2 years. Sequential grafts constructed of PTFE alone showed a 52% 12-month patency, which dropped to 47% at 24 months. None of the all-PTFE grafts remained patent for longer than 36 months. The conclusions then were obvious. Performing an intermediate popliteal anastomosis with reversed saphenous vein does nothing to increase patency, which will be predictably good, but may slightly prolong and complicate the operation. Patency with sequential grafts using PTFE alone are much less successful, not unlike the patency seen with femorotibial PTFE grafts reported elsewhere. The patency at 1 and 2 years for composite sequential grafting with a distal vein jump graft gave durability superior to PTFE alone and comparable with all-vein reconstruction. Numbers in this series were not sufficient to establish Life Table rates significant past the 2-year time frame.

Eleven years after their first description of the technique, Friedmann and DeLaurentis, now adding experience from the Pennsylvania Hospital, published an extensive review of composite sequential technique authored by Rosenfeld et al.[8] Patients were divided into 33 cases with sequential femoropopliteal-popliteal bypass and 22 cases with femoropopliteal tibial bypass. Patency rates were similar whether the distal anastomosis was at the popliteal or tibial level. Life Table analysis for the femoropopliteal tibial grafts showed 12-month accumulated patency of 65%, 2-year patency of 59%, and 42% patency thereafter. The paper also mentioned the situation in which portions of the bypass graft occluded while others remained patent. In commenting on Rosenfeld's paper, Bergan of Chicago recalled an experience at Northwestern where the distal limb of the composite sequential graft remained open after the proximal bypass had occluded, concluding, "We have no explanation for why that happened."[8]

Interest in composite sequential bypassing at Northwestern, for reasons of patency, has remained generally optimistic. As more expertise with the use of all-venous bypasses using cephalic vein, lesser saphenous vein, and other sources has increased, the composite sequential graft has not been used as frequently. However, a review of a 7-year period identified 67 reconstructions using femoropopliteal with popliteal to tibial venous jump grafts. With this number of patients and a mean follow-up of 33 months (1 to 91 months), a significant Life Table analysis was possible, and the work was presented to the Midwestern Vascular Surgery Society in 1991.[9] Six-millimeter PTFE material was used in every case from the common femoral to popliteal artery. The intermediate anastomosis was placed above the knee for 44 patients and below the knee for 23 patients. Extension grafts of greater saphenous vein were used for 57 individuals, and the lesser saphenous vein was used for 10. The

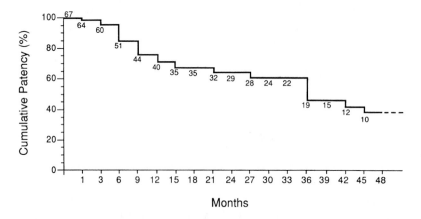

Figure 22–2. Cumulative Life Table patency of 72% for 1 year, 64% for 2 years, and 48% for 3 years was calculated. This is primary patency, and the standard error exceeds 10% after 48 months, as indicated by the *dotted line*. (*Reprinted with permission* from: McCarthy WJ, Pearce WH, Flinn WR, et al. Long-term evaluation of composite sequential bypass for limb-threatening ischemia. *J Vasc Surg.* 1992;15:766.)

tibial artery in 26, and to the peroneal artery in 21 patients. Cumulative Life Table primary patency of 72% at 1 year, 64% at 2 years, and 48% after 3 years was calculated (Fig. 22–2). The Life Table was significant with a standard error less than 10% at 4 years. An interesting finding was that two of the grafts were functioning well after 7 years, the longest being patent 91 months after its initial placement. Limb salvage was 84% at 2 years and 70% at 4 years. Of interest in this review were five cases in which the proximal portion of the bypass failed but the distal venous remnant remained patent, allowing fairly straightforward reconstruction. Two patients had the reverse, with distal vein failure and proximal PTFE patency.

SUMMARY

Conclusions from these admittedly few reports suggest that composite sequential bypass is a useful solution when sufficient autologous vein is not present to allow tibial bypass for limb salvage. The technique appears to provide superior patency to an all-prosthetic femoral-to-tibial artery bypass graft.

Acknowledgments

This work was supported in part by the Alyce F. Salerno Foundation, the Gaylord Freeman Aneurysm Research Fund, and the Veterans Administration Research Service.

REFERENCES

1. Sottiurai VS, Yao JST, Flinn WR, et al. Intimal hyperplasia and neointima: an ultrastructural analysis of thrombosed grafts in humans. *Surgery.* 1983;93:809–817.
2. DeLaurentis DA, Friedmann P. Arterial reconstruction about and below the knee: another look. *Am J Surg.* 1971;121:392–397.
3. Dale WA, Pridgen WR, Shoulders HH. Failure of composite (Teflon and vein) grafting in small human arteries. *Surgery.* 1962;51:258–262.
4. Bliss BP, Fonseka N. "Hitch-hike" grafts for limb salvage in peripheral arterial disease. *Br J Surg.* 1976;63:562–564.
5. Flinn WR, Flanigan DP, Verta MJ Jr, et al. Sequential femoral-tibial bypass for severe limb ischemia. *Surgery.* 1980;88:357–365.
6. Verta MJ Jr. Composite sequential bypasses to the ankle and beyond for limb salvage. *J Vasc Surg.* 1984;1:381–386.
7. Flinn WR, Ricco J-B, Yao JST, et al. Composite sequential grafts in severe ischemia: a comparative study. *J Vasc Surg.* 1984;1:449–454.
8. Rosenfeld JC, Savarese RP, Friedmann P, et al. Sequential femoropopliteal and femorotibial bypasses: a ten-year follow-up study. *Arch Surg.* 1981;116:1538–1543.
9. McCarthy WJ, Pearce WH, Flinn WR, et al. Long-term evaluation of composite sequential bypass for limb-threatening ischemia. *J Vasc Surg.* 1992;15:761–770.

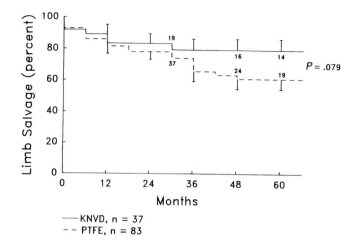

Figure 23–2. Limb salvage with knitted nonvelour Dacron (KNVD) and expanded polytetrafluoroethylene (PTFE).

certainly be stated that the retrospective data are compelling enough to recommend a prospective, randomized comparison of Dacron versus PTFE for femoropopliteal reconstruction.

REFERENCES

1. Mathisen SR, Wu HD, Sauvage LR, et al. An experimental study of eight current arterial prostheses. *J Vasc Surg.* 1986;4:33–41.
2. Camilleri JP, Phat VN, Bruneval P, et al. Surface healing and histologic maturation of patent polytetrafluoroethylene grafts implanted in patients for up to 60 months. *Arch Pathol Lab Med.* 1985;109:833–837.
3. Christenson JT, Eklof B. Sparks mandril, velour Dacron and autogenous saphenous vein grafts in femoropopliteal bypass. *Br J Surg.* 1979;66:514–517.
4. Stephen M, Loewenthal J, Little JM, et al. Autogenous veins and velour Dacron in femoropopliteal arterial bypass. *Surgery.* 1977;81:314–318.
5. Clifford PC, Gazzard V, Lawarance RJ, et al. Below knee femoropopliteal bypass in severe ischemia: results using EXS Dacron and human umbilical vein. *Ann Coll Surg Eng.* 1986;68:319–321.
6. Kenney DA, Sauvage LR, Wood SJ, et al. Comparison of noncrimped, externally supported (EXS) and crimped, nonsupported Dacron prostheses for axillofemoral and above-knee femoropopliteal bypass. *Surgery.* 1982;92:931–946.
7. Matsubara J, Nagasue M, Tsuchishima S, et al. Clinical results of femoropopliteal bypass using externally supported (EXS) Dacron grafts: with a comparison of above- and below-knee anastomosis. *J Cardiovasc Surg.* 1990;31:731–734.
8. Yashar JJ, Thompson R, Burnard RJ, et al. Dacron vs vein for femoropopliteal arterial bypass. *Arch Surg.* 1981;116:1037–1040.
9. Pevec WC, Darling RC, L'Italien GJ, et al. Femoropopliteal reconstruction with knitted, non-velour Dacron versus expanded polytetrafluoroethylene. *J Vasc Surg.* 1992. In press.
10. Rosenthal D, Evans D, McKinsey J, et al. Prosthetic above-knee femoropopliteal bypass for intermittent claudication. *J Cardiovasc Surg.* 1990;31:462–468.
11. Rutherford RB, Flanigan DP, Gupta SK, et al. Suggested standards for reports dealing with lower extremity ischemia. *J Vasc Surg.* 1986;4:80–94.

To evaluate both early and late operative results, it is necessary to stratify the procedures into profundaplasty, which was used as an adjunct to an inflow procedure and procedures where only profundaplasty is constructed. In our study, 237 profundaplasties were evaluated in 209 patents.[6] The procedures were classified as profundaplasty alone (PA) or inflow and profundaplasty (IP). The IP group consisted of patients who underwent profundaplasty combined with aortofemoral, femoral-femoral, or axillary-femoral grafts, as well as reconstructions combined with thrombectomy of an occluded limb of an aortofemoral bypass graft. Indications for revascularization were either incapacitating claudication or limb salvage, which was defined as rest pain or ischemic necrosis. In the PA group, the indications were claudication in 17.6% and limb salvage in 82.4%. In the IP group, indications were claudication in 42% and limb salvage in 58%.

The operative mortality rate was 2%, all occurring in the limb salvage group. Five-year patency rate in the claudication group was 77% and was only 23% in the limb salvage group. The limb salvage rate in IP patients calculated by a Life Table method was 89% at 1 year, which decreased to 80% at 6 years. In contrast, the cumulative PA limb salvage rate varied from 51% at 1 year to 36% at 7 years. I have previously demonstrated that this difference was a result of more advanced tibial occlusive disease in the PA group. With 104 limbs of patients in the limb salvage group who were alive at the end of the follow-up period, 41% ultimately required amputation, and of these, 79% required amputation within the first postoperative year. An additional 13% required additional vascular procedures during the follow-up period to maintain limb viability. There were 19 above-knee amputations, of whom 89% had failure of the profunda repair. All 24 successful below-knee amputations had a patent profundaplasty at the time of amputation. Six patients had profundaplasty to lower the level from above-knee to below-knee. Eighteen percent of the patients in the claudication group went on to limb salvage in the follow-up period, and all were successfully treated with additional vascular reconstruction. An additional 10% had deterioration of their walking distance. The remaining 72% maintained their postoperative improvement throughout the course of the follow-up.

Long-term patient survival rates of the claudication group and limb salvage groups were calculated by a Life Table method. Cumulative survival rate at 6 years in the claudication group was 77% compared with 35% in the limb salvage group.

When patients are evaluated by the operative indication (limb salvage or claudication), those with claudication have less severe disease and better long-term prognosis, as compared with those who require profundaplasty for limb salvage. At 5 years, patient survival was 77% in the claudication group compared with 25% in the limb salvage group. This statistically significant difference in the cumulative patent survival rate was present at all postoperative intervals. The cause of death in both groups of patients was primarily caused by widespread atherosclerosis. Fifty-seven percent of these patients had documented atherosclerotic causes of death, including myocardial infarction in 33%, congestive heart failure in 15%, and stroke in 9%.

The difference between the claudication and limb salvage groups was also reflected in the cumulative patency rate. The patency rate of profundaplasty performed for claudication was 73% at 5 years, compared with 30% for the limb salvage group. This differential persisted at more than 84 months, with a patency rate in the claudication group of 73% and only 13% of patients with limb salvage, demonstrating a more rapid progression of occlusive disease in the limb salvage patient.

The only amputation in the claudication group was a result of an operative complication. Most claudication patients did not develop significant progressive occlusive disease in the follow-up interval, which would have put them in the limb salvage category. Only 18% progressed to a limb salvage status, all of whom were successfully treated with additional vascular reconstructive procedures. An additional 10% had deterioration of walking ability during the course of the follow-up, indicating mild progression of the occlusive disease. The benign course for the remaining 72% of patients in the claudication group was an unexpected finding and gives further support to the concept of patients with claudication having a milder form of atherosclerotic disease.

The importance of collateral flow through the profunda system for healing a below-knee amputation was demonstrated by the high incidence of failure of profunda repairs in patients who required thigh amputations. Seventeen of 19 above-knee amputations were in patients who had failure of their profundaplasties. In the below-knee amputation group, all 24 patients who had successful wound healing maintained patency of their profunda repairs. This emphasizes the importance of profunda circulation for stump healing at the below-knee level to maintain a functional knee joint. It is clear from my experience that the status of profunda circulation should be evaluated, and if significant occlusive disease is found, a profundaplasty should be performed on all patients requiring major limb amputation. Most amputations were required within the first postoperative year, demonstrating the advanced stage of atherosclerotic disease in the limb salvage group. Those patients surviving the first postoperative year without amputation obviously have a less virulent form of occlusive disease.

The only measurable effect of diabetes mellitus in our study was a cumulative limb salvage rate.[7] The 5-year limb salvage rate was 38% in diabetic patients and 60% in nondiabetic patients. This difference approached but did not obtain statistical significance. This was most likely due to the small number of diabetic patients followed longer than 36 months. Profundaplasty for claudication is a durable procedure; however, when performed for limb salvage it only temporarily forestalls the ravages of atherosclerosis, resulting in poor long-term patient survival, limb salvage, and graft patency.

Some insight into why IP is a more durable procedure can be gleaned from the measurement of operative flow after reconstruction, which provides interesting physiologic correlations.[4] The volume of flow after IP (238 mL/min) was higher than after PA (162 mL/min). In a similar study, Cotton et al[8] measured 279 mL/min after IP, compared with 163 mL/min for PA. The volume of flow after IP was higher in patients with claudication (319 mL/min) than those in the limb salvage category (189 mL/min). When I examined the segmental pressure indices to explain this difference, the most significant pressure decrease occurred across the popliteal segment, which suggests that increased resistance across the profunda popliteal collateral bed in patients operated on for limb salvage counted for lower operative flows than were found in patients with claudication. The tibial grading index was the same and did not account for the difference in flows. This agrees with data by Morris-Jones and Jones,[9] who noted after reviewing arteriograms of patients undergoing profundaplasty that the most significant difference in limbs with claudication and severe ischemia was the quality of the collateral bed in the thigh.

Measurable flow with extended profundaplasty was the same as with standard profundaplasty, giving comparable degrees of ischemia and levels of disease. This further supports the concept that when profundaplasty is properly performed, the proximal profunda stenosis is corrected over whatever distance is necessary; the critical difference in terms of results lies in the runoff bed and not to the length of the profundaplasty.

Kalman et al,[10] in a more recent study of isolated profundaplasty, reported excellent results with a cumulative clinical success rate considered as both a patent repair and clinical improvement of 83% at 30 days, 67% at 1 year, 57% at 2 years, and 49% at 3 years. Cumulative limb salvage in this group of patients was 76%. The most significant determinant in this series was that good tibial outflow correlated with greater success than those who had poor tibial outflow. Good tibial outflow is defined as two to three patent tibial arteries, poor was considered zero to one. Ouriel et al[11] reported 2- and 4-year patency rates of 83% and 76% when the middle and distal profunda arteries were used for distal anastomosis of an inflow procedure.

There is a tendency for early results of profundaplasty to be dependent on the length of the endarterectomized patch and the length of the profundaplasty. I analyzed my profundaplasty results according to the length of profundaplasty, dividing it into short (<2 cm), standard (8 cm or beyond the lateral circumflex branch to the first perforator), and extended (>8 cm or beyond the first perforator). In a study comparing standard and extended profundaplasties using autogenous material, 12- and 24-month results generally indicated that the more extensive the patch angioplasty, the lower the cumulative patency.[12] For standard-length profundaplasties using saphenous vein, the 12-month patency was 90%, compared with 80% for endarterectomized superficial femoral artery use as a patch. This is compared with 48% for extended vein angioplasties at 12 months and 60% for extended profundaplasties for use of endarterectomized superficial femoral artery as a patch. These differences tended to decrease with time but were still present at 24 months, where standard-length profundaplasties reconstructed with saphenous vein had a 78% cumulative patency and standard-length profundaplasties reconstructed with endarterectomized superficial femoral artery had an 80% cumulative patency, compared with 60% and 50% for extended profundaplasties. There was no significant difference between endarterectomized superficial femoral artery and autogenous vein used as a patch material. Endarterectomy of an occluded superficial femoral artery can be a reasonable source of patch material, allowing the conservation of what is often a limited amount of vein available for surgical repair.

The results of profundaplasty often are related to the indications for operation. My success with isolated profundaplasty and limb salvage situations was best in patients with ischemic ulcers as the cause, with 53% of profundaplasties being successful, compared with only 32% in rest pain and 35% in patients with ischemic necrosis. These results have caused profundaplasty to take a lesser role to tibial and popliteal artery bypasses in the treatment of critical limb ischemia. If a distal bypass can be performed, certainly with autogenous tissues, results are much better than can be obtained with PA. This limited role of profundaplasty was emphasized by Howard et al.[13] The role of profunda artery reconstruction becomes more important in patients who do not have an adequate vein for distal bypass or who have infected prosthetic grafts originating or terminating in the groin that require removal and as a means of revascularizing legs after failure of prior autogenous lower-leg revascularizations. Profundaplasty remains an important tool in the care of patients with lower-limb occlusive disease, and all vascular surgeons should have a knowledge of the anatomy and physiology of the profunda femoris system to allow proper selection of patients who can benefit by this procedure.

REFERENCES

1. Haimovici H, Shapiro JH, Jacobson HG. Serial femoral arteriography in occlusive disease: clinical-roentgenologic considerations with a new classification of occlusive patterns. *Am J Roentgen.* 1960;83:1042.

2. Mitchell RA, Bone GE, Bridges R, et al. Patient selection for isolated profundaplasty. Arteriographic correlates of operative results. *Am J Surg.* 1979;138:912–919.

3. Boren CH, Towne JB, Bernhard VM, et al. Profundapopliteal collateral index. A guide to successful profundaplasty. *Arch Surg.* 1980;115:1366–1372.

4. McCoy DM, Sanchek AP, Schuler JJ, et al. The role of isolated profundaplasty for the treatment of rest pain. *Arch Surg.* 1989;124:441–444.

5. Sladen J, Burgess JJ. Profundaplasty: expectations and ominous signs. *Am J Surg.* 1980;140:242–245.

6. Towne JB, Bernhard VM, Rollins DL, et al. Profundaplasty in perspective: limitations in the long-term management of limb ischemia. *Surgery.* 1981;90:1037–1046.

7. Towne JB, Rollins DL. Profundaplasty: its role in limb salvage. *Surg Clin North Am.* 1986;66:403–414.

8. Cotton L, Roberts C, Cane F. Valve and the electromagnetic flow meter in arterial reconstruction. In: Roberts VC, ed. *Blood Flow Measurement.* London: Sector Publishing Ltd; 1972:107–110.

9. Morris-Jones W, Jones CDP. Profundaplasty in the treatment of femoropoliteal occlusion. *Am J Surg.* 1974;127:680–686.

10. Kalman PG, Johnston KW, Walker PM. The current role of isolated profundaplasty. *J Cardiovasc Surg.* 1990;13:107–111.

11. Ouriel K, DeWeese JA, Ricotta JJ, et al. Revascularization of the distal profunda femoris artery in the reconstructive treatment of aortoiliac occlusive disease. *J Vasc Surg.* 1987;6:217–220.

12. Rollins DL, Towne JB, Bernhard VM, et al. Endarterectomized superficial femoral artery as an arterial patch. *Arch Surg.* 1985;120:367–369.

13. Howard TR, Bergan JJ, Yao JS, et al. The demise of primary profundaplasty. *Am J Surg.* 1988;156:126–130.

25

Operative Repair of Popliteal Aneurysms:

Twenty-Five Years Experience

*James A. DeWeese, MD, Cynthia Shortell, MD,
Richard Green, MD, and Kenneth Ouriel, MD*

Popliteal arterial aneurysms are uncommon. Dent et al[1] reported only a 2.4% incidence of popliteal aneurysms in 1,488 patients seen with aneurysms of the abdominal aorta and its peripheral branches. During 1958 to 1990, when 1,431 patients underwent operations for abdominal aortic aneurysms at the University of Rochester, only 42 patients with popliteal aneurysms were operated on. However, if a popliteal aneurysm is found, there is a 43% chance that an abdominal aortic aneurysm will be present and also a 43% chance that there is an aneurysm in the opposite popliteal artery.[1-8]

PATHOGENESIS

In the past, syphilis was a frequent cause of popliteal aneurysms, but currently almost all popliteal aneurysms are secondary to arteriosclerosis. Gedge et al[9] pointed out that they usually occur just distal to the tendinous hiatus of the adductor magnus muscle or distal to a fibrous band and the arcuate popliteal ligament at the level of the knee joint. It is therefore possible that these aneurysms are another example of a post-stenotic dilatation of an artery as described and studied by Halsted.[10]

NATURAL HISTORY

Complications of popliteal aneurysms include thrombosis, distal embolization, venous or nerve compression, and rupture. Thrombosis and embolization are responsible for 68% to 80% of the symptoms and pathologic changes seen in untreated aneurysms.[6,11,12] Occlusion of the popliteal artery by thrombus, or the distal vessels by emboli, may result in claudication, rest pain, blue toe syndrome, or gangrene.

Venous compression is seen in less than 10% of symptomatic aneurysms.[6] It may be responsible for distal edema or thrombosis. Nerve compression with pain or neurologic deficit is also described in 8% to 12% of symptomatic patients.[6,12] Rupture is a rare complication but has been described in 3% to 6% of symptomatic patients in recent series.[6,12]

The natural history of all aneurysms is enlargement and finally development of complications. In a collected series of 177 patients with uncomplicated aneurysms followed for less than 4-years average time, 31% became complicated.[7,8,11,12] In general, the development of complications is related to the size of the aneurysms. Whitehouse et al[7] described symptoms in only one (9%) of 11 aneurysms less than 2.0 cm in diameter as compared with 23 (66%) of 35 greater than 2.0 cm in diameter. Gifford et al[11] described the complications in 62 popliteal aneurysms, most of which were greater than 3 cm in diameter. Multiple complications were seen, including 68% thromboembolic, 39% venous compression, 20% nerve compression, and 26% rupture.[11] However, Inahara and Toledo[3] reported nine limbs with acute ischemia secondary to thrombosis of popliteal aneurysms, which were all less than 2.5 cm in diameter.

It is generally agreed that an operation is indicated for a popliteal aneurysm greater than 2 cm in diameter in a medically sound patient.

DIAGNOSIS

The diagnosis may be suspected after palpation but must be confirmed. Computed tomography scans can be definitive. Color duplex scanning is less expensive and can accurately determine the diameter of the vessel and the presence of thrombus in the vessel. Arteriography should be performed and should include visualization of all distal vessels. Although it does not help to determine the size of the aneurysm because of the thrombus lining, it does provide information regarding the vessels proximal and distal to the aneurysm for planning of the operation.

SURGICAL MANAGEMENT

Antyllus, a Greek surgeon in the second century AD, ligated the artery proximal and distal to a popliteal aneurysm and then opened and packed the aneurysm sac.[13] Anel performed proximal ligation of popliteal aneurysms in 1710, and DeSault, a French surgeon, performed a superficial femoral artery ligation for a popliteal aneurysm on June 22, 1785.[13] Hunter performed the same operation on December 12, 1785, and must be credited with popularizing the technique.[13] Matas[14] was the first to treat popliteal aneurysms and still maintain blood flow by performing endoaneurysmorrhaphy as reported in 1920. Linton[15] in 1949 reported successful treatment of 15 patients by performing a lumbar sympathectomy followed by excision of the aneurysm. All these methods of treatment quickly became obsolete with the flourishing of direct arterial reconstructive techniques in the past three decades.

Isolated reports of successful direct reconstructions before the present era were available. In 1907 Enderlen of Wurzburg excised a popliteal aneurysm and was able to perform an end-to-end anastamosis of the cut ends of the popliteal artery. (This method of repair is still possible in some patients with ectatic vessels.[16]) In 1913 Pringle of Glasgow excised a popliteal aneurysm and then restored continuity with an interposition graft.[17] This technique, usually through a posterior approach, was the most common operation performed during the 50s and early 60s.[16,18] In the 60s, however, a number of surgeons began to ligate the popliteal artery and then bypass the excluded aneurysm through a medial approach with end-to-side anastomoses. We performed our first bypass of a doubly ligated aneurysm in 1964. Edwards[19] reported six similar successful operations in 1969 that served to popularize the technique. Various modifications of the method include end-to-end anastomoses proximally, or distally, or both. Towne et al[20] and Wylie[21] have not ligated the artery proximal to the aneurysm in patients where the superior geniculate vessels are patent in hopes of preserving these collateral vessels should graft thrombosis occur.

The type of graft used has changed through the years. Initially autologous veins and arterial homografts were available.[16] Homografts and nylon grafts proved unsatisfactory because of the development of aneurysms.[20,22] Teflon, Dacron, bovine heterografts, umbilical vein grafts, and more recently, polytetrafluoroethylene grafts have been used. Autologous veins remain the graft of choice.

RESULTS OF OPERATION

Patency Rates

Long-term patency rates of grafting procedures reported by the Life Table method are available. Cumulative patency rates of 5 years for series evaluating 40 to 62 operations were 50% to 76%[3-5,12,23] (Table 25–1). Ten-year patency rates were 26% to 76%[3-5,12] (Fig. 25–1). Fifteen-year patency rates were 16% to 64% in two series.[5,12] The wide variation in the 10- and 15-year experiences may be the result of a small number of cases available for observation. Another series of 99 reconstructions who were followed 1 to 14 years (average, 37 months) had a patency rate of 68%.[6]

Patency rates for different types of grafts used for reconstructions were compared in four series, and significant differences between veins and nonvein grafts were found in all series. Five-year patency rates for vein grafts were 77%, 94%, and 89%(1°), and for nonvein grafts were 30%, 43%, and 29%(1°).[23-25] Ten-year patency rates for vein grafts were 94% and 84% and for nonvein grafts were 27% and 40%.[12,25] Vermilion et al[6] reported patency of 7 of 13 polytetrafluoroethylene grafts followed an average of 11 months and of 27 of 39 Dacron grafts followed an average of 53 months. McCollum et al[26] reported good results with Dacron grafts used for popliteal artery reconstruction in 87 patients.

Patency rates were also compared between patients who were symptomatic, had complicated aneurysm, or had limb-threatening findings (usually caused by thrombosis of the aneurysm or peripheral embolization) and those patients who were asymptomatic, had uncomplicated aneurysm, or were operated on electively. Five-year patency rates for reconstructions performed for complicated problems were 54%, 53%(1°) and 39% compared with 82%, 77%(1°) and 92% for uncomplicated problems[4,23,25] (Fig. 25–2). At 10 years, the patency rate was 48% for symptomatic patients and 82% for asymptomatic patients.[25] The differences in Anton's series and the difference in primary patency rates in Schellack's series were not significant. The differences in secondary patency rates at 5 years were significant in Schellack's series.

It has been presumed by many that the decreased patency rate in patients with complicated problems was secondary to peripheral embolization from the thrombus-lined aneurysm.[27] This concept is supported by Shortell et al.[4] Their 5- and 10-year patency rates for 30 patients with two to three vessel runoff was 89% and 64%,

TABLE 25–1. RESULTS OF OPERATION

Reference	Date	Type	No.	Graft (%) Patency			Limb Salvage		
				5 yr	*10 yr*	*15 yr*	*5 yr*	*10 yr*	*15 yr*
Overall									
Inahara and Toledo[3]	1963–1977		40	76	76	—	—	—	—
Szilagyi et al[5]	1964–1979		50	50	26	16	—	—	—
Schellack et al[23]	1965–1985		62	61(1°)	—	—	—	—	—
Dawson et al[12]	1958–1985		57	75	64	64	95	95	95
Shortell et al[4]	1964–1990		51	67	47	—	94	94	—
Type of graft									
Reilly et al[24]	1958–1982	Vein	114	77	—	—	—	—	—
		Dacron	40	30	—	—	—	—	—
Anton et al[25]	1952–1984	Vein	57	94	94	—	98	98	—
		Other	49	43	27	—	75	67	—
Dawson et al[12]	1958–1985	Vein	25	—	84	—	—	—	—
		Other	17	—	40	—	—	—	—
Schellack et al[23]	1965–1985	Vein	32	89(1°)	—	—	—	—	—
		Other	28	29(1°)	—	—	—	—	—
Complicated aneurysm									
Anton et al[25]	1952–1984	Asymptomatic	55	82	82	—	93	93	—
		Symptomatic	68	54	48	—	82	79	—
Shellack et al[23]	1965–1985	Uncomplicated	20	77(1°)	—	—	—	—	—
		Complicated	42	53(1°)	—	—	—	—	—
Shortell et al[4]	1964–1990	Elective	32	92	—	—	100	—	—
		Limb threatening	19	39	—	—	84	—	—
Runoff									
Shortell et al[4]	1964–1990	Good runoff	30	89	64	—	93	—	—
		Poor runoff	11	24	0	—	91	—	—

respectively, compared with 24% and 0% for 11 patients with one or less vessel runoff.[4]

Amputations

The limb salvage rate has also been evaluated by Life Table methods (Table 25–1). The overall salvage rate for 57 patients reported by Dawson et al[12] was 95% 5, 10, and 15 years after operation. The limb salvage rates for 51 patients reported by Shortell et al[4] was 94% at 5 and 10 years. These rated are significantly better than the graft patency rates in the same series (Fig. 25–1). This indicates that only 5% to 6% of the patients in these two series required amputation despite thrombosis of 36% to 53% of their grafts.

Limb salvage was decreased, however, in certain subgroups. Anton et al[25] reported limb salvage rates of 98% at 5- and 10-year follow-up when vein grafts were used for reconstruction as compared with 5- and 10-year salvage rates of 75% and 67% when other grafts were used. In their series, therefore, amputation rates for patients with nonvein grafts at 5 years were 25% at a time when 57% of the grafts were

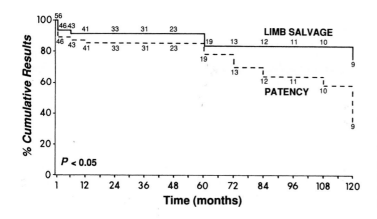

Figure 25–1. Cumulative Life Table patency and limb salvage rates for all bypass grafts. The difference between patency and salvage reaches significance *P*<.05 at 72 months.

thrombosed.[25] They reported similar correlations in asymptomatic and symptomatic aneurysms. Amputation rates at 5 years were 7% for asymptomatic patients when 18% of grafts were thrombosed, but amputation rates were 18% for patients operated on for symptomatic aneurysms when 46% of the grafts were thrombosed.[25] Many patients thrombose their grafts without loss of limb. The discrepancy between patency of grafts and limb salvage may be explainable. There is good collateral circulation consisting primarily of the geniculate arteries around the midpopliteal artery. It is true the amputation rate for acute popliteal artery injuries with the associated trauma in World War I was 43% and World War II was 73%.[28] However, Delhet reported an incidence of gangrene in only 2.77% of 86 cases of popliteal aneurysm treated by "extirpation" without arterial reconstructions between 1888 and 1895.[13] During the same period there was a 7.65% incidence of gangrene after ligation of the aneurysm.[13] An 8.33% incidence of amputation was reported after the Antyllus method consisting of incision and packing of aneurysms.[13] Linton[15] reported no amputations after lumbar sympathectomy and excision of aneurysm in 15 patients. More recent series of aneurysm resections and graft replacement suggested that such good long-term results occur only in patients operated on before embolization and/or progression of distal arteriosclerosis, or associated soft tissue injury prevents collateralized or bypassed popliteal arteries from remaining patent.[27] In some instances where the popliteal artery aneurysm is gradually occluding, the collateral circulation is improving, and severe ischemia is avoided after thrombosis of the artery or graft.

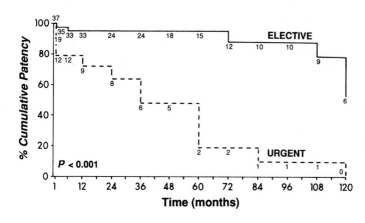

Figure 25–2. Cumulative Life Table patency for patients undergoing operation on an elective basis and those operated on for limb-threatening ischemia. The difference between the two groups reach significance *P*<.001 at 12 months.

New Aneurysms

Towne et al[20] performed 69 graft reconstructions on popliteal aneurysms and observed the development of six new aneurysms involving the popliteal artery proximally or distally to the graft. These were recognized 5 months and 10 years (average, 5.5 years) after the original operations. This unusual occurrence points out the need for continued careful follow-up of these patients.

Enlargement

Schellack et al[23] reported on two patients who continued to complain of discomfort after the ligation and bypass of large popliteal aneurysms. One patient was being followed for "mild discomfort." An "obliterative aneurysmorrhaphy" was performed on the other patient. At operation, "it was evident that well developed geniculate collaterals were responsible for persistent patency and continued enlargement of his aneurysm."[23]

Flynn and Nicholas[29] described two similar patients. One patient had proximal and distal ligation and bypass of a 7 × 10-cm aneurysm and returned 3.5 years later with "aching" in his calf and a 9 × 13-cm nontender aneurysm. An arteriogram showed a patent graft and no contrast material entering the aneurysm. At operation the aneurysm was incised and clot removed. "A small geniculate artery was seen to be feeding the aneurysm distally."[29] The vessel was ligated, and aneurysm walls were plicated. The second patient had similar exclusion procedure of a 5 × 8-cm aneurysm. He returned 13 months later for "painless" swelling. The aneurysm was 7 × 10 cm in size. An arteriogram showed a patent graft with no visualization of the aneurysm. "On opening the aneurysm a large amount of clot and *serum* was removed. A single geniculate artery was found back-bleeding into the aneurysm."[29] The vessel was ligated, and walls of the aneurysm were opposed.[29] Other cases of late enlargement or appearance of compression symptoms of veins or nerves have been described in which no feeding collaterals were identified from outside of the aneurysm.[4] Roberts[30] described a patient with enlargement of a thrombosed popliteal aneurysm from which he aspirated 700 mL of a lymphatic-type fluid. This would suggest that in some patients the enlargement is a result of continued hematoma formation with serous replacement, as is seen in subcutaneous hematomas.

PATIENT SURVIVAL

As true with all peripheral arterial reconstructions, the survival rates after popliteal arterial reconstruction is lower than that of the normal population of similar ages. Five- and 10-year survival rates of about 60% and 40% are reported.[6,12,25] Cardiac deaths usually related to coronary artery disease are responsible for 30% to 50% of the deaths. Stroke is responsible for 6% to 20% of deaths and ruptured aneurysm 3% to 6% of the deaths.[6,12,25]

REFERENCES

1. Dent TL, Lindenauer SM, Ernst CB, et al. Multiple arteriosclerotic arterial aneurysms. *Arch Surg.* 1972;105:338–344.
2. Baird RJ, Sivasankar R, Hayward R, et al. Popliteal aneurysms: a review and analysis of 61 cases. *Surgery.* 1966;59:911–917.

3. Inahara T, Toledo AC. Complications and treatment of popliteal aneurysms. *Surgery.* 1978;84:775–783.
4. Shortell CK, DeWeese JA, Ouriel K, et al. Popliteal artery aneurysms: a 25-year surgical experience. *J Vasc Surg.* 1991;14:771–779.
5. Szilagyi DE, Schwartz RL, Reddy DJ. Popliteal arterial aneurysms. *Arch Surg.* 1981;116: 724–729.
6. Vermilion BD, Kimmins SA, Pace WG, et al. A review of one hundred forty-seven popliteal aneurysms with long-term follow-up. *Surgery.* 1981;90:1009–1014.
7. Whitehouse WM Jr, Wakefield TW, Graham LM, et al. Limb-threatening potential of arteriosclerotic popliteal artery aneurysms. *Surgery.* 1983;93:694–699.
8. Wychulis AR, Spittell JA Jr, Wallace RB. Popliteal aneurysms. *Surgery.* 1970;68:942–952.
9. Gedge SW, Spittel JA Jr, Ivins JC. Aneurysm of the distal popliteal artery and its relationship to the arcuate popliteal ligament. *Circulation.* 1961;24:270–273.
10. Halsted WS. An experimental study of circumscribed dilation of an artery immediately distal to a partially occluding band, and its bearing on the dilation of the subclavian artery observed in certain cases of cervical rib. *J Exp Med.* 1916;24:271.
11. Gifford RW Jr, Hines E Jr, Janes JM. An analysis and follow-up study of one hundred popliteal aneurysms. *Surgery.* 1953;33:384–393.
12. Dawson I, van Bockel JH, Brand R, et al. Popliteal artery aneurysms. *J Vasc Surg.* 1991;13:398–407.
13. Matas R. Surgery of the vascular system. *Keen's Surg.* 1912;5:256–268.
14. Matas R. Endo-aneurismorrhaphy. *Surg Gynecol Obstet.* 1920;30:456–459.
15. Linton RR. The arteriosclerotic popliteal aneurysm. *Surgery.* 1949;26:41–58.
16. Julian OC, Dye WS, Javid H, et al. The use of vessel grafts in the treatment of popliteal aneurysms. *Surgery.* 1955;38:970–980.
17. Pringle JH. Two cases of vein-grafting for the maintenance of a direct arterial circulation. *Lancet.* 1913;1:1795–1796.
18. Austin DJ, Thompson JE. Excision and arterial grafting in the surgical management of popliteal aneurysms. *South Med J.* 1958;51:43–48.
19. Edwards S. Exclusion and saphenous vein bypass of popliteal aneurysms. *Surg Gynecol Obstet.* 1969;128:829–830.
20. Towne JB, Thompson JE, Patman DD, et al. Progression of popliteal aneurysmal disease following popliteal aneurysm resection with graft: A twenty year experience. *Surgery.* 1976;80:426–432.
21. Wylie EJ (discussion in Wychulis AR). Popliteal aneurysms. *Surgery.* 1970;68:951–952.
22. Barner HB, DeWeese JA, Dale WA, et al. Aneurysmal degeneration of femoropopliteal arterial homografts. *JAMA.* 1966;631–634.
23. Schellack J, Smith RB III, Perdue GD. Nonoperative management of selected popliteal aneurysms. *Arch Surg.* 1987;122:372–375.
24. Reilly MK, Abbott WM, Darling, RC. Aggressive surgical management of popliteal artery aneurysms. *Am J Surg.* 1983;145:498–502.
25. Anton GE, Hertzer NR, Beven EG, et al. Surgical management of popliteal aneurysms. *J Vasc Surg.* 1986;3:125–134.
26. McCollum CH, DeBakey ME, Myhre HO. Popliteal aneurysms: results of 87 operations performed between 1957 and 1977. *Cardiovasc Res Cen Bull.* 1983;21:93–100.
27. Bouhoutsos J, Martin P. Popliteal aneurysm: a review of 116 cases. *Br J Surg.* 1974;61: 469–475.
28. DeBakey ME, Simone FA. *Vascular Surgery in World War II.* Washington, DC: US Government Printing Office; 1955.
29. Flynn JB, Nicholas GG. An unusual complication of bypassed popliteal aneurysms. *Arch Surg.* 1983;118:111–113.
30. Roberts B. (discussion in Shortell CK). Popliteal artery aneurysms: a 25-year surgical experience. *J Vasc Surg.* 1991;14:771–779.

26

Influence of Warfarin Therapy on Infrainguinal Polytetrafluoroethylene Bypass

B. Timothy Baxter, MD, Walter J. McCarthy, MD, William H. Pearce, MD, James S. T. Yao, MD, PhD, and William R. Flinn, MD

Direct arterial bypass remains the most commonly used, hemodynamically effective, and most durable treatment for infrainguinal arterial occlusive disease.[1–4] The long-term patency of these grafts may be influenced by a variety of factors including patient age, underlying disease process, and distal arterial anatomy[5,6]; however, no factor is more identifiably influential on infrainguinal graft patency than whether the graft material used is autogenous vein or a prosthetic material. The presence of a biologically active endothelium makes autogenous vein grafts less thrombogenic than any prosthetic material throughout the lifetime of the graft. The superior performance of autogenous grafts is most evident when bypass is performed to vessels below the knee, and prospective studies have confirmed the statistically superior long-term patency for autogenous vein compared with expanded polytetrafluoroethylene (PTFE) for below-knee bypass.[7,8] This recognition has led some surgeons to abandon the use of prosthetic bypass to infragenicular vessels but has also stimulated the more aggressive pursuit of techniques for increased use of autogenous materials such as *in situ* grafting,[9] upper extremity veins,[10,11] nonreversed vein grafts, and composite grafts.[12] Despite these recognized differences in performance and innovative techniques to maximize autogenous graft usage, vein of adequate length and diameter for more distal bypasses is simply not clinically available in some cases. Although primary amputation may be an alternative for "limb salvage" in such cases, most would consider this therapeutic and philosophic approach inconsistent. It has seemed logical, therefore, to investigate whether the durability of infrainguinal PTFE bypass grafts could be improved with the adjuvant use of some regimen of antithrombotic therapy.

It was initially believed that the administration of antiplatelet medications such as aspirin (ASA) and/or dipyridamole would improve the patency of infrainguinal prosthetic grafts because of their early antithrombotic effect and the late prevention of perianastomotic fibrous hyperplasia, the pathologic process that is most frequently associated with intermediate PTFE graft failure (3 to 24 months). Despite the routine administration of these medications to all patients in their study, the 4-year patency of PTFE bypass grafts to tibial and peroneal vessels was only 12% in the study of Veith et al.[7] Low-molecular-weight Dextran (Dextran-40), a hemorrheologic agent with antiplatelet activity, has also been investigated as a means of improving early infrainguinal bypass graft patency. Rutherford et al[13] noted an improvement in early prosthetic distal bypass patency in patients treated with perioperative Dextran-40; however, the observed therapeutic effect was short-lived. This observation led the authors to speculate about the use of extended antithrombotic therapy with agents such as warfarin, especially in nonvein distal bypass grafts.

Experience in our own institution with patients requiring repetitive distal bypass procedures[14] led to the identification of a group of patients with infragenicular PTFE grafts that had been maintained on long-term warfarin therapy empirically because of repeated graft failures. A retrospective review of this subgroup[15] revealed a statistically significant improvement in 4-year graft patency compared with similarly matched historic controls (37% versus 12%; $P<.05$). Obvious concern existed about the validity of this comparison because this was not a prospective study of patients undergoing *primary* (surgical and pharmacologic) therapy. These observations, however, stimulated the investigation of the routine prospective use of postoperative antithrombotic therapy with heparin and warfarin in all patients requiring below-knee PTFE bypass grafts in hopes of more accurately documenting the use and potential risks of this therapeutic approach. This chapter examines the clinical course and late graft patency of patients who had *primary* below-knee bypass with PTFE bypass and were treated with this regimen of long-term anticoagulant therapy.

PATIENT POPULATION

A total of 45 patients (32 men, 13 women) had 47 primary PTFE bypass grafts to the popliteal or infragenicular (anterior tibial, posterior tibial, or peroneal) arteries below the knee and were prospectively placed on long-term systemic warfarin postoperatively. Bypass was to the below-knee popliteal artery in 24 cases and to infrapopliteal vessels in 23 cases (AT = 12, PT = 9, peroneal = 2). Polytetrafluoroethylene grafts used included straight (6-mm popliteal) and tapered (6.5- to 4.5-mm crural) at the discretion of the operating surgeon. Procedures were considered *primary* when no previous infrainguinal surgical revascularization procedure had been attempted in the ipsilateral extremity. This group represented only 5% of all distal bypass procedures performed at our institution during this period, reflecting our commitment to autogenous vein bypass whenever possible.

The risk factors for peripheral vascular disease included diabetes mellitus (38%), hypertension (36%), and tobacco use (47%). Limb-threatening ischemia was the indication for operation in 45 cases (96%), whereas in two cases, patients (4%) were severely limited by claudication. The manifestations of severe ischemia included 23 with rest pain, 11 with nonhealing ulcers, and 11 with gangrene. The mean preoperative ankle/brachial index was 0.4 ± 0.04 for this group of patients.

SURGICAL MANAGEMENT

All grafts originated from the common femoral artery (43) or the femoral limb of an aortobifemoral graft (4). Standard operative administration of intravenous heparin

(100 U/kg) before arterial clamping was used routinely, and protamine reversal was not used in any case. The technical adequacy of the distal anastomosis was examined by completion angiography, angioscopy, or both, and direct exploration was performed when any abnormality was suggested by one of these studies.

A continuous heparin infusion (500 to 1,000 U/h) was begun in the recovery room, and the dose was subsequently titrated to maintain the partial thromboplastin time 2 to 2.5 times control values (60 to 80 seconds). Warfarin therapy was initiated once the PTT was controlled and the patient had resumed oral intake, usually within 48 hours after operation. The therapeutic goal of the warfarin was to increase the prothrombin time (PT) to 50% above control values (18 to 22 seconds) before discharge. None of the patients in this study had an identifiable coagulation disorder (protein C, protein S, or antithrombin III deficiency) where the use of warfarin therapy would clearly have been essential to maintain graft patency, making results appear more favorable. Additionally, all grafts were performed entirely with PTFE; no sequential or composite grafts were included.

Patients were seen in follow-up at least every 3 months after discharge for the first 2 years and every 6 months thereafter unless new ischemic symptoms arose. The mean follow-up for the 47 distal bypass grafts was 24 months (range, 7 to 72 months). Graft patency was determined in every case by serial noninvasive testing in addition to the direct patient examination, and only *primary* patency of these grafts was assessed.

OBSERVATIONS

The cumulative Life Table (Kaplan-Meier) patency rates for all grafts studied were 53% at 2 years and 44% at 4 years (Fig. 26–1). Although the patency for below-knee femoropopliteal and infragenicular bypass grafts were not different at 2 years (56% and 62%, respectively), there was continued attrition in the infrapopliteal bypass group, resulting in an observed patency rate of 36% at 4 years, whereas patency remained stable in the below-knee popliteal group (56%) (Fig. 26–2). When compared with historic controls treated with antiplatelet medications from the multicenter study involving this institution, patency was improved by anticoagulant therapy in patients

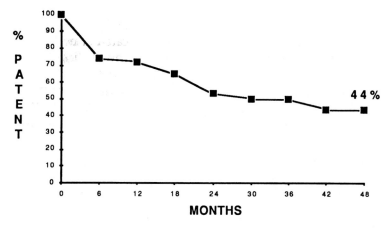

Figure 26–1. Cumulative patency rate for all primary below-knee polytetrafluoro-ethylene (PTFE) bypass grafts treated with long-term anticoagulation was 53% at 2 years, whereas the 4-year patency rate was 44%.

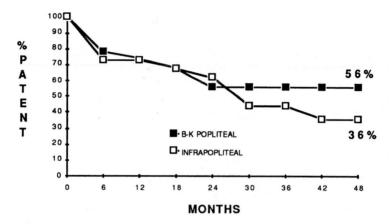

Figure 26–2. Cumulative graft patency rate for primary polytetrafluoroethylene (PTFE) bypass to the below-knee (BK) popliteal and infrapopliteal vessels in patients treated with long-term warfarin therapy was 56% and 36%, respectively, at 4 years.

with primary infragenicular grafts. The 2- and 4-year patency rates for below-knee popliteal bypasses (56%) did not differ from ASA-treated historic controls (54%). The ankle–brachial index increased significantly in all limbs from a preoperative mean value of 0.4 ± 0.02 to 0.9 ± 0.03 postoperative ($P<.01$).

At the time of clinically documented graft occlusion, PT was measured in 18 patients and found to be subtherapeutic (<15 seconds) in eight (44%). This observation led us to logically question whether graft thrombosis in such cases was more the result of a lack of pharmacologic control of the medication than a failure of the antithrombotic therapy to provide benefit. If these patients were excluded from the statistical analysis of primary patency, the 2- and 4-year cumulative patency rates for all below-knee PTFE grafts in this study would have been 63% and 49%, which are quite respectable primary patency rates for below-knee bypass with any graft material.

COMPLICATIONS

The morbidity and mortality of the study group is shown in Table 26–1. Anticoagulation in the immediate postoperative period was implicated in the development of five wound hematomas (11%) that required operative evacuation. There were three

TABLE 26–1. MORBIDITY AND MORTALITY OF THE STUDY GROUP

Complication	Patients	%
Early		
Hematoma	5	11
Wound infection	3	6
Minor amputation	2	4
Death	1	2
Late		
Graft infection	0	0
Bleeding	2	4
Death	5	11

wound infections in this series, all of which developed in patients with postoperative hematomas; however, no patient in this study developed a graft infection.

Warfarin therapy had to be discontinued in two patients (4% of the study group) 1 month and 9 months postoperatively because of serious bleeding complications. One patient developed significant gastrointestinal hemorrhage and one had a spontaneous retroperitoneal hematoma. Both required transfusion and reversal of anticoagulation. Shortly thereafter, graft thrombosis occurred in both limbs, and ultimately major amputation was required in one patient. In both patients the PT was in excess of 25 seconds when bleeding occurred.

Two patients failed to heal foot ulcers despite patent grafts and required transmetatarsal amputations, which healed successfully. After thrombosis of the primary bypass, revision was attempted in 11 of 23 cases, and secondary patency was achieved in eight of these limbs (73%). Fourteen patients eventually required major amputation (above-knee or below-knee) after ultimate failure of reconstructive attempts. The 2- and 4-year cumulative limb salvage rates were 74% and 65% for the period of this study (Fig. 26–3).

There was one postoperative death (2%) caused by myocardial infarction, which was unrelated to postoperative anticoagulation, and five late deaths related to coronary (3) and cerebrovascular (2) disease. All but one of these late deaths occurred well after graft thrombosis and *cessation* of warfarin therapy. The overall mortality in this study group was thus 13% over the 6-year period of this review, and the long-term warfarin treatment did not identifiably contribute to an increased risk of late mortality.

DISCUSSION

Through the synthesis and elaboration of specific vasoactive proteins, the confluent, biologically active endothelial surface of normal arteries and veins naturally resists thrombus formation. It is, therefore, understandable that autogenous vein is the most durable conduit for infrainguinal arterial bypass. Autogenous vein may not be available, however, in as many as 20% to 40% of patients[9] because of previous

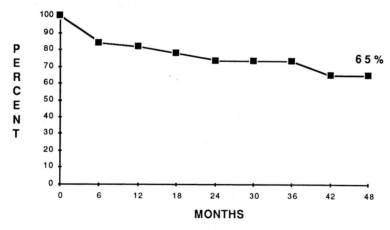

Figure 26–3. Cumulative limb salvage for polytetrafluoroethylene (PTFE) grafts to below-knee (BK) popliteal and crural vessels in patients treated with long-term warfarin therapy was 74% and 65% at 2 and 4 years, respectively.

coronary or lower extremity bypass or because it is morphologically inadequate. In these cases, when the limb is threatened with critical ischemia, the use of revascularization with a prosthetic graft has logically been questioned. Veith et al[7] reported a 12% 4-year patency rate for prosthetic infrapopliteal grafts, and a similarly compromised 5-year patency rate of 18% was reported by Kent et al.[16] These observations led us to adopt the empiric use of systemic anticoagulation in patients with previous graft failures who required repetitive distal prosthetic bypass. We noted an observed improvement in 4-year patency (37%) for infrapopliteal PTFE grafts,[15] but this original patient group was extremely nonhomogeneous and was retrospectively reviewed. In the present review, the 4-year cumulative patency for prospectively studied, *primary* infragenicular PTFE grafts was 36%. The similarity of these patency figures suggests that this is an effect of the therapy rather than a function of some unknown component of patient selection.

Early experimental work suggested that ASA and dipyridamole, through the inhibition of platelet-derived growth factors, could reduce the formation of fibrous hyperplastic lesions that compromised the patency of prosthetic distal bypass grafts.[17,18] However, there has been inconsistent clinical documentation of a beneficial effect of this therapy in femoral-distal bypass grafting in humans.[19–21] Aspirin may improve the *early* patency rates in both aortocoronary grafts and lower extremity bypass grafts when it is started preoperatively and continued in the early postoperative period.[19,21–25] This suggests that the benefit is related to the *antithrombotic* effect of these medications rather than an *antiproliferative* effect on fibrous hyperplasia. Additionally, there has been an increasing uncertainty about the precise role of platelets and platelet-derived growth factor in the development of fibrous hyperplasia.[26]

Warfarin has no known pharmacologic effect on any of the growth factors thus identified nor on the development of fibrous hyperplasia. Nevertheless, in our two separate studies this therapy has resulted in improved patency rates in infragenicular PTFE grafts compared with similar grafts in the study of Veith et al,[7] in which all patients were treated with antiplatelet medications. Clearly it would be necessary to perform a randomized prospective comparison of these treatment regimens to be scientifically sound, but the inconsistent therapeutic effect of ASA and dipyridamole to date may not justify such a study in infragenicular grafts.

Dicumarol, a warfarin-like anticoagulant, has been shown by Kretschmer et al[27] to improve the intermediate patency (30 months) of femoropopliteal vein grafts in a randomized, prospective clinical comparison. The prospective treatment of below-knee femoropopliteal PTFE grafts with warfarin in the present study produced *no* identifiable improvement in graft patency compared with historic controls (56% versus 54%). It is uncertain why similar therapy would not have the same beneficial effect observed by Kretschmer et al[27] on the more thrombogenic PTFE grafts studied here. One possible explanation for this discrepancy is that the control group in the study of Kretschmer et al apparently received no antiplatelet medications postoperatively, which may have served to widen the discrepancy in observed patency rates for the two groups in their study.

In the present study of primary PTFE bypasses, it is interesting to note that the 2-year patency for infragenicular grafts was 62% compared with the 45% 2-year patency observed in our previous study.[15] This may reflect our current, more aggressive approach to the adequate maintenance of therapeutic warfarin levels because this appeared to have an impact on graft failure in the original study. Still, however, 44% of the patients in the prospectively treated group who presented with graft occlusion had *subtherapeutic PT*. The maintenance of therapeutic levels of warfarin therapy clearly remains a critical clinical problem among patients in whom this therapeutic strategy is used. Continued follow-up over extended periods will be necessary to more accurately delineate its true effect.

The 4-year patency rate of 56% for PTFE grafts to the below-knee popliteal in this study was similar to the 54% reported by Veith et al[7] for identical procedures treated with ASA and dipyridamole alone. The more dramatic effect on crural bypass patency (36% versus 12%) may in part be explained by an assumption that infragenicular PTFE grafts may function much closer to the functionally critical level of blood flow velocity[28,29] below which thrombus formation would normally occur in untreated patients. Although a randomized comparison of antiplatelet and anticoagulant therapy in the specific group of patients requiring below-knee femoropopliteal PTFE grafts would seem justified (because the impact of warfarin therapy on the patency of these grafts appears less certain), the small numbers of primary prosthetic grafts performed would require multicenter participation.

The reluctance to use anticoagulant therapy postoperatively in this elderly population has been based on obvious concern about hemorrhagic complications. Early postoperative bleeding complications continue to be a problem and occurred in 11% of cases in this study. The incidence of wound infection continues to be higher in these patients, but no graft infections occurred. The morbidity of long-term anticoagulation in the elderly has been studied extensively in patients with deep venous thrombosis and prosthetic heart valves. In a study of 321 patients of various ages on warfarin, Gurwitz et al[30] demonstrated that age alone was not a significant risk factor for bleeding complications. Although the late mortality rate (22%) in the study of Kretschmer et al[27] using postoperative dicumarol was substantial, none of the deaths was identifiably related to the anticoagulant therapy, a finding similar to that of our own first report.[15] As demonstrated by the two late hemorrhagic complications in the present study, the risk of bleeding is increased significantly when the PT exceeds twice control values. Frequent monitoring of the PT, especially in the first several months after initiation of therapy, is critical to both the safety and efficacy of the therapy. Both graft failure and bleeding complications were associated with PTs outside the desired therapeutic range.

In this unselected, consecutive series of patients undergoing primary below-knee PTFE bypass, long-term anticoagulation with warfarin was effective in improving patency in grafts to the infrapopliteal vessels when compared with historic controls treated with antiplatelet medications. Patency was not improved in the below-knee femoropopliteal grafts in this study when compared with these same historic controls. Overall, limb salvage rates were 74% and 65% at 2 and 4 years in patients treated with postoperative warfarin therapy. Although autogenous vein remains the conduit of choice, infrainguinal bypass grafting with PTFE should be considered a viable option when vein is not available, even if bypass is carried to the below-knee levels. Early anticoagulation with heparin followed by long-term anticoagulation with warfarin should be considered in all prosthetic grafts to the crural vessels. The benefit of this therapy in below-knee femoropopliteal bypass is less clear, but it may be indicated in selected cases where poor runoff would be expected to severely limit graft flow rates.

Acknowledgment

This work was supported in part by the Alyce F. Salerno Foundation.

REFERENCES

1. Harrington ME, Schwartz ME, Sanborn TA, et al. Expanded indications for laser-assisted balloon angioplasty in peripheral arterial disease. *J Vasc Surg.* 1990;11:146–154.

2. Hewes RC, White RI, Murray RR, et al. Long-term results of superficial femoral artery angioplasty. *AJR.* 1986;146:1025–1029.

3. Simpson JB, Selmon MR, Robertson GC, et al. Transluminal atherectomy for occlusive peripheral vascular disease. *Am J Cardiol.* 1988;61:96G–101G.

4. Dalman RL, Taylor LM. Basic data related to infrainguinal revascularization procedures. *Ann Vasc Surg.* 1990;4:309–312.

5. O'Mara CS, Flinn WR, Neiman HL, et al. Correlation of foot arterial anatomy with early tibial bypass patency. *Surgery.* 1981;89:743–752.

6. Imparato AM, Kim GE, Madayag M, et al. Angiographic criteria for successful tibial arterial reconstructions. *Surgery.* 1973;74:830.

7. Veith FJ, Gupta SK, Ascer E, et al. Six-year prospective multicenter randomized comparison of autologous saphenous vein and expanded polytetrafluoroethylene grafts: infrainguinal arterial reconstruction. *J Vasc Surgery.* 1986;3:104–114.

8. Veteran Administration Cooperative Study Group 141. Comparative evaluation of prosthetic, reversed, and *in situ* vein bypass grafts in distal popliteal and tibial-peroneal revascularization. *Arch Surg.* 1988;123:434–438.

9. Leather RP, Shah DM, Karmody AM. Infrapopliteal arterial bypass for limb salvage: increased patency and utilization of saphenous vein *in situ. Surgery.* 1981;90:1001–1008.

10. Harris RW, Andros G, Dulawa LB, et al. Successful long-term limb salvage using cephalic vein bypass grafts. *Ann Surg.* 1984;200:785–792.

11. Graham JW, Lusby RJ. Infrapopliteal bypass grafting: use of upper limb vein alone and in autogenous composite grafts. *Surgery.* 1982;91:646–649.

12. LaSalle AJ, Brewster DC, Corson JD, et al. Femoropopliteal composite bypass grafts: current status. *Surgery.* 1982;92:36–39.

13. Rutherford RB, Jones DN, Bergentz SE, et al. The efficacy of Dextran-40 in preventing early postoperative thrombosis following difficult lower extremity bypass. *J Vasc Surg.* 1984;1:765–772.

14. Bartlett ST, Olinde AJ, Flinn WR, et al. The reoperative potential of infrainguinal bypass: long-term limb and patient survival. *J Vasc Surg.* 1987;5:170–179.

15. Flinn WR, Rohrer MJ, Yao JST, et al. Improved long-term patency of infragenicular polytetrafluoroethylene grafts. *J Vasc Surg.* 1988;7:685–690.

16. Kent KC, Whittemore AD, Mannick JA. Short-term and mid-term results of an all-autogenous tissue policy for infrainguinal reconstruction. *J Vasc Surg.* 1989;9:107–114.

17. Hobson RW, Lynch TG, Jamil Z, et al. Results of revascularization and amputation in severe lower extremity ischemia: a five year clinical experience. *J Vasc Surg.* 1985;2:174–185.

18. Rutherford RB, Jones DN, Bergentz SE, et al. Factors affecting the patency of infrainguinal bypass. *J Vasc Surg.* 1988;8:236–246.

19. Green RM, Roederscheimer R, DeWeese JA. Effects of aspirin and dipyridamole on expanded polytetrafluoroethylene graft patency. *Surgery.* 1982;92:1016–1026.

20. Kohler TR, Kaufman JL, Kacoyanis G, et al. Effect of aspirin and dipyridamole on the patency of lower extremity bypass grafts. *Surgery.* 1984;96:462–466.

21. Clyne CAC, Archer TJ, Atuhaire LK, et al. Random control trial of a short course of aspirin and dipyridamole for femorodistal grafts. *Br J Surg.* 1987;74:246–248.

22. Mayer JE, Lindsay WG, Castaneda W, et al. Influence of aspirin and dipyridamole on patency of coronary artery bypass grafts. *Ann Thorac Surg.* 1981;31:204–210.

23. Chesebro JH, Clements IP, Fuster V, et al. A platelet-inhibitor-drug trial in coronary-artery bypass operations: benefit of perioperative dipyridamole and aspirin therapy on early post-operative vein-graft patency. *N Engl J Med.* 1982;307:73–78.

24. Lorenz RL, Schacky CV, Weber M, et al. Improved aortocoronary bypass patency by low dose aspirin (100 mg daily): effects on platelet aggregation and thromboxane formation. *Lancet.* 1984;1:1261–1264.

25. Brown BG, Cukingnan RA, DeRouen T, et al. Improved graft patency in patients treated with platelet inhibiting therapy after coronary bypass surgery. *Circulation.* 1985;72:138–146.

26. Clowes AW. The role of aspirin in enhancing arterial graft patency. *J Vasc Surg.* 1986;3:381–385.

27. Kretschmer G, Wenzl E, Piza E, et al. The influence of anticoagulant treatment on the probability of function in femoropopliteal vein bypass surgery: analysis of a clinical series (1970–1985) and interim evaluation of a controlled clinical trial. *Surgery.* 1987;102:453–459.
28. Bandyk DF, Cato RF, Towne JB. A low flow velocity predicts failure of femoropopliteal and femorotibial bypass grafts. *Surgery.* 1985;98:799–807.
29. Sauvage LR, Walker MW, Berger KG, et al. Current arterial prosthesis. *Arch Surg.* 1979;114:687–691.
30. Gurwitz JH, Goldberg RJ, Holden A, et al. Age-related risks of long-term oral anticoagulation therapy. *Arch Int Med.* 1988;148:1733–1736.

V

Visceral Artery Reconstruction

27

Chronic Visceral Ischemia

Ronald J. Stoney, MD, and
Christopher G. Cunningham, LCDR, MC, USNR

HISTORY

The early clinical experience with chronic visceral ischemia was marked by controversy. This began nearly a century ago, when Councilman[1] reported three patients with chronic occlusion of the superior mesenteric artery associated with abdominal pain. His suggestion that the gradual occlusion of the major visceral arteries could lead to intestinal ischemia causing abdominal pain was not widely accepted. The remarkable capacity of the mesenteric circulation to form collateral networks had been carefully studied by Chiene[2] in 1869. He described these collaterals in a patient with complete occlusion of the origins of the major visceral arteries, without concomitant intestinal infarction. The relationship between chronic visceral arterial occlusion and abdominal pain was dismissed by Osler[3] as a variant of angina pectoris, the result of coexisting coronary artery disease.

More than 40 years later in 1936, Dunphy[4] correctly established the relationship between chronic intestinal ischemia resulting from atherosclerotic obstruction of the major visceral branches and abdominal pain. He recognized the clinical syndrome of chronic postprandial abdominal pain, weight loss, and altered intestinal motility in seven of 12 patients dying of intestinal infarction. It was this symptom complex Mikkelson[5] termed *intestinal angina*. One year later, in 1958, Shaw and Maynard[6] reported the first successful surgical treatment for intestinal angina: superior mesenteric artery (SMA) thromboendarterectomy. Subsequently, reimplantation and the popular bypass techniques were also introduced for visceral revascularization. In 1962 Morris et al[7] described retrograde prosthetic bypass grafting from the infrarenal aorta to the mesenteric arteries and Fry and Kraft,[8] concerned about prosthetic graft thrombosis or erosion of adjacent viscera resulting in the dreaded complication of infection or prosthetic-enteric fistula, used autogenous vein bypass. In 1966, Stoney and Wylie[9] introduced both transaortic visceral thromboendarterectomy and antegrade aortovisceral bypass originating from the supraceliac aorta. Transaortic visceral endarterectomy provided durable inflow for the short high flow ensured a complete simultaneous revascularization of both major visceral branches, and antegrade aortovisceral bypass provided durable inflow for the short, high-flow grafts.

The history of chronic visceral ischemia from its recognition as a clinical entity to current surgical management concepts has been accompanied by improvements in diagnostic imaging, anesthesia, surgical nutrition, and critical care. As we approach a half century of surgical treatment of chronic visceral ischemia, we must examine not only our clinical results but also challenge concepts that may inadvertently limit the expansion of our knowledge in clinical science of visceral ischemia.

ETIOLOGY

Although there are numerous possible causes for chronic occlusion of the mesenteric arteries, atherosclerosis is responsible for more than 95% of cases. Atherosclerotic plaque of the anterior paravisceral aortic surface (ventral) encroaches on the orifice and appears to spill over into the proximal visceral branches. These so-called ostial lesions are proximal, which allows for the development of a protective distal collateral arterial network. Usually, at least two of the three major visceral branches [celiac axis (CA), SMA, and inferior mesenteric artery (IMA)] are severely stenotic or occluded, which causes splanchnic circulatory insufficiency leading to intestinal ischemia.

The ischemic basis of intestinal angina is widely accepted; however, the precise mechanism by which ischemia mediates this pain remains unclear. Severe pain occurs only after meals, implying that postprandial increased oxygen demands are greater than the collaterals can supply. Most patients experience this pain within 15 to 20 minutes of eating, suggesting that food ingestion increases the demand for gastric blood flow, thereby creating a steal from the remaining gastrointestinal tract.

Other infrequent cases of chronic visceral ischemia include "coral reef" atheroma, an unusual exophytic, calcific, polypoid lesion in the lumen of the paravisceral aorta that produces chronic intestinal ischemia by obstructing the orifices of the major visceral branches.[10] Although most patients with this pattern of atherosclerosis present with renovascular hypertension and claudication, almost one-fourth have chronic visceral ischemia.

Rare nonatheromatous causes of chronic visceral ischemia include radiation and autoimmune arteritis, fibromuscular hyperplasia,[11] coarctation of the abdominal aorta, and celiac artery compression by the median arcuate ligament.[12] The pathophysiology of this latter syndrome is unclear, and its potential for causing chronic visceral ischemia remains controversial. This chapter will discuss only atherosclerosis, which is the major cause of visceral branch obstruction and chronic visceral ischemia.

CLINICAL PRESENTATION

Chronic visceral ischemia has an insidious onset that quietly starves the affected patient and, if not detected, leads to inanition and fatal intestinal gangrene. It is caused by the gradual atherosclerotic occlusion of the major visceral branches of the aorta. When the demands for splanchnic blood flow during digestion exceed the capacity of the visceral collateral network, intestinal angina ensues.

The clinical syndrome may be gradual in onset and subtle in character. Abdominal pain that is typically midabdominal in location, postprandial in time, and crampy in nature associated with aversion to eating and weight loss are the hallmarks of this disorder. A substantial number may also complain of gastrointestinal motility disturbances (nausea, occasional vomiting, diarrhea, or constipation). Patients are predominantly women in the sixth and seventh decade of life. Physical findings are not diagnostic, although most patients will have an epigastric bruit. Laboratory studies are nonspecific.

The vague presentation and progressive nature of chronic visceral ischemia suggest a differential diagnosis ranging from malignancy to malingering. The index of suspicion for this disorder rises dramatically if a thorough evaluation of weight loss and postprandial abdominal pain fails to provide an etiology.

Biplane aortography is essential to confirm the diagnosis. The anterior–posterior projections demonstrate visceral collateral pathways; the lateral aortic projections visualize the proximal SMA and CA in profile and the aortic origins of these branches. Magnetic resonance angiography of the paravisceral aorta is currently being developed and, in the future, may supplant aortography as the preferred noninvasive imaging study.

The goal of therapy is restoration of normal mesenteric blood flow. This usually provides long-term relief of symptoms, restoration of gastrointestinal function, and freedom from the threat of fatal visceral infarction. The realization of these goals begins with early recognition of this syndrome by the astute clinician. Profound wasting and malnutrition seen in the advanced stages of this disease increase the risks of treatment morbidity.

VISCERAL REVASCULARIZATION EVOLUTION

The surgical treatment of chronic visceral ischemia began with transarterial endarterectomy.[6] Although reimplantation was introduced, it was a difficult option to master. Retrograde prosthetic autogenous bypass became the preferred visceral revascularization. The reasons were obvious. Exposure of distal trunks or branches of the major visceral arteries was simple, and infrarenal exposure was a familiar region of the aorta and at low risk for clamping. However, Williams[13] correctly noted that the early reports of these retrograde grafts lacked any significant follow-up data. This suggested that this method of visceral revascularization would not protect the patient against the threat of fatal visceral infarction if late graft failure occurred.

There was a clear challenge to develop durable methods of visceral revascularization among those surgeons interested in this rare problem. However, the desire to introduce direct approaches for the repair of the CA and SMA was not supported by some who suggested that direct repair was dangerous, unnecessary, and technically ambitious.[7,8,14] Visceral artery reconstruction began at the University of California, San Francisco in 1959, and during the early years, transarterial endarterectomy and reimplantation were the favored techniques. However, the endarterectomy technique restricted the resection of the para ostial aortic atheroma. This contributed to the early recurrence of visceral ischemia because progression of the unresected aortic disease impaired flow again into the operated visceral branch. This was previously observed in transrenal endarterectomy and led to our introduction of transaortic renal endarterectomy,[15] which eliminated these concerns.

The transaortic endarterectomy technique demands an unrestricted access to the paravisceral aorta and the ability to mobilize and control this segment and all involved branches. This required that our initial approach to the upper abdominal aorta combine transthoracic and retroperitoneal abdominal (Pillsbury) incisions. This provided complete unrestricted aortic access and circumferential mobilization and control of the upper abdominal aorta and branches as required.[16] This approach facilitates transaortic visceral endarterectomy, as well as combined transaortic visceral and renal endarterectomy, when indicated. More recently, we have introduced left medial visceral rotation for elective transaortic visceral endarterectomy.[17] This is accomplished entirely through an abdominal incision and avoids the morbidity of left thoracotomy. It does not compromise aortic exposure or the technical maneuvers required for extraction endarterectomy of the visceral or renal branches. It is now our preferred approach to the upper abdominal and distal thoracic aorta for any recon-structive procedure.

At about the same time, our experience with managing patients with failed retrograde aortovisceral prosthetic bypass performance elsewhere heightened our concern about the concept of retrograde bypass, which Williams had also emphasized. It was anticipated that the transabdominal exposure of the supraceliac, subdiaphrag-matic aorta occasionally required for aortic control in redo procedures and aneurysm rupture would provide an ideal site for the aortic implantation of a visceral bypass graft. Using this approach, with mobilization and caudad displacement of the pancreas, it was consistently possible to expose the celiac axis and superior mesenteric artery in soft undiseased portions beyond the orifice atheroma. This allowed the creation of an antegrade aortovisceral bypass using small straight or bifurcated Dacron prostheses to revascularize one or both of the major visceral branches.[18] The procedure was reserved for those high-risk patients who were disabled and nutrition-ally crippled by neglected chronic intestinal ischemia. This techinque appeared to present a low-risk, less-threatening procedure than the more demanding exposure for endarterectomy, which could be extended to renal as well as visceral branches and often is combined with infrarenal aortic reconstruction. Aortovisceral bypass was purposely restricted, because of its limited exposure, only to those patients requiring visceral revascularization.

Transaortic Visceral Endarterectomy

Transaortic visceral endarterectomy was used in 48 patients in the past two decades at UCSF.[17] The medial visceral rotation to expose the upper abdominal aorta is the

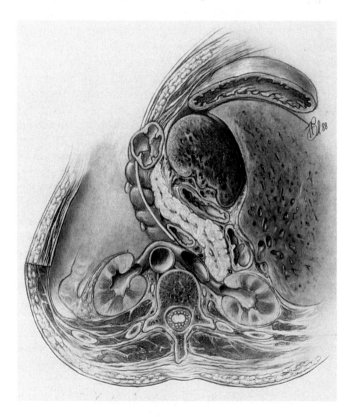

Figure 27–1. Medial visceral rotation approach to aorta. Note that the kidney remains in its anatomic location while other abdominal viscera are displaced medially after mobilization from the left.

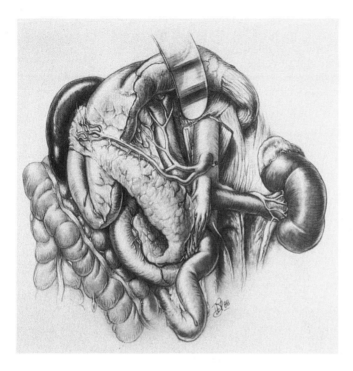

Figure 27–2. Extent of the aorta that can be exposed easily after medial visceral rotation is shown. Note that exposure is essentially the same as that provided by the thoracoretroperitoneal approach.

preferred approach and is described as follows: The left kidney remains in its anatomic position, while the plane behind the left colon, spleen, pancreas, and stomach is developed to allow displacement of these structures toward the midline (Fig. 27–1). The entire aorta, from the distal thoracic level inferiorly, can be completely exposed in this manner (Fig. 27–2). During complete aortic occlusion and with control of any intervening intercostal branches, a "trap-door" aortotomy is placed to circumscribe the orifices of the CA and SMA (Fig. 27–3A) and an endarterectomy is performed, removing the aortic wall lesion and its extensions into the visceral orifices (Fig. 27–3B). In half of our patients, the atheroma was confined to the ventral surface of the aorta involving the CA and SMA orifices. The transaortic endarterectomy was limited to the ventral surface and visceral orifices. However, in the other half, more diffuse aortic disease, frequently in the setting of associated renal artery occlusive lesions, required extension of the aortotomy caudally to allow removal of a cylinder of the aortic atheroma and bilateral (three-quarter) or unilateral (one-quarter) renal endarterectomy (Fig. 27–4). After completion of the endarterectomy, the aortotomy is closed with a running suture.

Antegrade Aortovisceral Bypass

Aortovisceral bypass grafts originating from the supraceliac, subdiaphragmatic aorta were performed in 25 patients at UCSF during the past two decades.[17] A transabdominal, transcrural approach was used in 23 cases, but medial visceral rotation has been successfully used recently in two cases. The proximal anastomosis, placed in the disease-free supraceliac aorta, requires temporary total aortic occlusion. However, circumferential aortic mobilization is not routinely performed unless there is an intervening pair of intercostal arteries that need to be controlled. A small ellipse of aorta, oriented obliquely, is excised to facilitate the end-to-side anastomosis (Fig. 27–5) using braided Dacron. The aortic clamps are removed, restoring flow with the

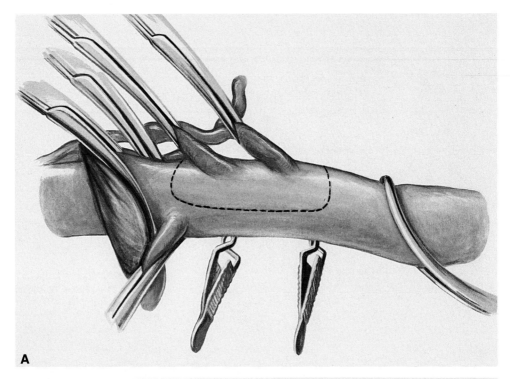

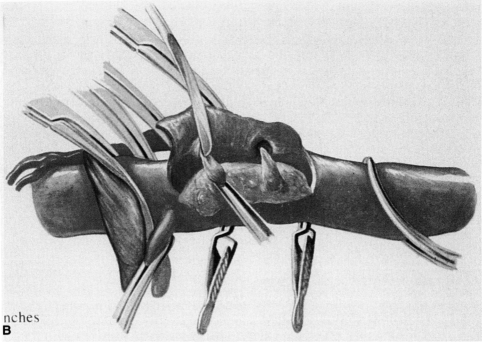

Figure 27–3. (A) Trap-door aortotomy circumscribing the visceral orifices. Note total proximal and distal aortic occlusion and control of individual intercostal arteries. **(B)** Trap-door aortotomy has been opened and hinged on right aortic wall. Endarterectomy is proceeding with removal of the SMA lesion.

TABLE 27–2. PERIOPERATIVE RESULTS

	Antegrade Bypass (*n* = 26)		Transaortic Endarterectomy (*n* = 48)	
	No.	*%*	*No.*	*%*
Outcome				
Alive	24	92.3	41	85.4
Dead	2	7.7	7	14.6
Complications (all patients)				
None	16	61.5	23	47.9
One	8	30.8	12	25.0
Two or more[a]	1	3.8	11	22.9
Complications (surviving patients)				
None	16	61.5	23	47.9
One	8	30.8	11	22.9
Two or more[a]	0	0.0	7	14.6

[a] *P* = .03 (Fisher's exact test, one-tailed).

TABLE 27–3. OPERATIVE DETAILS

	Antegrade Bypass (*n* = 26)		Transaortic Endarterectomy (*n* = 48)	
	No.	*%*	*No.*	*%*
Approach				
Transabdominal[a]	23	88.5	5	10.4
Thoracoretroperitoneal[a]	1	3.8	36	75.0
Medial visceral rotation	2	7.7	7	14.6
Arteries repaired				
Celiac	26	100.0	47	97.9
SMA[a]	12	46.2	45	93.8
IMA[b]	1	3.8	9	18.8
Mean repaired arteries[b]	1.50 ± 0.58		2.10 ± 0.43	
Associated vascular repairs				
Visceral + aorta	2	7.7	2	4.2
Visceral + renal[c]	0	0.0	12	25.0
Visceral + renal + aorta[d]	1	3.8	11	22.9
Ischemia times				
Visceral[e]	26.0 ± 15.8		30.5 ± 15.5	
Renal[e]	25.2 ± 16.8		30.4 ± 16.0	

[a] *P* = 0.001 (chi square)
[b] *P* = 0.07
[c] *P* < .001 (unpaired Student's *t* test).
[d] *P* = .01.
[e] *P* = .003 (Fisher's exact test, one-tailed).
[f] Mean ± SD.
P = .0001 (χ^2).
SMA, superior mesenteric artery; IMA, inferior mesenteric artery.

use aggressive intraoperative cardiac monitoring, and achieve technical perfection in the revascularization.

DISCUSSION

The surgical correction of chronic visceral ischemia is a challenge for the vascular surgeon. Selection of the most appropriate operation depends on the pattern and distribution of disease, the need for simultaneous repair of adjacent arterial lesions, and the concern regarding the overall (operative) risk. Antegrade aortovisceral bypass uses straight or bifurcation prosthetic grafts in these high-flow applications. Aortic inflow is ensured by end-to-side anastomosis of the prosthesis to the undiseased supraceliac aorta, and the distal anastomosis is constructed end-to-end to the visceral branch to optimize flow. The short straight course of the graft avoids the potential for kinking and early graft failure seen with retrograde grafts. Aortovisceral bypass is performed transabdominally with limited aortic and visceral artery exposure. Trans-aortic visceral endarterectomy is the preferred operation for patients that require simultaneous repair of other adjacent vascular beds. Unrestricted supraceliac and paravisceral aortic control are easily obtained through a transabdominal incision and left-to-right medial visceral rotation. These complex exposures are maintained with a self-retaining retraction device, allowing the surgeon and assistant to concentrate their efforts on the operation rather than retraction. Transaortic endarterectomy is performed through an anterolateral trap-door aortotomy. Simultaneous renal endarterectomy or removal of an aortic coral reef atheroma is easily accomplished, and the wide exposure also facilitates infrarenal aortic repair if required.

Adjunctive perioperative measures may include correcting nutritional deficiencies by instituting preoperative hyperalimentation. Maintaining adequate hydration, particularly during evaluation and aortography, is critical because dehydration may lead to intestinal infarction secondary to the hemoconcentration and hypotension that causes critical organ ischemia. Intraoperatively, the use of transesophageal two dimensional ultrasound allows for precise, real-time monitoring of intracardiac performance, which is crucial during supraceliac aortic clamping. Renal ischemia is better tolerated when preceded by mannitol diuresis. The technical adequacy of the repair must be evaluated intraoperatively to prevent catastrophic early failures. Duplex ultrasonography is our preference.

CONCLUSION

Chronic visceral ischemia remains a formidable challenge in diagnosis and treatment. An understanding by primary care and family physicians of the hallmarks of this disorder is an important key to early recognition, diagnosis, and referral to the vascular surgeon for definitive care. The vascular surgeon who is prepared to execute transaortic visceral endarterectomy and aortovisceral bypass can safely restore normal visceral circulation. This will provide durable relief from the physically and psychologically crippling symptoms of chronic visceral ischemia, restore nutritional well-being, and prevent fatal intestinal gangrene.

Acknowledgment
This work was supported in part by Pacific Vascular Research Foundation.

REFERENCES

1. Councilman WT. Three cases of occlusion of the superior mesenteric artery. *Boston Med Surg.* 1894;130:4.
2. Chiene J. Complete obliteration of celiac and mesenteric arteries: viscera receiving their blood supply through extra-peritoneal system vessels. *J Anat Physiol.* 1869;3:65.
3. Osler W. The lumleian lectures on angina pectoris. *Lancet.* 1910;i:839i.
4. Dunphy JE. Abdominal pain of vascular origin. *Am J Med Sci.* 1936;192:109.
5. Mikkelson WP. Intestinal angina: its surgical significance. *Am J Surg.* 1957;94:262.
6. Shaw RS, Maynard EP III. Acute and chronic thrombosis of mesenteric arteries associated with malabsorption. Report of two cases successfully treated by thromboendarterectomy. *N Engl J Med.* 1958;258:874–878.
7. Morris GC Jr, Crawford ES, Cooley DA, et al. Revascularization of the celiac and superior mesenteric arteries. *Arch Surg.* 1962;84:113–125.
8. Fry WJ, Kraft RO. Visceral angina. *Surg Gynecol Obstet.* 1963;117:417–424.
9. Stoney RJ, Wylie EJ. Recognition and surgical management of visceral ischemic syndromes. *Ann Surg.* 1966;164:714–722.
10. Qvarfordt PC, Reilly LM, Sedwitz MM, et al. "Coral reef" atherosclerosis of the suprarenal aorta: a unique clinical entity. *J Vasc Surg.* 1984;1:903.
11. Palubinskas AJ, Ripley HR. Fibromuscular hyperplasia in extra-renal arteries. *Radiology.* 1964;82:451.
12. Dunbar JD, Molner RL, Berman FF, et al. Compression of the celiac trunk and abdominal angina: preliminary report of 15 cases. *Am J Roentgenol.* 1965;95:731.
13. Williams LF Jr. Vascular insufficiency of the bowels. *Dis Mon.* August 1970.
14. Rob CG. Surgical diseases of the celiac and mesenteric arteries. *Arch Surg.* 1966;93:21–31.
15. Wylie EJ. Endarterectomy and autogenous arterial grafts in the surgical treatment of stenosing lesions of the renal artery. *Urol Clin North Am.* June 1975.
16. Stoney RJ, Wylie EJ. Surgical management of arterial lesions of the thoracoabdominal aorta. *Am J Surg.* 1973;126:157–164.
17. Cunningham CG, Reilly LM, Rapp JH, et al. Chronic visceral ischemia: three decades of progress. *Ann Surg.* 1991;214:276–288.
18. Rapp JH, Reilly LM, Qvarfordt PC, et al. Durability of endarterectomy and antegrade grafts in the treatment of chronic visceral ischemia. *J Vasc Surg.* 1986;3:799–806.
19. Roizen MF, Beaupre PN, Alpert RA, et al. Monitoring with two-dimensional transesophageal echocardiography. *J Vasc Surg.* 1984;1:300–305.
20. Okuhn SP, Reilly LM, Bennett JB III, et al. Intraoperative assessment of renal and visceral artery reconstruction: the role of duplex scanning and spectral analysis. *J Vasc Surg.* 1987;5:137–147.
21. Hollier LH, Bernatz PE, Pairolero PC, et al. Surgical management of chronic intestinal ischemia: a reappraisal. *Surgery.* 1981;90:940–946.

28

Late Results of Renovascular Surgery

Richard H. Dean, MD

Operative management of renovascular hypertension by renal revascularization was introduced by Freeman and associates[1] more than 40 years ago when they cured a patient of hypertension by aortic and bilateral renal artery thromboendarterectomy. Although the date of the first aortorenal bypass is unknown, controversy over the preferential use of operation and renal revascularization by the respective method has continued during the ensuing decades. There is little argument regarding the theoretic superiority of relieving the source of the rein-angiotensin-dependent hypertension in renovascular hypertension by revascularization. Nevertheless, significant controversy continues regarding the practical role of operative intervention in its treatment. Much of the controversy stems from reports that show a low rate of blood pressure benefit, a high technical failure rate of revascularization, or a high operative risk. Current results in centers having a larger operative experience with the management of renovascular hypertension, however, demonstrate the practical value of such inter-ventional management. Although the risk of operation is affected by the patient population submitted to operation, reports now show operative mortality rates can be less than 1%, early patency of revascularization in excess of 95%, and initial beneficial blood pressure response rates in excess of 90%.[2] Unfortunately, few centers collected their data for review regarding the long-term benefit to blood pressure and late fate of the reconstruction in patients who have undergone renovascular surgery.

Because hypertension is most commonly a silent process and is manifested only by late sequelae of acceleration in the rate of atherosclerosis and frequency of cardiovascular morbid and mortal events, the need for long-term clinical, functional, and anatomic follow-up patients treated by operation is even more acute.

Late follow-up of patients who have undergone renal revascularization entails examination of the durability of the reconstruction itself, the permanency of the initial beneficial blood pressure response, and the effect on morbid event-free survival. Discussion of the late fate of renal revascularization procedures focuses on both of these variables.

LATE FATE OF BYPASS GRAFTS

Several factors affect the late fate of aortorenal bypass grafts. Principal among these are the graft material used by bypass and the flow through the conduit. Renal artery

TABLE 28–1. RENAL ARTERY GRAFT FLOWS (ML/MIN)

Group	No. of Patients	Before Papaverine	After Papaverine
Atherosclerosis	13	30–400	145–545
Range		168 ± 35	294 ± 62
Mean ± SE		(*P*<.10)	(*P*<.02)
Fibromuscular dysplasia	7	110–600	190–780
Range		302 ± 35	485 ± 69
Mean ± SE		(*P*<.10)	(*P*<.02)
Cure	6	125–600	364–780
Range		333 ± 58	549 ± 57
Mean ± SE		(*P*<.02)	(*P*<.001)
Improved	14	30–400	145–450
Range		148 ± 33	267 ± 27
Mean ± SE		(*P*<.02)	(*P*<.001)

grafts seldom exceed 5 cm in length and more commonly are as short as 3 cm. In addition, although renal artery graft flows are variable, they are usually relatively high. In a study of graft flows in 20 patients before and after papaverine hydrochloride augmentation, we found that resting flows ranged from 30 cc/min in a patient with severe intrarenal disease to 600 cc/min in a patient with isolated main renal artery fibromuscular dysplasia. Papaverine augmentation produced flows ranging from 145 cc/min to 780 cc. Review of these graft flows in relationship to type of lesion and response to operation are shown in Table 28–1. Because long-term patency of the graft is affected by both its length and flow rate, these combine to render characteristics such as graft surface thrombogenicity relatively unimportant and provide a high probability of long-term patency, regardless of the graft material selected.

In contrast to the favorable characteristics of short length and high flow rates, the practical aspects of graft anastomosis to the small distal renal artery magnify the importance of technical precision and the consequence of technical errors on long-term patency. Similarly, the physical characteristics of the graft material in regard to its ease of suturing and handling in small vessel anastomoses are of more practical than theoretic concern. Without question, in such short grafts with high flow rates, technical skill in performing the anastomoses and positioning of the graft are of much greater importance than are theoretic concerns over rapidity of graft endothelialization, graft compliance, and late degenerative changes in autogenous grafts. I believe that technical misadventures have produced far more failures of renal revascularization than have all late sequelae of graft material selection combined.

Discussion of the late fate of the respective conduits available for aortorenal bypass is best approached by reviewing data concerning each of the respective conduits. Sequential follow-up angiography for 1 to 20 years after operation in 196 patients is available in the author's experience for review. Overall results of these studies are shown in Table 28–2.

AUTOGENOUS ARTERY

Theoretically, an arterial autograft should represent the ideal substitute for any diseased arterial segment. The limited availability of donor arterial segments for use as autografts and their inaccessibility make them impractical for most arterial recon-

TABLE 28–2. RESULTS OF SEQUENTIAL 1- TO 20-YEAR POSTOPERATIVE ANGIOGRAPHY

	No. of Grafts	%
No adverse change	174	88
Graft thrombosis	4	2
Graft stenosis	10	5
Graft dilatation	7	3
False aneurysm	3	2

structive procedures, however. Nevertheless, the size and length of the renal artery and the presence of neighboring donor vessels make the use of autogenous arterial grafts a feasible method of renal revascularization. Although the splenic artery is an acceptable donor as a renal artery bypass graft, the hypogastric artery matches the renal artery in size, is relatively easily exposed, and at least on one side, can be sacrificed without sequelae.

Wylie and his group[3] have the greater experience with use of hypogastric autografts for renal revascularization. In a 1975 review of 49 patients who underwent renal artery bypass using the iliac artery system, they reported a 98% early patency rate and no late degenerative changes in the grafts during follow-up through 5 years. Their favorable experience has led them to believe it to be the graft of choice in any age group when the bypass technique is used.

The greatest use of hypogastric arterial autografts is in the management of children with renal artery stenoses. In this age group, potential sources of venous autografts are diminutive and may have a propensity for late aneurysmal degeneration. The structural similarity and dimensions of the hypogastric artery are particularly suitable for use in this age group. Similarly, follow-up angiography by Wylie's group showed that hypogastric autografts usually appropriately enlarge with age in proportion to the increased demands for flow.

The observed enlargement of autogenous grafts is advantageous when it parallels renal perfusion requirements but becomes pathologic if enlargement progresses to a point of aneurysmal dilatation. Certainly, the structural integrity of an arterial autograft is superior to a venous autograft in this regard. Nevertheless, the peculiarities of the disease causing renal artery stenosis in children bears comment. Although Wylie and associates have seen no instances of hypogastric artery graft aneurysmal degeneration during follow-up, my experience has included such a child. This 10-year-old child underwent a left renal artery bypass using a hypogastric artery graft and a superior mesenteric artery bypass using an iliac vein. Progressive aneurysmal dilatation of both grafts was noted during sequential follow-up arteriography (Fig. 28–1). These two grafts were replaced after 7 years. Retrospective review of sections taken from the hypogastric artery at the original operation revealed fibromuscular dysplasia similar to that seen in the renal artery. A second child with a diffuse fibrodysplastic angiopathy involving renal arteries and carotid arteries also had mild dilatation of his hypogastric renal artery graft during the 2 years of angiographic follow-up. Similar review of sections taken from his hypogastric artery also revealed histologic evidence of fibromuscular dysplasia. Although I concur that the hypogastric artery is the graft material of choice in small children, my experience tempers my enthusiasm for the conviction that such an arterial autograft is the ideal substitute. Further, it is argued that children who have undergone renal artery surgery using any conduit should be followed indefinitely, for no graft material is immune to pathologic changes during follow-up.

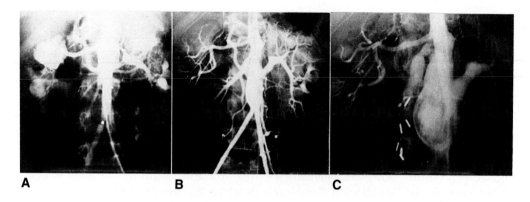

A   **B**   **C**

Figure 28–1. Sequential arteriogram showing progressive aneurysmal dilatation of a hypogastric artery left aortorenal bypass and an iliac vein aortosuperior mesenteric artery bypass in a child. (**A**) pre-op, 1970; (**B**) post-op, 1970; (**C**) post-op, 1973.

Finally, the uncertainty of long-term stability of even arterial autografts suggests that the surgeon should not compromise perfusion to other areas when harvesting a donor autograft. In this regard, the technique of harvesting the common, internal, and external iliac arteries for use as a bifurcation graft in the management of bilateral renal artery lesions and the re-establishment of perfusion to the lower extremity with a synthetic conduit, as described by Wylie, unnecessarily accepts the probability that the patient will require subsequent repeat replacements of the lower extremity grafts during the decades for long-term follow-up. Because follow-up studies of renal artery procedures in childhood are relatively short when compared with the potential durability required of these grafts, the concept of complicating this unknown by also disturbing lower extremity perfusion would appear to be inappropriate.

VENOUS AUTOGRAFTS

The venous system represents the most readily available source for autogenous replacement of diseased arterial segments. Although frequently overlooked, the use and durability of venous autografts depend on the structural integrity of the donor vein and the flow characteristics of the recipient arterial system.

The structural characteristics of the venous system limit potential sources of arterial substitutes to veins of the extremities. Several intra-abdominal veins, such as gonadal, inferior mesenteric, and iliac veins, are expendable and, thereby, are potential sources of arterial substitutes. Their structural weakness when compared with extremity veins, however, increases the risk of their aneurysmal degeneration when subjected to arterial pressures and flow rates. This unacceptable tendency for aneurysmal dilatation is illustrated in the child depicted in Figure 28–1. The iliac vein used to bypass his superior mesenteric artery stenosis underwent greater than a 300% enlargement within a 3-year period. For this reason, the autogenous saphenous vein is the single venous source with acceptable structural characteristics for use in renal revascularization.

Related to structural characteristics are the hemodynamic parameters of flow and their effect on vessel wall structure. Teleologically, growing vessels enlarge in response to demand for flow. The mechanisms providing this controlled enlargement, however, remain unknown. Nevertheless, even arteries may ultimately degenerate when faced with unusually high flow rates. Donor arteries in long-standing large arteriovenous fistulas may pathologically degenerate into aneurysms even after the fistulous communication is closed. Therefore, it is not surprising that when the saphenous vein is structurally immature or is faced with very high flow rates that it also may aneurysmally degenerate. The actual incidence of aneurysmal degeneration of saphenous vein autografts, however, is quite low. Ernst et al[4] reported only five cases (7%) of 75 saphenous vein aortorenal grafts. Five years later, Stanley and Fry[5] updated that experience and reported seven cases (4%) of aneurysmal dilatation in 181 such grafts. In our center, we have identified graft aneurysmal dilatation in four (3%) of 157 saphenous vein grafts followed for at least 1 year.

Examination of the factors increasing the risk of aneurysmal dilatation of saphenous vein grafts demonstrates the predisposition of this adverse change in children. In my experience, all patients with aneurysmal degeneration were less than 25 years of age, and all were cured by operation. Although the overall incidence of aneurysmal degeneration was only 3%, all four instances occurred in this subgroup, for an incidence of 67%. The occurrence only in young patients who were cured by operation suggests an interesting hypothesis. Specifically, when the vessel and kidney beyond the stenosis are normal, cure of hypertension and relatively higher flow rates should be expected. In this situation, and in children whose saphenous vein is structurally less mature, flow through the graft is disproportionately higher and aneurysmal degeneration more likely. Further circumstantial support for this hypothesis is drawn from the fact that aneurysmal degeneration of saphenous vein aortorenal grafts in patients with atherosclerotic lesions has not been seen in my experience. Because most of these patients have some intrarenal arteriolar nephrosclerosis, which results in lower graft flow rates, this group would be at reduced risk for aneurysmal degeneration of the graft.

In addition to the small potential for aneurysmal dilatation, saphenous vein aortorenal grafts may develop fibrotic stenosis at the site of venous valves (Fig. 28–2) and subendothelial fibroblastic proliferation with secondary tubular stenosis (Fig. 28–3). Venous valves assume a neutral position in the reversed venous autograft. If such valves become fibrotic in that position and undergo contracture, a web-like stenosis of the vein graft will ensue. Although this has been demonstrated in only two of our saphenous vein grafts followed at least 1 year, it suggests that the valveless segment of vein should be used if possible.

Three instances of subendothelial fibroblastic proliferation of saphenous vein aortorenal grafts have been identified in follow-up angiographic studies of the 196 grafts. Two of these occurred in patients having complex branch renal artery repairs, and the final one occurred in a patient who underwent bilateral renal artery grafts. In these instances, the vein was subjected to a prolonged ischemia time without the benefit of any specific measure designed to provide protection against intimal damage. Whether use of cold, heparinized blood or other preservative solutions would have prevented late tubular stenosis in these patients, however, is conjectural.

Notwithstanding the small risk of aneurysmal dilatation and late graft stenosis (<10%), the saphenous vein remains a valuable source of graft material. Except in small children and other special circumstances, the autogenous saphenous vein is our graft choice for most patients undergoing aortorenal bypass. Nevertheless, follow-up angiography should be performed to assess long-term durability. Interestingly, in my experience with sequential angiographic follow-up studies, no graft shown to be normal after 1 year has subsequently undergone degenerative changes. For this reason, even centers not interested in study of the long-term consequence of renal

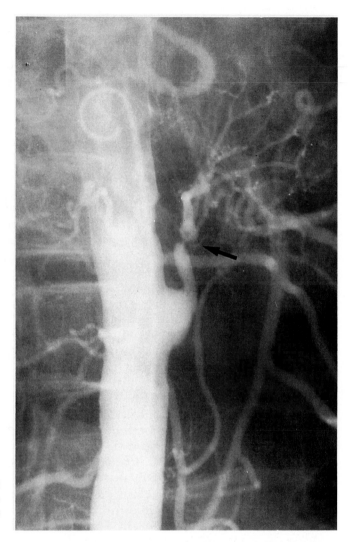

Figure 28–2. Arteriogram of stenosis of a saphenous vein aortorenal bypass at a site of a venous valve.

revascularization should, at least, study patients 1 year postoperatively to exclude the development of late graft abnormalities.

SYNTHETIC GRAFTS

The use of synthetic graft material for aortorenal bypass has the theoretic advantage of instant availability in a variety of sizes; also, it requires no additional operative dissection for its acquisition. In contrast, the obvious disadvantages include desirability of autogenous tissue for small vessel anastomoses and the potential for progressive neointimal proliferation on a thrombogenic graft surface.

For many years, the term *synthetic graft* has been synonymous with *Dacron graft*. Recently, however, expanded polytetrafluoroethylene grafts have also become a popular synthetic conduit for arterial replacement. Before 1978, our experience with synthetic grafts in the aortorenal position was limited to 42 6-mm knitted Dacron grafts. Since that time, we have preferentially used 6-mm polytetrafluoroethylene

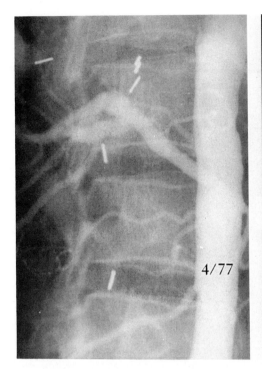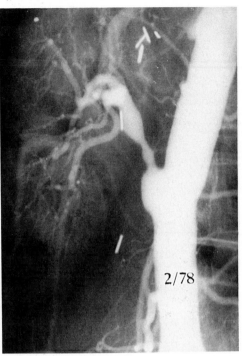

Figure 28–3. Sequential arteriogram showing development of tubular subendothelial fibroblastic proliferation in a saphenous vein aortorenal bypass.

(goretex) grafts as the synthetic conduit of choice. Such synthetic grafts can exhibit excellent adaptation over follow-up. Sequential arteriograms in a 7-year-old child who underwent a 6-mm knitted Dacron graft demonstrated excellent incorporation during follow-up (Fig. 28–4). Unfortunately, because such grafts are not autogenous, they continue to be at risk for adverse changes. Whereas the results of angiographic follow-up in our overall experience have shown a small incidence of autogenous graft aneurysmal degeneration and fibrous stenoses, all such lesions have developed during early follow-up within 18 months. In contrast, recurrence of hypertension secondary to suture line neointimal proliferation and the appearance of anastomotic false aneurysms occurred even after late follow-up in patients with synthetic grafts. Figure 28–5 shows bilateral false aneurysms of the aortic anastomoses in a patient with bilateral aortorenal bypasses uncovered at follow-up arteriography 20 years after their insertion. Because the anastomosis between a synthetic graft and the native vessel never acquires significant strength other than that determined by the integrity of the suture line, it is not surprising that such anastomotic false aneurysms occur even after many years. This suggests that autogenous material is preferable, especially when the durability of reconstruction is measured in decades, as it is when children and young adults require renal revascularization. In addition, it demonstrates the need for empiric serial angiographic follow-up of the asymptomatic patient, for the first clinical presentation of such false aneurysms would be rupture.

LATE FATE OF PATIENTS

As stated earlier, safety of operation, technical success of revascularization, and the blood pressure response to successful revascularization are only the initial consider-

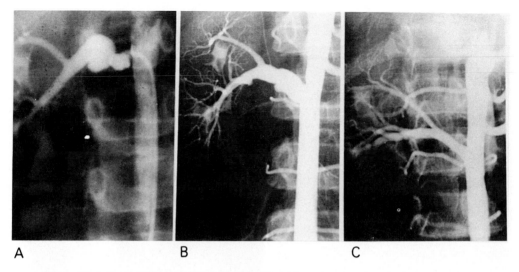

A   B   C

Figure 28–4. Sequential arteriogram showing **(A)** right renal artery stenosis and poststenotic dilatation; **(B)** early postoperative appearance of a 6-mm Dacron aortorenal bypass; and **(C)** 2-year postoperative study showing incorporation.

ation regarding the value of operative management or renovascular hypertension. Because long-term relief of hypertension and its differential benefit on symptom-free survival is the most pertinent aspect of any intervention, evaluation of the late fate of patients submitted to operative management in the remote past is valuable. In this regard, we reviewed the late follow-up status of 71 patients who underwent operative therapy for renovascular hypertension from 15 to 23 years ago and evaluated factors that might have been of value in predicting long-term symptom-free survival.[2,6]

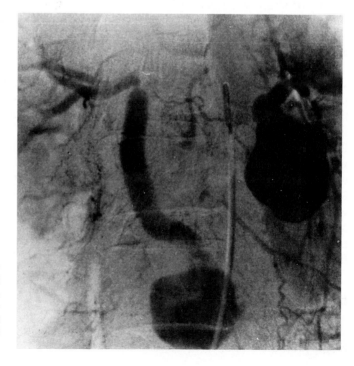

Figure 28–5. Arteriogram obtained 20 years after bilateral Dacron aortorenal bypasses, demonstrating bilateral false aneurysm at the aortic anastomoses and stenosis at the site of distal anastomosis on the right.

TABLE 28–3. PATIENT POPULATION

Demography	Fibromuscular Dysplasia	Atherosclerosis	Other
Number of patients	27	39	5
Male	8	23	2
Female	19	16	3
Age (yr)			
Range	4 mo–58 yr	37–68	
Mean	29	51	

That review included follow-up information on 66 of the 68 patients surviving operation. Preoperative clinical characteristics of the 71 patients evaluated in the report are summarized in Tables 28–3 and 28–4. Ages ranged from 4 months to 68 years at the time of operation. The renovascular lesion was fibromuscular dysplasia in 27 patients (38%) and the atherosclerosis in 39 (55%). Patients with atherosclerosis were considered to have either diffuse or focal disease. Diffuse atherosclerotic disease was defined as at least moderate aortoiliac disease as seen on the abdominal aortogram. Atherosclerotic disease was considered focal only if the only significant anatomic lesion seen was the renal artery lesion. According to this definition, 16 patients had focal disease (41%), and 23 patients had diffuse disease (59%). Five additional patients were judged to have hypertension due to other causes, including pyelonephritis, radiation arteritis, and trauma.

The atherosclerotic group of patients ranged in age from 37 to 68 years (mean, 51.7 ± 8.4 years). Those with diffuse involvement were significantly older (mean, 54.5 ± 8.5 years) than those with focal disease (mean, 47.7 ± 6.5 years), $P<.0005$. In contrast, the group with fibromuscular dysplasia ranged in age from 4 months to 58 years (mean, 29.4 ± 15.0 years).

Figure 28–6 shows the overall early blood pressure response to operative treatment in the 68 surviving patients of the study. Of all patients with fibromuscular dysplasia, 74% were cured and 21% improved. For comparison, only 30% of patients with atherosclerosis were cured and 49% were improved. These differences were statistically significant ($P >.01$, χ^2 contingency table test). However, there were no statistical differences in the frequency of benefit when patients with focal and diffuse atherosclerosis lesions were compared. Interestingly, among the 11 patients who did not benefit from operation were two patients with residual technical failures of reconstruction, one patient on whom no preoperative functional studies to prove the presence of renovascular hypertension were performed, five patients whose preoperative functional studies were negative, two patients with significant residual contralat-

TABLE 28–4. CLINICAL CHARACTERISTICS

	Number	%
Birth control pills	12	32
Smoking	37	52
Hyperlipidemia	28	39
Diabetes	11	15
History cerebrovascular disease	14	20
History cardiac disease	47	66
Obesity	23	32

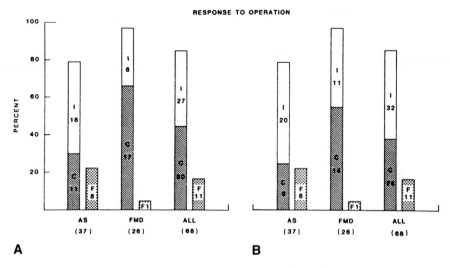

Figure 28–6. Comparison of initial benefit with late blood pressure response in the respective types of lesions. (**A**) Early result (1–6 months follow-up); (**B**) Late result(1–23 years follow-up). AS, atherosclerosis; FMD, fibromuscular dysplasia, ALL,both AS and FMD combined; C, cured; I, improved; F, failed.

eral disease and documented progression, and one patient who was rendered anephric.

Follow-up to time of death or the date of the report showed that overall benefit from operation persisted, as also depicted in Figure 28–6. Although there was a decrease in the percentage of patients who sustained a cure in both the fibromuscular dysplasia and the atherosclerosis groups, the percentage who had a beneficial response (cured and improved) remained unchanged over long-term follow-up. Comparison of the initial blood pressure response to operation (1 to 6 months postoperatively) with the blood pressure status at the time of death or current date (up to 23 years later) in patients reveals that the effect of operative treatment is maintained over long-term follow-up. In those patients who required repeat renovascular surgery for recurrent renovascular hypertension during follow-up, most were performed for the management of contralateral lesions that had progressed to functional significance (produced renovascular hypertension).

Table 28–5 identified the incidence and cause of death from any cause during follow-up of all patients in relation to disease type. Interestingly, two of the three

TABLE 28–5. MORTALITY BY DISEASE

	Diffuse Atherosclerotic Disease	Focal Atherosclerotic Disease	Fibromuscular Dysplasia	Other	Total
Cardiovascular deaths					
Myocardial infarction	8	4			12
Cerebrovascular accident	2				2
Congestive heart failure	3	1	1		5
Sudden death	3				3
Other vascular	3	1	1		5
Noncardiovascular deaths					
Cancer	1	1	3		5

deaths from cardiovascular events in the group with fibromuscular dysplasia occurred in patients who had concomitant diffuse atherosclerosis. The remaining death was in a 4-year-old child who after primary nephrectomy had persistent hypertension caused by progressive contralateral disease. Death from cardiovascular morbid events primarily occurred in the group with atherosclerosis. Figure 28–7 displays survival by Life Table analysis in relation to blood pressure benefit in the 37 patients with atherosclerosis who survived operation. Because response to operation currently is predictable, follow-up information about the patients who benefited by operation 15 to 23 years ago is the more valuable. Study of this subgroup is more informative because operative failures reflect the less-effective patient selection and treatment during this earlier period and are of less relevance to current results of operative management. Figure 28–8 shows the cumulative proportion of patients who benefited and survived relative to disease type (deaths from cardiovascular causes). Although the difference in survival between the three groups has statistical significance ($P <$ .00005), the ages of the groups are also significantly dissimilar, as described earlier.

The age-adjusted differences in survival of patients with focal and diffuse atherosclerosis were also statistically significant. This suggests that early intervention for renovascular hypertension in the atherosclerotic process has a more pronounced effect on subsequent cardiovascular mortality than does later intervention. Alternatively, differences in actual survival may only reflect the higher probability of cardiovascular death in patients with a later, more advanced stage of atherosclerosis. Because the cohort of failures in each of the two subgroups is so small, the effect of blood pressure control on survival in these subgroups (focal and diffuse atherosclerotic disease) is difficult to assess at this time. Thus, patients with diffuse atherosclerotic disease and uncontrolled hypertension may have died even more precipitously than other subgroups of patients with atherosclerosis.

The results of the evaluation of morbid event data were similar to those of

SURVIVAL VERSUS RESPONSE TO OPERATION

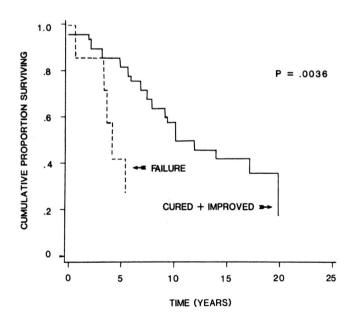

Figure 28–7. Kaplan-Meier Life Table analysis. Survival by response to operation in 37 atherosclerotic patients (deaths from cardiovascular causes).

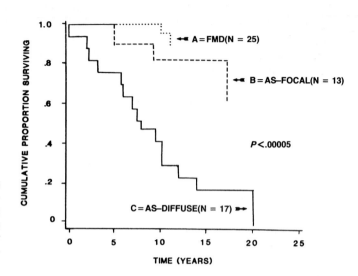

Figure 28–8. Kaplan Meier Life Table analysis. Survival of 55 patients benefited from operation by type and stage of disease (deaths from cardiovascular causes). FMD, fibromuscular dysplasia; AS, artheriosclerosis.

survival. There was a statistically significant difference in the time to the first cardiovascular morbid event when comparing patients among the respective disease types and stages (fibromuscular dysplasia and focal and diffuse atherosclerotic disease). After differences in the times to first morbid event were adjusted for age, they did not retain significance when patients with focal and diffuse atherosclerotic disease were compared. However, significantly more cardiovascular morbid events per patient per unit time occurred in the group with diffuse atherosclerotic disease (median 0.269 cardiovascular morbid event per patient per year) than in the group with focal atherosclerotic disease (median 0.057 cardiovascular morbid event per patient per year; $P < .02$). Because of the limited number of individuals having any specific risk factor(s) in the respective disease (atherosclerotic versus fibromuscular dysplasia) or stage of disease (diffuse versus focal atherosclerotic disease) groupings, stastical analysis for identification of factors predictive of early morbid events or death or, alternatively, of long-term morbid event-free survival was unrewarding.

Finally, because this study was not a comparative study of different treatment regimens and because no disease-matched group of medically treated patients is currently available, the report has limited pertinence to the broader issue of the relative merits of surgical versus medical therapy of renovascular hypertension.

In summary, late follow-up of patients previously submitted to operative management of renovascular disease suggests that both the initial anatomic and functional results are sustained. Further, the durability of operative correction has resulted in a sustained benefit in hypertension and renal function in most properly selected patients.

REFERENCES

1. Freeman N. Thromboendarterectomy for hypertension due to renal artery occlusion. *JAMA.* 1954;157:1077.
2. Dean RH. Surgery for renovascular hypertension. In: Bergan JJ, Yao JST, eds. *Operative Techniques in Vascular Surgery.* New York, NY: Grune and Stratton; 1980.

3. Wylie EJ. Endarterectomy and autogenous arterial grafts in the surgical treatment of stenosing lesions of the renal artery. *Urol Clin North Am.* 1975;2:351.
4. Ernst CA, Stanley JC, Marshall FF, et al. Autogenous saphenous vein aortorenal grafts. *Arch Surg.* 1972;105:855.
5. Stanley JC, Fry WJ. Surgical treatment of renovascular hypertension. *Arch Surg.* 1977;112:1291.
6. Dean RH, Krueger TC, Whiteneck JM, et al. Operative management of renovascular hypertension: results after a follow-up of 15–23 years. *J Vasc Surg.* 1984;1:234–242.

29

Long-Term Results in Surgery for
Renovascular Hypertension in a
Pediatric Population

James C. Stanley, MD

Renal artery occlusive disease is second only to thoracic aortic coarctation as the most common form of surgically correctable hypertension in the pediatric population. The precise incidence of this form of hypertension is unknown, although its clinical importance has been firmly established.[1-7] Although this entity has been the subject of many reports, only three centers have an experience with more than 25 patients treated surgically.[1,4-6] Because of the paucity of cases, the long-term results of primary surgical procedures for renovascular hypertension in the pediatric population are poorly defined and often anecdotal. The outcomes for reoperation in this subset of hypertensives are even less well established.[8] Nevertheless, the limitations as well as benefits of specific surgical procedures have allowed a number of conclusions to be made regarding the operative management of pediatric renovascular hypertension.

SURGICAL TECHNIQUES

Any definition of the durability of the various forms of pediatric renal revascularization necessitates an introductory discussion on the basic arterial reconstructions in children. Optimal operative interventions remain highly individualized, although certain general approaches have become relatively well standardized during the past decade.

Exposure is important to successful pediatric renal revascularization. A supraumbilical transverse incision is preferred, being carried from the opposite midclavicular line to the posterior axillary line on the side of the affected renal artery. Extension of such an incision into both flanks is performed for bilateral repairs. Transverse abdominal incisions offer distinct technical advantages over vertical midline abdominal incisions. The renal vessels, as well as the abdominal aorta, are exposed by incising the lateral parieties adjacent to the colon, allowing separation of the mesocolon and duodenum from the retroperitoneal structures by both blunt and sharp dissection. This retroperitoneal approach facilitates better visualization of the renal arteries than is possible through an incision in the posterior peritoneum at the base of the mesentery. Routine *ex vivo* revascularization with autotransplantation of the kidney is often preferred by those with special expertise in renal transplantation[9] but has not been contemporary practice at most centers treating large numbers of children with renovascular hypertension. Before clamping the aorta or renal arteries, the patients are systemically anticoagulated with heparin, 150 IU/kg. Anticoagulation should be reversed with administration of protamine at the conclusion of the arterial reconstruction.

Aortorenal Bypass and Aortic Reimplantation of the Renal Artery

The internal iliac artery is used most often for pediatric renal revascularizations requiring aortorenal bypass (Fig. 29–1). The excised internal iliac artery should include a branch at its distal end. This allows creation of a wide branch-patch aortic orifice by incising the crotch between the branch and trunk of the artery. Prosthetic grafts, because of technical limitations in sewing them to small renal arteries, and vein grafts, because of the propensity for late aneurysmal changes in children,[10] are rarely recommended for renal artery reconstructive procedures in these young patients.

Aortic reimplantation of the renal artery is a reasonable alternative to aortorenal bypass in a child whose stenotic disease is limited to the origin of the vessel (Fig. 29–2). In these circumstances, the proximal renal artery should be spatulated on opposite sides to create a generous anastomotic orifice. A lateral aortotomy with its length usually being a little over twice the diameter of either the iliac artery graft or spatulated renal artery allows for sufficient growth of the graft's anastomosis. The aortic anastomosis is performed in an end-to-side manner using interrupted or continuous monofilament suture, depending on the size and age of the patient.

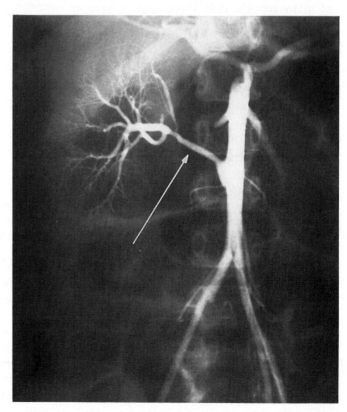

Figure 29–1. Internal iliac artery aortorenal graft (*arrow*) in a child who presented with midrenal artery stenosis. (*Reproduced with the permission of Mosby-Year Book, Inc., from Stanley JC, Brothers TE. Surgical treatment of renovascular hypertension in children. In: Ernst CB, Stanley JC, eds.* Current Therapy in Vascular Surgery, *2nd ed. 1991: 877.*)

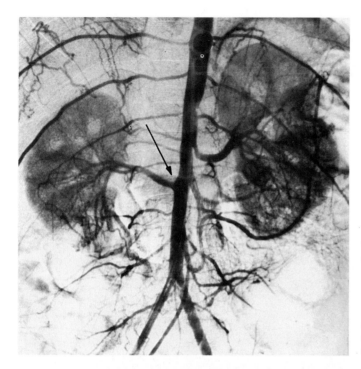

Figure 29–2. Renal artery aortic reimplantation (*arrow*) in an infant who presented with a proximal ostial stenosis. (*Reproduced with the permission of Mosby-Year Book, Inc., from Stanley JC, Brothers TE. Surgical treatment of renovascular hypertension in children. In: Ernst CB, Stanley JC, eds.* Current Therapy in Vascular Surgery, *2nd ed, 1991:878.*)

Distal renal artery-to-graft anastomoses are fashioned in an end-to-end manner. These anastomoses are facilitated by spatulation of both the renal artery and the graft. The anastomosis is completed in most children using three or four running monofilament sutures in a discontinuous manner to allow for later growth. In vessels 2 mm or less in diameter, individual interrupted sutures are placed about the entire anastomotic circumference. Anastomoses using a spatulation technique are ovoid and have relatively lengthy circumferences that are less apt to develop later strictures when compared with nonspatulated anastomoses (Fig. 29–3). Occasionally, when stenoses affect multiple renal arteries, the transected vessels are anastomosed to each other to form a common orifice to which an aortorenal graft may then be anastomosed.

Operative Arterial Dilation

Alone or in concert with a bypass procedure, operative arterial dilation is a less-often used means of renal revascularization in the pediatric population. It is most applicable to intraparenchymal intimal webs. Rigid metal dilators are advanced through the stenosis by way of a transverse arteriotomy in the main renal artery. It is important that these dilators be thoroughly lubricated with a substance such as silicone solution to lessen the potential for intimal drag and disruption. The stenotic area should be dilated progressively by passage of increasingly larger dilators, usually in increments of 0.5 mm, not exceeding the predicted normal diameter of the artery by more than 1.0 mm.

Thoracoabdominal Bypasses

Thoraco abdominal bypasses using expanded Polytetrafluoroethylene or fabricated Dacron prostheses, in conjunction with renal or splanchnic arterial repairs, have in the past been the most common operations performed in the management of abdominal aortic narrowings and concomitant renal artery stenoses. Extraperitoneal reflection of the abdominal viscera through a thoracoabdominal incision provides generous access

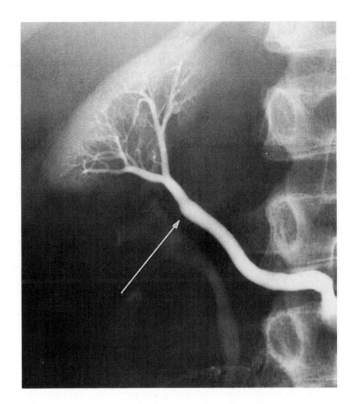

Figure 29–3. Ovoid appearance of a spatulated autogenous saphenous vein–segmental renal artery anastomosis (*arrow*) during immediate postoperative period. (*Reproduced with the permission of the American Medical Association from Fry WJ, Ernst CB, Stanley JC. Renovascular Hypertension in the pediatric patient. Archives of Surgery. 1973;107:695.*)

to the proximal abdominal aorta and its renal branches. End-to-side graft-to-aorta anastomoses are constructed with the thoracic anastomosis usually completed before the infrarenal anastomosis. Autogenous internal iliac artery is preferred for renal artery reconstructions. The most common site from which these grafts usually originate is the thoracoabdominal prosthesis. However, the native aorta may be a better site of origin, in that late anastomotic neointimal hyperplasia will be less likely to occur with such an autologous arterial-to-aortic anastomosis than with one involving the synthetic thoracoabdominal graft.

Primary Patch Aortoplasty

Prosthetic graft material, combined with reimplantation of the renal arteries onto the normal aorta, has recently been preferred over thoracoabdominal bypass for most combined renal and aortic reconstructions in young children (Fig. 29–4). The patch should be generous enough to not be constrictive as the patient grows into adulthood. Similarly, caution must be taken not to overcorrect the narrowing, resulting in an aneurysmal aortic segment that might be the source of mural thrombus formation and distal embolization. Avoidance of competitive parallel flow within the native aorta and the bypass, absence of individual renal grafts, and a reduction in the number of anastomoses that must be performed represent advantages of this technique.

RESULTS OF SURGICAL THERAPY

Blood Pressure Response

Cumulative surgical experience with pediatric-aged renovascular hypertensive patients reveals excellent results (Table 29–1). A beneficial outcome should be anticipated in almost all patients treated operatively. Although certain discrepancies exist

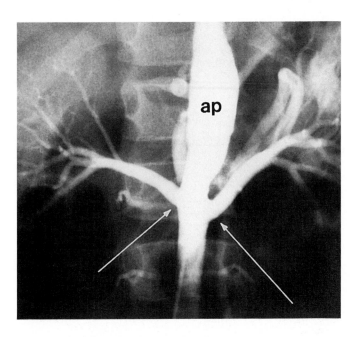

Figure 29–4. Aortoplasty (*ap*) of midabdominal aortic coarctation (ePTFE patch) with bilateral reimplantation of renal arteries (*arrows*) in a 5-year-old patient who had a suprarenal abdominal aortic coarctation and bilateral renal artery ostial stenotic disease.

from one center to the next regarding the number of primary arterial reconstructions versus primary nephrectomies, improved vascular surgical techniques have increased the likelihood of successful renal revascularizations with lesser risks to the kidney.

Outcomes from operations for pediatric renovascular hypertension must be judged by carefully defined criteria, including (a) *cured*, if no antihypertensive medications were administered for the preceding 6 months and blood pressures are below the 95th percentile for age and sex; (b) *improved*, if pressures are within normotensive ranges on drug therapy (excluding angiotensin converting enzyme inhibitors) or if their diastolic pressures are greater than normal but at least 15% lower than preoperative levels; and (c) *failure*, when diastolic pressures remain greater than established normal levels but are not 15% lower than preoperative values, or when angiotensin converting enzyme inhibitors are required to normalize the blood pressure.

Results from the largest reported series of surgically treated pediatric renovascular hypertensives, followed an average of 42 months postoperatively, support an aggressive surgical approach.[5] Among the 40 children in the former experience, 85% were cured of their hypertension, 12.5% were improved, and only 2.5% failed to benefit from operative therapy. Persistent hypertension among improved children was attributed to untreated contralateral disease. The only failure in this former series occurred in a patient with extensive intraparenchymal stenoses in whom operative dilation was unsuccessful.

Durability of Aortorenal Bypass with Vein Grafts

Late stenoses affect less than 5% of aortorenal vein grafts placed in children.[11] These are usually recognized during the first postoperative year and may represent sequelae of operative graft trauma or technical errors in fashioning an anastomosis. Reoperation in these circumstances has led to nephrectomy in more than half the children.[8] Although the incidence of graft occlusions in these patients is similar to that of other complex renal revascularizations using vein, the morbidity associated with reoperation and other complications attending vein graft usage has led to abandonment of these conduits in most practices. Nevertheless, there are certain circumstances when vein proves to be the only option available for renal revascularization. In such a

TABLE 29-1. PEDIATRIC RENOVASCULAR HYPERTENSION: COMPARATIVE RESULTS OF SURGICAL TREATMENT

Medical Center	No. Patients	Primary Procedures		Secondary Procedures	Postoperative (%) Status[a]			Operative Mortality (%)
		Reconstruction	Nephrectomy		Cured	Improved	Failure	
University of Michigan[b] (1963–1980)[5]	40	49	2	6	85	12.5	2.5	0
Cleveland Clinic (1955–1977)[1,4]	27	22	11	5	59	18.5	18.5	4
University of California Los Angeles (1967–1977)[6]	26	19	11	7	84.5	7.5	4	4
Vanderbilt University[c] (1962–1977)[3]	21	15	8	4	68	24	8	0
University of Pennsylvania (1974–1987)[2]	17	30	0	1[d]	76.5	23.5	0	0
University of California San Francisco (1960–1974)[7]	14	10	4	2	86	7	0	7

[a] Criteria for blood pressure response defined in cited publications. Operative mortality not included in failure category. Data expressed to nearest 0.5%.
[b] Includes 34 cases from University of Michigan and six cases from University of Texas, Southwestern.
[c] Results included data from four patients with parenchymal disease treated by nephrectomy.
[d] Two revascularized kidneys considered to have become infarcted postoperatively were not removed in this series.

setting, the surgeon must be particularly fastidious in maintaining close follow-up of the patient.

Aneurysmal dilatation of autogenous saphenous vein aortorenal grafts represents a second and major detriment to the long-term durability of vein grafts in the treatment of pediatric renovascular hypertension (Fig. 29–5). Aneurysmal grafts affected nearly 20% of aortorenal vein grafts studied in the early Michigan experience,[5,8] and the actual frequency of this complication may be closer to 75%. Aneurysmal changes were recognized an average of 14 months postoperatively and as early as 6 months after operation. Half the dilated grafts in this group remained stable, with continued expansion or thrombus accumulation being the basis for removing the other vein grafts. Peripheral embolization of microthrombi from the graft surface causing renal infarction is the greatest concern attending progressive vein graft dilation in these children.

Recently, it has been recommended that an external Dacron mesh be placed about aortorenal vein grafts in children to prevent aneurysmal dilation[2] and, once an uncomplicated dilation is recognized, that the graft be plicated to reduce its diameter.[11] However, concern exists that the synthetic mesh may not be strong enough to prevent eventual graft dilation, such as has been observed in like circumstances with human umbilical vein grafts. Similarly, the long-term outcome of vein graft plication has not been established.

Deleterious effects of disrupting vasa vasorum when removing vein segments for grafting in children are of more than theoretic importance. Transmural injury of veins during their removal has been well recognized. Devascularization of a vein graft is

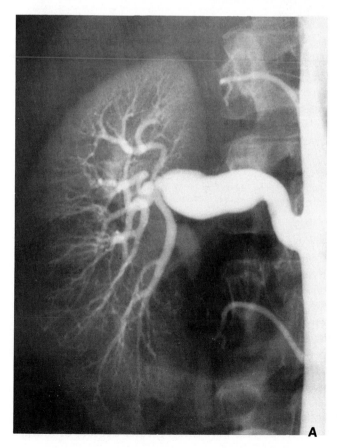

Figure 29–5. (A) Aneurysmal autogenous saphenous vein aortorenal graft in an adolescent 18 months **A** postoperative. (*Figure continues*)

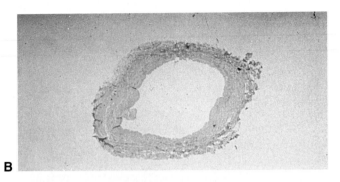

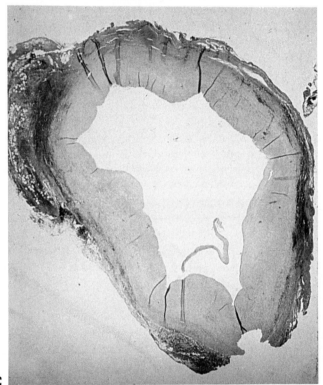

Figure 29–5. (*continued*) (**B**) Microscopic sections of saphenous vein segment removed at time of original operation. (**C**) Aneurysmal graft removed at the time of the aforenoted arteriogram (hematoxylin-eosin stain, x9). (*Reproduced with the permission of the American Medical Association from Ernst CB, Stanley JC, Marshall FF, et al. Autogenous saphenous vein aortorenal grafts, a ten-year experience. Archives of Surgery. 1972;105:857.*)

primarily a result of disrupting vasa vasorum, not interrupting blood flow through its lumen. Circulation within the vasa vasorum does not resume until 48 to 72 hours after transplantation. Overdistention of vein segments and injudicious dissection of periadventitial tissue containing the vasal elements undoubtedly worsens graft ischemia.

That younger patients develop aneurysmal vein grafts is perhaps quite significant. This age-related complication has been apparent in all large operative experiences with pediatric renovascular hypertension. Extensive adventitial networks of vasa vasorum and simple loops penetrating deep into the media nourish the normal vein in young individuals.[12] As adulthood is entered, attenuation of the adventitial plexuses occur and the simple afferent-efferent loops in the media develop into complex and more superficial plexuses connecting neighboring vasal loops. This suggests that transluminal diffusion of nutriments is operative in adult veins. These differences in the nutrient blood supply of veins may cause greater degrees of mural ischemia during transplantation of vein segments from younger patients compared with older adults.

Durability of Aortorenal Bypass with Arterial Grafts

Late stenoses are uncommon when the hypogastric artery is used for renal reconstructions in children.[7,11] Nevertheless, diffuse excentric narrowings of arterial grafts have been noted in two cases cared for by the author, with the initial procedure undertaken at the University of Michigan in one case and at the Cleveland Clinic in the second case. In both instances, the arterial autografts were carefully procured, with no obvious departures from standard operative handling. Recognition of graft failure in these cases occurred within 6 months of operation, being manifest by severe recurrent hypertension. Both children underwent successful reoperative surgery with replacement of the abnormal arterial graft. The removed stenotic conduits exhibited a panfibrotic process involving both the intima and media.

Aneurysmal dilation of internal iliac artery grafts used for aortorenal bypasses in the pediatric age group is rare.[3,7,11] The author has treated only one such patient, whose primary procedure was performed at the University of California, San Francisco. In this case, histologic examination of an arterial segment left over from the initial procedure revealed dysplastic changes. A similar case has been described in the Vanderbilt experience.[3] Thus, in these patients, a contributing factor may have been that the artery was already abnormal at the time of its implantation. Because of the very high frequency of aneurysmal deterioration of autologous vein grafts, autologous artery grafts are still preferred over vein for bypass procedures in children. Nevertheless, arterial autografts are not immune from subsequent pathologic changes in children, and their handling at the time of implantation should be performed with great care and caution to lessen vessel trauma that might compromise later graft function.

The use of the arterial grafts *in situ* when treating childhood renovascular hypertension deserves special note. Performance of a splenorenal bypass by direct anastomosis of the proximal or midportion of the splenic artery to the end of the left renal artery has not enjoyed favor in treating pediatric renovascular disease. The results of this type reconstruction in children are very poor.[4,13] This may reflect the rather small and vasospastic splenic artery found in children. Whatever the cause, early thrombotic complications have been surprisingly common with splenorenal bypasses in pediatric cases. In addition, many children have a normal-appearing celiac artery orifice at the time they are being subjected to renovascular reconstructive procedures, with later failure of this artery to grow as the child becomes older. This results in evolution of a functionally significant stenosis involving the parent vessel of the splenic artery, with an eventual outcome of recurrent hypertension. There is simply no current means of determining whether a celiac artery will become stenotic at an older age in a child being treated for developmental renal artery stenoses.

Durability of Renal Artery Reimplantation

Renal artery-aortic implantations in adults are not commonly performed because of a high incidence of technical complications, especially early thromboses. It is likely that many of these occlusions relate to the presence of thickened intima and atherosclerotic tissue within the aorta. Aortic reimplantations for renal ostial disease in the pediatric population are, to the contrary, unlikely to be complicated by the problems accompanying similar adult reconstructions. In the author's experience, no late stenotic or aneurysmal changes have been noted with implantation of segmental vessels onto each other in five cases and aortic reimplantations of the main renal artery an additional eight times. Segmental resection and direct arterial reanastomosis has not enjoyed the same success as reimplantations.[9,11] Excessive anastomotic tension and development of late fibrotic stenoses preclude routine resectional therapy with reanastomoses. Reimplantation reconstructions demand a high degree of technical expertise and competence. They may become more widely used in the future, given the recognized problems accompanying other forms of pediatric renal artery reconstruction.

Durability of Renal Artery Dilatations

Operative dilation of renal artery stenotic disease has a reasonable but limited role in treating pediatric renovascular hypertension.[5] No long-term studies exist documenting the durability of such interventions, but the failure rate may be excessive.[11] At the University of Michigan, dilation alone or in concert with some other form of renal revascularization has been undertaken in five children. In two instances, dilation resulted in early vessel occlusion and subsequent nephrectomy. In a third case, late fibrotic narrowing of the dilated artery resulted in loss of the kidney. Because of this experience, the author has favored reimplantation of a stenotic segment vessel onto an adjacent artery rather than transluminal dilation. An exception is the treatment of an isolated web-like lesion or intraparenchymal stenosis. In the latter setting, balloon dilation or even alcohol-induced renal infarction may be as reasonable as operative dilation. Lastly, subtotal nephrectomy may be appropriate in certain instances of polar segmental renal artery stenotic disease not amenable to convential arterial reconstruction.

Durability of Combined Aortic and Renal Artery Reconstruction

Although some have advocated staged treatment of abdominal aortic coarctation and renovascular hypertension, it has been the author's usual practice to undertake single-stage procedures in these circumstances. The technical difficulties encountered at secondary operations may be formidable. Despite the magnitude and complexity of definitive primary procedures, contemporary surgical experience supports such an approach in treating these patients.[14–17] The major concern with these complex reconstructions is development of anastomotic narrowings if autologous vein or artery conduits to the kidney are originated from the synthetic thoracoabdominal graft.

The long-term durability of primary aortoplasty with a synthetic patch graft has not been defined, but on theoretic grounds such should be at least as good as that of a thoracoabdominal bypass. The author has treated one patient with aortic aneurysmal dilation, occurring after pregnancy in a young person who had undergone an earlier patch aortoplasty from the level of the celiac artery to the aortic bifurcation. Five other patients with patch graft aortoplasties have experienced no complications over an average follow-up of 38 months.

Performance of 42 thoracoabdominal bypasses, 13 aortoplasties, and 18 miscellaneous aortic reconstructive procedures, accompanied by concomitant renal artery reconstructive procedures or primary nephrectomy, has been associated with a reported operative mortality of 8% and excellent or good results regarding blood pressure control in 89% of the surviving patients.[14]

REFERENCES

1. Benjamin SP, Dustan HP, Gifford RW Jr, et al. Stenosing renal artery disease in children: clinicopathological correlation in 20 surgically treated cases. *Clev Clin Q.* 1976;43:197–206.

2. Berkowitz HD, O'Neill JA Jr. Renovascular hypertension in children. Surgical repair with special reference to the use of reinforced vein grafts. *J Vasc Surg.* 1989;9:46–55.

3. Lawson JD, Boerth R, Foster JH, Dean RH. Diagnosis and management of renovascular hypertension in children. *Arch Surg.* 1977;122:1307–1316.

4. Novick AC, Straffon RA, Stewart BH, et al. Surgical treatment of renovascular hypertension in the pediatric patient. *J Urol.* 1978;119:794–805.

5. Stanley JC, Fry WJ. Pediatric renal artery occlusive disease and renovascular hypertension: etiology, diagnosis and operative treatment. *Arch Surg.* 1981;116:669–676.

6. Stanley P, Gyepes MT, Olson DL, Gates GF. Renovascular hypertension in children and adolescents. *Radiology.* 1978;129:123–131.

7. Stoney RJ, Cooke PA, Strong ST. Surgical treatment of renovascular hypertension in children. *J Pediatr Surg.* 1975;10:631–639.

8. Stanley JC, Whitehouse WM, Zelenock GB, et al. Reoperation for complications of renal artery reconstructive surgery undertaken for treatment of renovascular hypertension. *J Vasc Surg.* 1985;2:133–144.

9. Jordan ML, Novick AC, Cunningham RL. The role of renal autotransplantation in pediatric and young adult patients with renal artery disease. *J Vasc Surg.* 1985;2:385–392.

10. Stanley JC, Ernst CB, Fry WJ. Fate of 100 aortorenal vein grafts: characteristics of late graft expansion, aneurysmal dilatation, and stenosis. *Surgery.* 1973;74:931–944.

11. Stanley JC. Renal revascularization: Errors in patient selection and complications of operation. In: Towne JB, Bernard VM, eds. *Complications in Vascular Surgery.* St. Louis, Mo: Quality Medical Publishing; 1991:180–203.

12. Short RHD. The vasa vasorum of the femoral vein. *J Pathol Bacteriol.* 1940;50:419.

13. Martinez A, Novick AC, Cunningham R, et al. Improved results of vascular reconstruction in pediatric and young adult patients with renovascular hypertension. *J Urol.* 1990;144:717–720.

14. Graham LM, Zelenock GB, Erlandson EE, et al. Abdominal aortic coarctation and segmental hypoplasia. *Surgery.* 1979;86:519–529.

15. Lewis VD III, Meranze SG, McLean GK, et al. The midaortic syndrome: diagnosis and treatment. *Radiology.* 1988;167:111–113.

16. Messina LM, Goldstone J, Farrell LD, et al. Middle aortic syndrome: effectiveness and durability of complex arterial revascularization techniques. *Ann Surg.* 1986;204:331–339.

17. Stanley JC, Brothers TE. Midabdominal aortic coarctation and hypoplasia associated with renal artery stenosis. In: Ernst CB, Stanley JC, eds. *Current Therapy in Vascular Surgery.* 2nd ed. Philadelphia, Pa: BC Decker; 1991:856–860.

18. Stanley JC, Brothers TE. Surgical treatment of renovascular hypertension in children. In: Ernst CB, Stanley JC, eds. *Current Therapy in Vascular Surgery.* 2nd ed. Philadelphia Pa: 1991:875–880.

19. Fry WJ, Ernst CB, Stanley JC. Renovascular hypertension in the pediatric patient. *Arch Surg.* 1973;107:692–698.

20. Ernst CB, Stanley JC, Marshall FF, et al. Autogenous sapenous vein aortorenal grafts. A ten-year experience. *Arch Surg.* 1972;105:855–864.

VI

Late Results for
Management of
Upper Extremity
Ischemia

30

Long-Term Outcome
of Raynaud's Syndrome

James M. Edwards, MD, and John M. Porter, MD

Raynaud's syndrome is a clinical condition characterized by episodic digital vasospasm occurring in response to cold or emotional stimuli. The prevalence in the population is surprisingly high, although most patients who have this condition do not seek medical attention. In contradistinction to most of the diseases regularly cared for by vascular surgeons for which the long-term outcome is known, the long-term outcome of patients with Raynaud's syndrome remains unclear. In fact, our knowledge of most aspects of Raynaud's syndrome including pathophysiology, epidemiology, and optimal treatment is incomplete. In this chapter we present the epidemiology, pathophysiology, clinical evaluation, and long-term outcome of patients with Raynaud's syndrome. Where necessary we divide Raynaud's syndrome patients into rather arbitrary groups when discussing outcome. We do not discuss the group of patients with vibration-associated Raynaud's syndrome (vibration white finger) in this chapter, thus limiting our discussion to spontaneously occurring digital vasospasm.

We feel that it is important to review the epidemiology, pathophysiology, and clinical evaluation of Raynaud's syndrome before discussing outcome because of the well-recognized important differences between all patients with Raynaud's syndrome and those patients with Raynaud's syndrome who present to a physician for evaluation and treatment. Most authors who have written on the subject correctly note that the outcome of those patients who present for treatment with severe vasospastic symptoms or Raynaud's syndrome, perhaps in association with a connective tissue disease, is likely to be measurably worse than the outcome in those patients with mild digital ischemia who have not sought medical attention.

EPIDEMIOLOGY

Although multiple studies have attempted to determine the incidence of Raynaud's syndrome in the general population, this work has been handicapped by the lack of a standardized definition or test for Raynaud's syndrome. The absence of a standardized diagnostic test continues to be a major hindrance to the conduct of research in this area. Thus, the various series presented below cannot be compared without the understanding that different definitions of Raynaud's syndrome were used for each.

TABLE 30–1. INCIDENCE OF RAYNAUD'S SYNDROME BY SEX

		No.		Incidence (%)	
Authors	Date	Female	Male	Female	Male
Lewis and Pickering[3]	1933	62	60	30	25
Taylor and Pelmear[4]	1976	0	254	—	5.3
Olsen and Nielsen[5]	1978	67	0	22	—
Heslop et al[6]	1983	229	221	17.6	8.3
Maricq et al[7]	1986	1,075	677	5.1	3.5
Leppert et al[8]	1987	2,705	0	15.6	—
Silman et al[9]	1990	182	231	19	11

Reports on Raynaud's syndrome appeared in the literature soon after Raynaud's initial report.[1,2] Hutchinson,[2] while noting in 1901 that "we are all subjects of Raynaud's phenomena in a greater or less degree," did not specifically discuss the incidence of Raynaud's syndrome in the general population. The first report that we are aware of that discussed the incidence of Raynaud's syndrome was that of Lewis and Pickering[3] in 1933. They found an incidence of Raynaud's syndrome in 25% of male and 30% of female medical and nursing students.

Since this initial report, many others have appeared with reported incidences of Raynaud's syndrome in the general population ranging from 3.5% to 25% in male patients and 5.1% to 30% in female patients. These reports are summarized in Table 30–1.[4–9] The number of patients with Raynaud's syndrome in these reports who seek medical attention for this condition is usually only a small fraction of those who experience Raynaud's attacks. There are many plausible explanations for the differences found in these studies such as choice of patient population, definition of Raynaud's syndrome, method of determining the diagnosis, and climate. We have concluded that the incidence of Raynaud's syndrome is significant in cool damp climates and varies widely around the world. It appears quite possible that if the incidence of Raynaud's syndrome varies from location to location, the long-term outcome in patients with Raynaud's syndrome may also be, at least in part, dependent on geographic localization. The incidence of connective tissue diseases such as scleroderma, a condition very frequently associated with Raynaud's syndrome, may also vary by location.[10,11]

PATHOPHYSIOLOGY AND CLASSIFICATION

The pathophysiology of Raynaud's syndrome remains unknown despite more than a century of study. Alterations in the sympathetic nervous system, adrenoceptor number and function, and most recently, alterations in naturally occurring vasoactive peptides such as endothelin and calcitonin gene–related peptide have been suggested. In part because the pathophysiology is unknown, the classification of patients with Raynaud's syndrome differs from report to report. As the classification of patient groups may have an apparent effect on outcome, we will briefly review the main classification systems presently in use.

The classification system used most frequently continues to be that of Allen and Brown.[12] In the early 1930s, they critically reviewed Raynaud's original thesis and proposed strict criteria for the separation and diagnosis of Raynaud's disease, which they considered a benign idiopathic form of intermittent digital ischemia, and

Raynaud's phenomenon, a similar complex seen in association with one or more of a wide variety of systemic diseases. Among the diagnostic criteria used to differentiate Raynaud's disease from Raynaud's phenomenon was the requirement that patients must have had the digital ischemic attacks for at least 2 years without the development of a disease known to be associated with Raynaud's phenomenon. In subsequent reports, it has become abundantly clear that patients may have Raynaud's attacks for many years before the development of an associated disease. This clearly shows that the diagnosis of Raynaud's *disease* can never be made with certainty, nor does the diagnosis of Raynaud's disease in anyway preclude the later diagnosis of Raynaud's *phenomenon* or an associated systemic disease process.

Although the cause of Raynaud's syndrome is unknown, we continue to believe that patients with Raynaud's syndrome may be divided into two groups based on the presence or absence of finger arterial obstruction. The physiologic basis for intermittent digital ischemia appears to differ in these groups.

The patients in the first group, termed *vasospastic*, have normal digital arteries and normal digital blood pressure at rest. These patients have an abnormally forceful contraction of the digital vessels in response to cold or emotional stimuli, which results in digital artery closure. The other group of patients, termed *obstructive*, have organic disease of the palmar and digital arteries, which results in a decrease in resting digital blood pressure. In these patients, a normal vasoconstrictive response to cold appears sufficient to overcome the decreased intraluminal pressure and to cause digital artery closure. This implies that all patients with severe digital artery occlusive disease will have Raynaud's attacks. Our experience indicates this is correct.

We feel that a division of Raynaud's syndrome patients into vasospastic and obstructive makes more sense than a division on the basis of the presence or absence of a currently diagnosable associated disease, as it is clear that the diagnosis of an associated disease may not become obvious until years later. For this reason, we use the term *Raynaud's syndrome* to describe all patients with episodic digital ischemia and then divide them into two groups based on the results of digital blood pressure and plethysmography. We recognize that all patients with Raynaud's syndrome are at an increased risk for developing an associated connective tissue disease. All patients with digital artery obstruction clearly already have an associated disease. It is not known if the division of patients into vasospastic and obstructive can be use to predict long-term outcome, as at least some patients initially correctly characterized as vasospastic will later develop obstruction and some patients with obstruction undoubtedly already have abnormally forceful vasospasm. It is equally clear that some patients with vasospastic Raynaud's syndrome do, in fact, have an associated connective tissue disease, although in our experience most patients with connective tissue disease have digital artery obstruction. Digital ischemic ulceration never occurs in patients with only vasospasm. In our experience, ulcer occurrence has universally indicated digital artery obstruction. It has also been our experience that patients with obstructive Raynaud's syndrome consistently have more severe digital ischemic symptoms than patients with vasospastic Raynaud's syndrome.

CLINICAL EVALUATION

The extent of the initial clinical evaluation depends in part on presenting symptoms. The basic evaluation consists of history and physical examination directed toward the signs and symptoms of connective tissue disorders including xerostomia, xerophalmia, dysphagia, telangiectasias, and sclerodactyly. Other studies include an immunology screen consisting of a complete blood count, sedimentation rate, antinu-clear antibody (ANA), and rheumatoid factor, a hand radiograph for the presence of calcinosis and tuft resorption, and a vascular laboratory evaluation including digital blood pressure measurement, digital plethysmographic waveforms, and a cold chal-lenge test. The cold challenge test that we use is the digital hypothermic challenge test described by Nielson and Lassen.[13] In our opinion this is the most accurate test for cold-induced digital vasospasm.[14] We have found that digital temperature recovery time after hand ice-water immersion, although quite specific, is insufficiently sensitive and therefore is not an accurate cold challenge test.[14] Microscopy of the nailfold capillaries is part of the routine evaluation in many centers and may contribute important information on associated connective tissue disease but not vasospastic disease.

Patients with digital artery occlusion in the absence of connective tissue disease, especially those with unilateral or single digit Raynaud's syndrome, should undergo further evaluation directed toward diagnosis of a hypercoaguable state or embolic disease source. This evaluation often includes a hypercoaguable screen (protein C, protein S, antiphospholipid antibody, lupus inhibitor, lipoprotein (a), and antithrom-bin III levels), echocardiography, and occasionally angiography. A few of these patients will prove to have distal distribution atherosclerosis, proximal arterial disease with embolization, or Buerger's disease. Hypercoaguable states plus the three condi-tions listed above are about the only causes of digital artery obstruction encountered in the absence of connective tissue disease.

LONG-TERM FOLLOW-UP

The risk of subsequent development of connective tissue disease in patients present-ing with Raynaud's syndrome appears significantly related to abnormalities detected at the time of initial presentation. In this section we will present the available data on the subsequent development of connective tissue disease in patients initially present-ing with Raynaud's symptoms.

As shown in Table 30–2, 0% to 25% of patients (mean, 6.3% at 3.3 years), who after appropriate serologic and clinical screening are initially diagnosed as Raynaud's syndrome without an associated disease, will develop an associated connective tissue disease over time.[15–22] The chance of patients with one or more clinical or serologic

TABLE 30–2. RISK OF SUBSEQUENT DIAGNOSIS OF A CONNECTIVE TISSUE DISEASE IN PATIENTS WITH RAYNAUD'S SYNDROME AND NO SEROLOGIC OR CLINICAL ABNORMALITIES

Authors	Date	No.	Mean Follow-up (yr)	Progression to Connective Tissue Disease (%)
Blain et al[15]	1951	100	5+	25
Gifford and Hines[16]	1957	280	2+	4.6
Harper et al[17]	1982	37	2	2.7
Gerbracht et al[18]	1985	75	3.7	2.7
Sheiner and Small[19]	1987	78	3.5	0
Priollet et al[20]	1987	49	4.7	0
Fitzgerald et al[21]	1988	33	2.7	9
Kallenberg et al[22]	1988	29	6	3.4
Wollersheim et al[23]	1989	51	3.5	7.8
Gentric et al[24]	1990	16	4	6.3
Weiner et al[25]	1991	40	4	0

abnormalities, in most series a positive ANA, abnormal nailfold capillary pattern, or sclerodactyly, developing a connective tissue diseases over time is much higher (11% to 65%; mean, 42% at 4 years) as shown in Table 30–3.[17–25]

Blain and co-workers[15] reported in 1950 their experience with 100 patients diagnosed as having Raynaud's syndrome without an associated disease followed for more than 5 years. Six percent of their patients experienced moderate symptomatic progression and 25% experienced severe symptomatic progression defined as development of ulceration and gangrene or worsening ischemia requiring dorsal sympathectomy. The incidence of associated disease in the group that worsened was not given. Because of the presence of digital ulceration/gangrene, we have assumed in Table 30–2 that all patients in this group did develop an associated disease.

Gifford and Hines[16] reviewed the experience of the Mayo Clinic with Raynaud's syndrome in 1956. They were able to find records on 756 female patients diagnosed as having Raynaud's disease between 1920 and 1945. Information on the initial evaluation and follow-up was available on 280 patients, although the length of follow-up is not specified. Thirteen patients developed a systemic disease process over time, including a prolonged febrile illness resulting in death in two patients, polyarteritis nodosa in one patient, biliary cirrhosis in one patient, scleroderma in four patients, and rheumatoid arthritis in five patients.

Harper et al[17] prospectively studied 56 patients with Raynaud's syndrome without connective tissue disease. Thirty-nine patients were classified as primary Raynaud's phenomenon and the remaining 17 were classified as undifferentiated connective tissue disorder, which these authors defined as Raynaud's phenomenon in association with one or more suggestive but not diagnostic features of connective tissue disease. Thirty-seven of the 39 primary Raynaud's patients had negative serologic testing initially, and the remaining two patients had a positive ANA. At a mean follow-up of 23.7 months, only one of the 37 primary Raynaud's patients who were serologically negative initially developed connective tissue disease (and this patient initially had abnormal nailfold capillaroscopy) whereas eight of the 19 patients with the original diagnosis of undifferentiated connective tissue disorder or a positive ANA developed a connective tissue disease under follow-up.

Gerbracht et al[18] re-examined 87 patients originally diagnosed as having no associated disease at a mean interval of 3.7 years. Two of 75 patients without and two of 12 patients with clinical or serologic abnormalities at the initial examination developed connective tissue disease during follow-up.

Sheiner and Small[19] followed 78 patients with Raynaud's syndrome and negative

TABLE 30–3. RISK OF SUBSEQUENT DIAGNOSIS OF A CONNECTIVE TISSUE DISEASE IN PATIENTS WITH RAYNAUD'S SYNDROME AND ONE OR MORE SEROLOGIC OR CLINICAL ABNORMALITIES

Authors	Date	No.	Mean Follow-up (yr)	Progression to Connective Tissue Disease (%)
Harper et al[17]	1982	17	2	35.3
Gerbracht et al[18]	1985	12	3.7	16.7
Sheiner and Small[19]	1987	19	3.5	15.8
Priollet et al[20]	1987	24	4.7	58.3
Fitzgerald et al[21]	1988	25	2.7	32
Kallenberg et al[22]	1988	35	6	25.7
Wollersheim et al[23]	1989	20	3.5	65
Gentric et al[24]	1990	9	4	11
Weiner et al[25]	1991	23	4	17.4

serology for a mean of 3.5 years. No patients developed a connective tissue disease during follow-up. An additional 19 patients with positive ANAs were followed, and three of these patients developed connective tissue disease.

Priollet and colleagues[20] reviewed the records of 73 patients with Raynaud's syndrome, of whom 49 had negative serology (which included ANA, anticentromere antibody, rheumatoid factor, and ribonucleoprotein). None of the 49 patients with negative serology and 13 of the 24 patients with positive serologies developed connective tissue disease at a mean follow-up of 4.7 years.

Fitzgerald et al[21] prospectively followed 58 patients with Raynaud's syndrome for a mean of 2.7 years. Three of 33 patients without any clinical or serologic abnormalities and eight of 25 patients with one or more nondiagnostic abnormalities developed connective tissue disease during follow-up.

Kallenberg et al[22] reviewed the records of 64 patients initially referred for evaluation of Raynaud's syndrome. All patients were followed for at least 6 years. One of 29 patients with an initially negative ANA and nine of 35 patients with an initially positive ANA developed a connective tissue disease during follow-up.

Wollersheim et al[23] prospectively evaluated 71 patients with Raynaud's syndrome who initially had no clinical evidence of a connective tissue disease. Four of 51 patients with an initially negative ANA and 13 of 20 patients with an initially positive ANA developed connective tissue disease during a mean of 3.5 years follow-up.

Gentric et al[24] prospectively followed 25 patients with Raynaud's syndrome for a mean of 4 years. Sixteen of these patients had negative ANAs at the time of the initial evaluation. Only one patient in the entire group developed a connective tissue disease during follow-up.

Weiner et al[25] followed 53 patients with Raynaud's syndrome for a mean of 4 years. No patient who was initially seronegative developed connective tissue disease, whereas 10 of 23 patients with initially positive serologies developed one or more definite features of connective tissue disease, including four patients with clearly diagnosable diseases. Three of 38 patients with either normal or borderline nailfold capillary patterns and six of eight patients with abnormal capillary patterns developed definite features of a connective tissue disease over time.

The reason for the differences in these studies is doubtless multifactorial and related in part to differences in the population enrolled as well as length of follow-up. The papers published in the 1950s were severely handicapped by the lack of serologic testing, and no clear conclusion can be drawn from them.[15,16] It is clear from the remaining reports that patients who have any clinical or laboratory abnormalities (e.g., serology, capillary nailfold microscopy, ulcers), although not diagnostic of any disease process at the initial evaluation, have a much higher relative risk of developing a diagnosable connective tissue disease during follow-up.[17–25] Unfortunately most of the studies have so few patients followed for more than 5 years that little information is available concerning the long-term risk of patients with Raynaud's syndrome developing connective tissue disease more than 5 years later. Several authors have attempted to increase the length of follow-up by presenting their data with a calculated "follow-up from the time the patient noted the onset of Raynaud's attacks," which gives mean follow-up of 8 to 15 years with the same percentage results as shown in Table 30–2.[18,20] We do not believe that these calculated follow-up times are sufficiently accurate to support clinical decision making and have chosen to not use them.

The most reliable markers for later development of connective tissue disease in an individual patient with Raynaud's syndrome appear to be a positive ANA or abnormal capillary patterns on nailfold microscopy. Positive ANAs have been reported to occur in 12% of an otherwise normal female population and no connective tissue disease developed in these patients after 5 years of follow-up.[26] Additionally, the development of a connective tissue disease does not mean that the patient will ever develop ischemic digital ulceration or require finger amputation. In our experience, digital ulcerations, although painful, are benign in the large majority in that they do heal, albeit slowly, with conservative care and with minimal tissue loss.[27]

We are not aware of any published information that specifically describes the long-term outcome of patients with Raynaud's syndrome who initially present with an associated connective tissue disease. Our anecdotal experience is that although these patients do fare worse than those Raynaud's patients without an associated disease, including recurrent digital ischemic ulceration in the most severely affected, even these patients rarely require significant digital amputation. We have never been convinced that thoracic sympathectomy conveys any benefit in these patients and do not recommend its use. We have evaluated and followed more than 1,000 patients with Raynaud's syndrome during the past 20 years and have performed fingertip débridement to speed healing in 20 to 30 patients and distal interphalangeal amputations in only two patients during this period. No more proximal amputations have ever been required.

OVERVIEW

Curiously, the long-term outcome of patients with Raynaud's syndrome is not known with certainty despite years of interest. Patients who present with Raynaud's syndrome without evidence of digital artery obstruction, serologic abnormalities, or nailfold capillary abnormalities appear to have low likelihood of ever developing digital artery obstruction, ischemic digital ulceration, or an associated connective tissue disease.

Patients who present with one or more signs or symptoms of an associated connective tissue disease including positive ANA, significant digital artery obstruction, or ischemic digital ulceration, or an abnormal capillary nailfold pattern have a significant risk of developing an associated connective tissue disorder over time. These patients and those presenting with an associated connective tissue disease have a higher incidence of digital ulceration, which is best managed with conservative measures and local wound care. Major finger amputation (one or more phalanges) is rarely, if ever, required. Upper extremity sympathectomy appears to be of no value. The prognosis of Raynaud's patients who develop connective tissue disease is determined entirely by that disease. Such diseases in our experience may unpredictably pursue virulently aggressive or quiescent courses. We have found participation by immunologists or rheumatologists in patient management quite helpful.

Acknowledgment
This work was supported in part by grant RR-00334, General Clinical Research Centers Branch, Division of Research Resources, National Institutes of Health, Bethesda, Maryland.

REFERENCES

1. Garland GM. Raynaud's disease. *JAMA.* 1889;13:837–839.
2. Hutchinson J. Raynaud's phenomenon. *Med Press Circular.* 1901;128:403–405.
3. Lewis T, Pickering G. Observations upon maladies in which the blood supply to the digits ceases intermittently or permanently and upon bilateral gangrene of the digits: observations relevant to so-called "Raynaud's disease." *Clin Sci.* 1934;1:327–366.

4. Taylor Q, Pelmear PL. Raynaud's phenomenon of occupational origin: an epidemiological survey. *Acta Chir Scand*. 1976;465(Suppl.):27–32.

5. Olsen N, Nielsen SL. Prevalence of primary Raynaud's phenomenon in young females. *Scand J Clin Lab Invest*. 1978;38:761–764.

6. Heslop J, Coggon D, Acheson ED. The prevalence of intermittent digital ischaemia (Raynaud's phenomenon) in a general practice. *J R Coll Gen Pract*. 1983;33:85–89.

7. Maricq HR, Weinrich MC, Keil JE, et al. Prevalence of Raynaud's phenomenon in the general population. *J Chronic Dis*. 1986;39:423–427.

8. Leppert J, Aberg H, Ringqvist I, et al. Raynaud's phenomenon in a female population: prevalence and association with other conditions. *Angiology*. 1987;38:871–877.

9. Silman A, Holligan S, Brennan P, et al. Prevalence of symptoms of Raynaud's phenomenon in general practice. *Br Med J*. 1990;301:590–592.

10. Maricq HR, Weinrich MC, Keil JE, et al. Prevalence of scleroderma spectrum disorders in the general population of South Carolina. *Arthritis Rheum*. 1989;32:998–1006.

11. Michet CJ Jr, McKenna CH, Elveback LR, et al. Epidemiology of systemic lupus erythematosus and other connective tissue diseases in Rochester, Minnesota, 1950–1979. *Mayo Clin Proc*. 1985;60:105–113.

12. Allen E, Brown G. Raynaud's disease: a critical review of minimal requisites for diagnosis. *Am J Med Sci*. 1932;83:187–200.

13. Nielson SL, Lassen NA. Measurement of digital blood pressure after local cooling. *J Appl Physiol*. 1977;43:907–910.

14. Gates KH, Tyburczy JA, Zupan T, et al. The noninvasive quantification of digital vasospasm. *Bruit*. 1984;8:34–37.

15. Blain A III, Coller FA, Carver GB. Raynaud's disease: a study of criteria for prognosis. *Surgery*. 1951;29:387–397.

16. Gifford RW Jr, Hines EA Jr. Raynaud's disease among women and girls. *Circulation*. 1957;16:1012–1021.

17. Harper FE, Maricq HR, Turner RE, et al. A prospective study of Raynaud's phenomenon and early connective tissue disease: a five-year report. *Am J Med*. 1982;72:883–888.

18. Gerbracht DD, Steen VD, Ziegler GL, et al. Evolution of primary Raynaud's phenomenon (Raynaud's disease) to connective tissue disease. *Arthritis Rheum*. 1985;28:87–92.

19. Sheiner NM, Small P. Isolated Raynaud's phenomenon—a benign disorder. *Ann Allergy*. 1987;58:114–117.

20. Priollet P, Vayssairat M, Housset E. How to classify Raynaud's phenomenon: long-term follow-up study of 73 cases. *Am J Med*. 1987;83:494–498.

21. Fitzgerald O, Hess EV, O'Connor GT, et al. Prospective study of the evolution of Raynaud's phenomenon. *Am J Med*. 1988;84:718–726.

22. Kallenberg CG, Wouda AA, Hoet MH, et al. Development of connective tissue disease in patients presenting with Raynaud's phenomenon: a six year follow-up with emphasis on the predictive value of antinuclear antibodies as detected by immunoblotting. *Ann Rheum Dis*. 1988;47:634–641.

23. Wollersheim H, Thien T, Hoet MH, et al. The diagnostic value of several immunological tests for anti-nuclear antibody in predicting the development of connective tissue disease in patients presenting with Raynaud's phenomenon. *Eur J Clin Invest*. 1989;19:535–541.

24. Gentric A, Blaschek MA, Le Noach JF, et al. Serological arguments for classifying Raynaud's phenomenon as idiopathic. *J Rheum*. 1990;17:1177–1181.

25. Weiner ES, Hildebrandt S, Senecal JL, et al. Prognostic significance of anticentromere antibodies and anti-topoisomerase I antibodies in Raynaud's disease. A prospective study. *Arthritis Rheum*. 1991;34:68–77.

26. Yadin O, Sarov B, Naggan L, et al. Natural autoantibodies in the serum of healthy women—a five-year follow-up. *Clin Exp Immunol*. 1989;75:402–406.

27. Mills JL, Friedman EI, Taylor LM Jr, et al. Upper extremity ischemia caused by small artery disease. *Ann Surg*. 1987;206:521–528.

31

Upper Extremity Bypass:

Five-Year Follow-Up

Charles L. Mesh, MD, and James S.T. Yao, MD, PhD

Upper extremity ischemia is a relatively infrequent occurrence, and arterial lesions of the upper extremity account for only 4% of all operations performed by the vascular surgeon.[1,2] Unlike lower extremity ischemia, the possible etiologies for upper extremity ischemia are often multiple. Although the long-term mortality of patients with upper extremity occlusive disease[3,4] is equivalent to that of patients with lower extremity disease,[5,6] the risk of major amputation in the patient with upper extremity ischemia[1,2,4,7–12] is significantly less than that of the patient with lower extremity disorders.[13] This dichotomy has been explained by the relatively rich collateral vascular pathways of the upper extremity.

Direct surgical treatment of upper extremity arterial ischemia was first described in 1956.[14] Reflecting the relative rarity of this disorder, the first report of upper extremity autogenous vein bypass grafting did not appear until 1965, when Garrett and co-workers[15] described their series of 11 patients. Since then, there have been many reports of surgical treatment of upper extremity ischemia.[1,3,4,7–12,16–19] From review of the literature, it is difficult to determine the long-term results of upper extremity bypass grafting, as reports often mix different operative procedures such as bypass, endarterectomy, direct repair, and embolectomy. Further, many reports are not large enough to provide meaningful information about site of distal anastomosis, type of conduit, or even long-term outcome.

This chapter will focus on proximal upper extremity occlusive lesions with the exception of those associated with the subclavian steal syndrome. Because of the wide variation in vascular anatomy of the upper extremity, a brief review of this anatomy is included. The important role played by bypass grafting in relief of upper extremity ischemia will be illustrated by the long-term patencies achieved in the surgical experience at Northwestern University.

ANATOMY

The major arterial supply to the upper extremity is the subclavian artery. This artery spans the thoracic outlet and is arbitrarily divided into three parts by the anterior scalene muscle. The first part is primarily intrathoracic but gives off its three major branches (the vertebral, the thyrocervical trunk, and the internal thoracic) as it breaks the plane of the thoracic inlet just proximal to the anterior scalene muscle. The second portion, deep to the anterior scalene, has only one branch (the costocervical trunk). The third part of the subclavian artery extends laterally to the anterior scalene, overlying the first rib, and gives rise to the dorsal scapular artery.

The axillary artery courses 15 cm, from the lateral border of the first rib to the inferior border of the teres major muscle. Six branches arise from it (the highest thoracic, the thoracoacromial, the lateral thoracic, the subscapular, and the anterior and posterior humeral circumflex arteries). These arteries provide an abundant collateral network about the shoulder.

The brachial artery begins at the lower border of the teres major muscle and terminates at the elbow into the radial and ulnar arteries. The deep brachial artery is the first and largest branch, supplying the deltoid and triceps muscles. The radial or ulnar artery may arise just distal to the deep brachial in 10% to 15% and 2% to 3% of patients, respectively. Collateral branches around the elbow include the middle collateral and radial collateral arteries arising from profunda brachii, and the superior and inferior ulnar collaterals arising directly from the brachial.

The terminal branches of the brachial artery supply the hand and collateralize around the elbow. The first branch of the ulnar artery is the common interosseous. This artery, likened to the peroneal artery in the calf, provides the interosseous recurrent artery for collateralization with the middle collateral. It also gives rise to the anterior and posterior interosseous arteries, which supply the anterior and posterior forearm musculature, respectively. The anterior and posterior recurrent ulnar arteries also arise from the ulnar artery and anastomose with the superior and inferior ulnar collateral arteries, respectively. Distally, the ulnar artery directly forms the superficial palmar arch of the hand, which in turn forms the common digital arteries and thus supplies the major source of blood to the digits.

The radial artery branch anastomosing about the elbow with the radial collateral is the recurrent radial artery. Distally, the radial artery predominantly supplies the thumb and radial aspect of the index finger through the first volar metacarpal artery but also gives rise to smaller, deep palmar arch. An incomplete superficial palmar arch, present in 20% of cases, is defined as one in which the superficial arch does not anastomose with any radial branch, and the ulnar artery does not supply the thumb and radial aspects of the index finger.[20] The common digital arteries and the volar metacarpal arteries split into proper digital arteries, which supply radial and ulnar aspects of each digit.

The abundant collateral networks about the shoulder and elbow are responsible for the lack of symptoms in patients with chronic, isolated, proximal upper extremity occlusions. The exception to this rule is digital occlusion. Multilevel arterial occlusions, which include forearm or digital arterial obliteration, are common in symptomatic individuals.

ETIOLOGY

The etiology of upper extremity occlusive disease amenable to surgical intervention can be broadly categorized into occlusive, embolic, and traumatic. Proximal occlusive lesions do not usually produce severe ischemic symptoms in the absence of concomitant forearm or digital disease[17] caused by microembolization. Proximal occlusive lesions in the subclavian artery occur most often on the left and most commonly result from atherosclerosis at the origin of the artery at the aorta.[1,2,4,7,12] Other causes of proximal occlusion are Takayasu's arteritis, giant cell arteritis, radiation injury,[21] and fibromuscular dysplasia. The distal hand arteries, not accessible to surgery, can be obliterated by Buerger's disease, by connective tissue disorders, and in diabetics and patients with end-stage renal disease, by calciphylaxis.[22]

Emboli are another major cause of upper extremity ischemia.[23,24] The site of embolization, proximal or distal, determines clinical behavior. Proximal emboli are macroemboli. Macroemboli originate predominantly in the heart and migrate to the upper extremity 30% of the time. Sixty percent lodge in the brachial position, 23% in the axillary position, and 12% in the subclavian position.[22] These emboli usually cause acute symptoms. In contrast, microemboli originate from axillary or subclavian aneurysms because of mechanical compression. Symptoms are chronic in nature because of multiple distal artery involvement.[25–27] The cumulative obliteration of the forearm and digital vasculature results in progressive severe ischemia.

Trauma can be classified into iatrogenic and noniatrogenic. Nearly all iatrogenic trauma is penetrating[28] and results primarily from catheter injury.[29] The sites of injury reflect catheterization sites (brachial and axillary). Other iatrogenic axillary artery injuries result when this vessel is the site for angio-access for chemotherapy[30] or inflow for axillary-femoral bypass grafts.[31] The former causes obliteration of the axillary artery, and the latter causes distal embolization when the axillofemoral graft thromboses. Noniatrogenic trauma is also penetrating and nonpenetrating. Penetrating noniatrogenic trauma is predominantly from violent force such as gunshot or stab wounds. With increasing use of illicit drugs, severe hand ischemia can be seen in drug users caused by inadvertent intra-arterial injection. Unlike the lower extremity, repetitive, exaggerated shoulder motion is a common cause of upper extremity ischemia. Among these conditions is thoracic outlet compression of the subclavian artery by cervical rib or anomalous first rib and subsequent aneurysm formation.[25,27] In these patients, distal embolization is common. Not only bony anomalies can cause arterial injury. Repetitive trauma from violent throwing motion in baseball pitchers can also produce hand ischemia caused by injury of the axillary or subclavian artery.[32] Another form of repetitive axillary artery trauma is crutch injury.[33] Similarly, hypothenar hammer syndrome with injury to the ulnar artery has been described in athletes such as catchers or karate experts.

MANAGEMENT

Treatment of the patient with upper extremity ischemia has three major components: diagnostic, surgical, and adjunctive. The studies associated with each component can be performed simultaneously. Evaluation is incomplete if all three areas are not explored.

Diagnostic Investigation

The most useful diagnostic investigation in the patient with upper extremity ischemia is the history and physical examination.[34] Patients with acute symptoms will usually complain of either a painful digit or hand, reflecting micro- or macroembolization, respectively. More chronic presentations of forearm fatigue, hand rest pain, hand and arm cold intolerance, and digital ulceration or gangrene all reflect either multilevel disease or distal digital occlusions.

More detailed historic investigation should focus on medical history, trauma history, pharmacologic history, occupational history, and athletic activities. Medical history will reveal previous invasive arterial diagnostic or therapeutic procedures, a history of radiation therapy, a history of bypass or angio-access using the axillary artery, and a history of previous bypass surgery. Trauma history will reflect recent penetrating trauma. Cardiac history with attention to the presence of a recent myocardial infarction or atrial fibrillation will suggest macroembolization. Occupational history will point to vibratory white finger. A survey of athletic activities will focus on injury to the subclavian or axillary artery in baseball pitchers and the ulnar artery in catchers.

Physical examination will usually localize the lesion and consequently imply its etiology. Bilateral brachial blood pressure will indicate proximal occlusions when present, and palpation for subclavian, axillary, brachial, radial, and ulnar pulses will help to localize the level. Subclavian artery aneurysms and cervical ribs can frequently be palpated in the supraclavicular fossa. Auscultation for supra- and infraclavicular bruits with the arm in neutral and provocative positions will often reveal thoracic outlet compression. Finally, inspection of the skin with particular emphasis on the hand and digits may detail findings of fingertip cyanosis and punctate hemorrhage consistent with microembolization. Examination of the upper extremity is incomplete unless Allen's test is performed to ascertain palmar arch patency.

Arteriography

Arteriography provides diagnostic confirmation and guides surgical therapy. Although investigators have clearly documented that angiographic study in the upper extremity can diagnose the etiology of the disease process,[35] angiography is often a secondary confirmation reached after a thorough history and physical examination.

Angiography determines the precise intervention necessary once the decision for therapy is affirmed. Upper extremity angiography defines the pathologic lesion, its extent, and the degree of distal runoff destruction. As such it determines the type of therapy (bypass or nonbypass), inflow and outflow sites, the need for vascular exclusion (embolic source), and the need for pre- or intraoperative thrombolytic therapy (obliteration of distal runoff). Arteriography must include proximal arch vessels with complete visualization of the hand vasculature. If thoracic outlet compression is suspected, exposure must be made with the arm in abduction and external rotation to delineate the exact site of compression.

Noninvasive Tests

Noninvasive diagnostic measures supply primarily diagnostic and follow-up information. These tests consist of duplex scanning, segmental pressure measurements, analog waveform analysis, and the recording of finger systolic pressures.[36] Because duplex scanning provides B-mode anatomic data, it is helpful to detect subclavian artery aneurysms.

Segmental pressures, analog waveform analysis, and spectral analysis all are used predominantly for objective postoperative surveillance of upper extremity bypass grafts. As discussed above, this technology is not required for the detection of upper extremity ischemia and is usually not necessary for diagnosis. Although these tests can provide preoperative confirmation of the diagnosis suspected from the history and physical examination, their most important application is to establish a baseline for postoperative surveillance. Postoperatively, the noninvasive techniques supplement clinical examination in the follow-up of bypass grafts.

Surgical Technique

The details of surgical techniques have been reported previously.[37] Briefly, the inflow originates from either the proximal subclavian, axillary, or brachial artery. The normality of these vessels is determined by angiography. In patients undergoing repeat bypasses, the common carotid artery is occasionally used for inflow.

The site for distal anastomosis is determined on the basis of disease location and detailed examination of hand anatomy as depicted by angiography. It should be placed in the most easily exposed, patent vessel in direct continuity with the hand. If there is no continuity, the interosseous artery is often patent and available for bypass.[7] In recent years, intraoperative, as well as preoperative, thrombolysis has proven useful in cases of poor runoff with multiple distal arterial occlusions.[38]

The conduit of choice in upper extremity bypass is autogenous vein.[1–3,7,12,15,18] Like exposures, this preference is modified by location of disease and history of previous bypass grafts. In terms of disease location, upper extremity bypass grafting can be divided relative to the brachial bifurcation. There is no satisfactory alternative to autogenous tissue in distal bypasses to the forearm vessels. In contrast, prosthetic proximal (ePTFE) is used in proximal outflow sites if autogenous vein is unavailable. The one exception to this practice is a carotid subclavian bypass, in which a prosthesis is the conduit of choice.[39] The most common source of autogenous conduits is the greater saphenous vein. Other reported sources include the lesser saphenous vein,[7] basilic vein,[12] cephalic vein,[12] and external iliac artery.[17] Recently, several investigators have described use of the *in situ* technique in the upper extremity.[40,41]

Adjunctive Procedures

Three adjunctive measures are frequently required in addition to standard vascular reconstructions in patients with upper extremity ischemia. They are thoracic outlet decompression, intraoperative thrombolytic therapy, and anticoagulation. These secondary procedures are critical to the success to upper extremity bypass for two reasons. First, most subclavian aneurysms are the result of a cervical rib and thoracic outlet compression.[26,27,42] Failure to remove the bony anomaly of the thoracic outlet will inevitably doom a technically perfect upper extremity bypass to failure. Second, the pathophysiology of most symptomatic upper extremity ischemia involves an index proximal lesion with secondary embolization to the forearm and hand vasculature. As such, thrombolytic therapy, pre- or intraoperative, may improve the distal runoff enough to support a bypass.[39] Postoperative anticoagulation is a natural complement to this approach in the patient with poor runoff. Its effectiveness in extending the patency of lower extremity bypass has been documented.[43,44]

Decompression of the myo-osseous structures of the thoracic outlet (supraclavicular scalenectomy, first-rib resection, and cervical rib resection) is a critical part of the treatment of subclavian aneurysms caused by bony anomaly. This decompression procedure is executed through a combined supra- and infraclavicular approach.[27] Unlike the transaxillary approach, this technique provides wide exposure of all neural and vascular structures in the thoracic outlet, a requirement for patients with vascular compression in this region.[7,26,27] A different form of decompression is required in athletes with humeral head compression of the axillary artery. In this situation, the head of the humerus, obviously, cannot be removed. Instead, the arterial branch tethering the axillary artery against the humerus, usually the anterior humeral circumflex artery, is divided and effectively provides mobility of the axillary artery. Concomitant vein patch of the axillary artery at the site of compression ensures wider lumen of the artery.

Because one of the fundamental problems in the patient with symptomatic upper extremity ischemia is obliteration of the distal vasculature, the application of thrombolytic therapy is a natural step in patients without classical contraindications.[39] A dose of 125,000 to 250,000 units of urokinase is infused into the vasculature distal to elbow before occlusion for distal anastomosis. Intraoperative administration uses direct infusion into the distal vasculature, often impossible preoperatively because of proximal occlusions. In addition, during intraoperative thrombolysis the washout of urokinase by collaterals is obviated by inflow occlusion.

A final useful adjuvant in upper extremity bypass surgery is postoperative anticoagulation. It is used in patients with distal grafts and poor runoff, in those with repeated bypass grafts, and in those with proven coagulation disorders.

NORTHWESTERN UNIVERSITY EXPERIENCE

During a 13-year period extending from 1978 to 1991, 43 patients with upper extremity ischemia underwent upper extremity bypasses. A total of 61 procedures were performed in this group of 22 men and 21 women with ages ranging from 16 to 74 years. Twenty patients smoked, four patients had diabetes mellitus, 12 patients were hypertensive, and three patients suffered from collagen-vascular disorders. Table 31–1 summarizes the etiology of upper extremity ischemia. Indications for bypass were forearm fatigue in 15%, rest pain in 48%, tissue loss in 20%, cold intolerance in 11%, aneurysmal degeneration of vein grafts in 3%, and assymptomatic subclavian aneurysms in 3%.

There were 36 primary operations and 25 redo secondary bypasses. Table 31–2 summarizes the placement of proximal and distal anastomosis. Seventy-five percent of distal anastomoses were proximal to the brachial artery bifurcation, and the remainder were placed distal to this site. Seventy-two percent of grafts were autogenous tissue and 24% were prosthetic. Intraoperative thrombolysis was used in 11% of patients, and postoperative anticoagulation was deemed necessary in 31%.

Follow-up ranged from 1 month to 8 years and consisted of physical examination and Doppler-derived segmental pressures. Operative mortality was zero. There were

TABLE 31–1. ETIOLOGY OF UPPER EXTREMITY ISCHEMIA

Etiology	No. of Patients
Bypass graft thrombosis	18
Emboli (thoracic outlet syndrome)	18
Atherosclerosis	8
Unknown	3
Radiation arteritis	2
Takayasu's arteritis	2
Aneurysm (thoracic outlet syndrome)	2
Vein graft aneurysm	2
Rheumatoid arthritis	1
Fibromuscular dysplasia	1
Infection	1
Ehlers-Danlos syndrome	1
Buerger's disease	1
Arteriovenous malformation	1

TABLE 31–2. PROXIMAL AND DISTAL ANASTOMOSES

Proximal Anastomosis		Distal Anastomosis
Aortic Arch	2	Subclavian 1 Axillary 1
Subclavian	18	Subclavian 1 Axillary 15 Brachial 1 Radial 1
Axillary	13	Brachial 8 Radial 1 Ulnar 1 Interosseous 3
Brachial	9	Brachial 2 Radial 4 Interosseous 3
Carotid	19	Subclavian 5 Axillary 1 Brachial 11 Ulnar 1 Radial 1

no major upper extremity amputations. Long-term mortality in this patient population was 76.6% (Fig. 31–1). Overall patency at 5 years was 52.2% (Fig. 31–2). The patency for anastomosis proximal to the brachial artery bifurcation was better than that for more distal placement (i.e., distal to the brachial bifurcation) (Fig. 31–3). In addition, autogenous grafts faired better than did prosthetic conduits (Fig. 31–4). Finally, the patency rate for secondary redo bypass grafts was worse than that for primary grafts (Fig. 31–5). This latter finding may reflect the use of prosthetic grafts

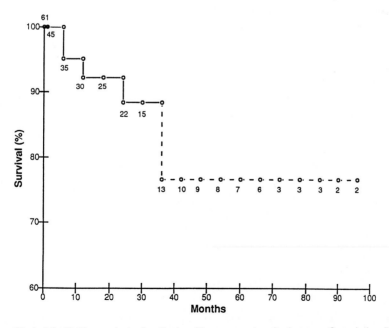

Figure 31–1. Life Table survival of patients with upper extremity bypass. Cumulative 5-year survival is 76.6%.

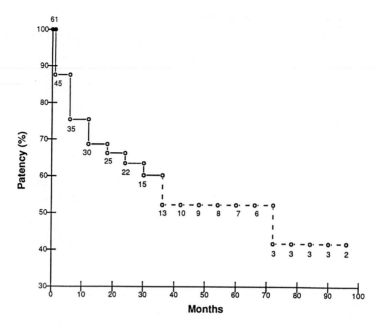

Figure 31–2. Life Table analysis of overall patency in patients with upper extremity bypass. Cumulative 5-year patency is 52.2%.

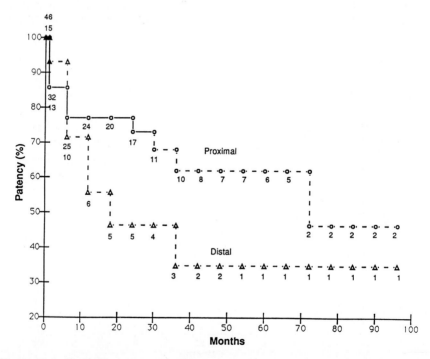

Figure 31–3. Life Table analysis of graft patency in upper extremity bypass grafts with distal anastomosis proximal to or beyond the brachial bifurcation. Cumulative 5-year patency for proximal bypass is 61.9% and that for distal bypasses is 34.8%.

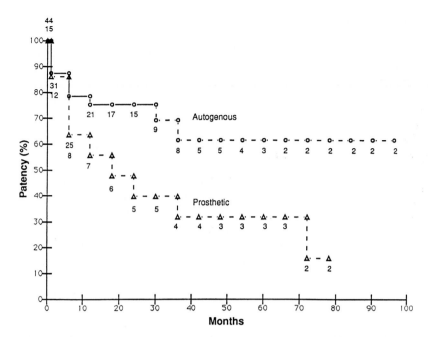

Figure 31–4. Life Table analysis of graft patency in autogenous and prosthetic upper extremity bypass grafts. Cumulative 5-year patency for autogenous conduits is 61.5% and that for prosthesis is 31.9%.

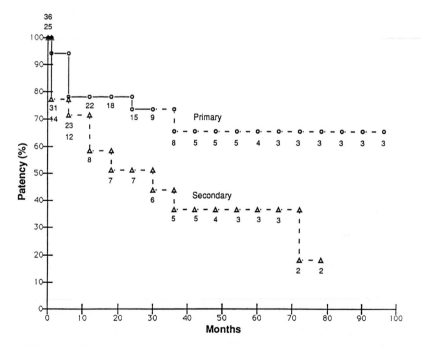

Figure 31–5. Life Table analysis of graft patency in primary and secondary "redo" upper extremity bypass grafts. The cumulative 5-year patency for primary grafts is 65.5%. Secondary, redo bypass grafts have a patency rate of only 36.6%. This difference is significant at $P<.05$ using log rank analysis.

for secondary bypasses. Finally, the secondary bypasses had a higher morbidity than did the primary procedures. Most complications were related to hemorrhage and hematoma in the secondary group and may reflect the higher rate of postoperative anticoagulation in this group.

COMMENTS

Since the report of Garrett et al[15] in 1965, there has been little discussion about the necessity of using vein as the graft to the axillary or more distal vessels. There is currently no more than anecdotal data available on the use of prosthetic bypasses to sites beyond the brachial artery bifurcation. We have previously reported a Life Table analysis of the Northwestern University experience with long vein grafts in the upper extremity and noted a 3-year overall patency rate of 67%.[7] Other workers have reported patency rates for long upper extremity autogenous bypasses ranging from 77% to 100% with follow-ups as long as 8 years.[1,3,4,8,12]

The mortality associated with upper extremity bypass can be divided into operative and long-term. The overall operative mortality of most reports is from 0% to 2%.[1,3,4,7,16] In these reports nearly all deaths occurred in patients subjected to intrathoracic procedures. This difference was clearly pointed out by the experience of Crawford et al[4] in 1969 with 108 intrathoracic and 177 extracavatary upper extremity bypasses for proximal subclavian or innominate artery disease. The operative mortalities were 5.6% and 2.3%, respectively. The discrepancy is certainly a reflection of the magnitude of the procedure and the age of the patients. The relative safety of extrathoracic repair of proximal subclavian artery occlusive disease has been confirmed in numerous other centers.[7,9,11] The long-term mortality reported in most series ranges from 10% to 50%.[3,9,11] Life Table analysis has been applied in three studies. Two studies found the 5-year survival rate to be 80%[3,11] and the other reported a rate of 50%.[9]

Patency rates in upper extremity bypass reflect the location of distal anastomosis (proximal to brachial bifurcation versus distal), length of bypass graft, and indications for surgery (upper extremity symptoms versus subclavian steal cerebrovascular symptoms). There are four available reports that have used Life Table analysis to interpret data.[2,3,10,11] Of those four studies, only McCarthy et al[7] have reported on patients with purely upper extremity symptoms. They found an overall 3-year patency for upper extremity bypass of 67%. They further analyzed their data based on site of distal anastomosis and noted that grafts at or above the brachial bifurcation and those distal to the brachial bifurcation had 2-year patency rates of 83% and 53%, respectively. Harris et al[3] also provided Life Table analysis of bypass in 28 patients for pure upper extremity ischemia and reported 2-year patencies of 88%. Although there was no Life Table, this group noted a 94% and an 84% patency for distal anastomosis located proximal and distal to the brachial bifurcation. The other two Life Table reports by Moore et al[10] and Kretschmer et al[11] dealt solely with proximal location of the distal anastomosis, mixed bypasses for pure upper extremity ischemia with those for subclavian steal, and reported patency rates of 84% and 78%, respectively, at 2 years. The figure that balances the patency rates for upper extremity bypass is the rate of major amputation. The aforementioned four reports noted that no major amputations were required.[2,3,10,11] Other workers have noted major upper extremity amputation rates of 1% to 6%.[1,12]

In contrast to long vein grafts, a large body of information exists regarding relatively short upper extremity grafts placed in the more proximal carotid-subclavian position. In this location, the differences in prosthetic versus autogenous conduit are striking. Diethrich et al[45] described the largest series in 1967 with 125 grafts. They used only Dacron tubes for conduits and reported more than 98% long-term patency with only one graft infection. Vogt et al[46] reported the largest series of autogenous conduits consisting of 36 veins. They noted only an 83% long-term patency rate, with two grafts requiring replacement (one for aneurysmal degeneration and one for stricture). Ziomek et al[39] compared 18 prosthetic and 13 autogenous carotid-subclavian bypasses using Life Table methods and noted a pronounced difference at 5 years of 91% and 57% patency rates, respectively. We reported a lower 2-year proximal patency of 88%, but included both vein and prosthesis, only two carotid-subclavian bypasses (both polytetrafluoroethylene), and no patients with subclavian steal.[7] All other available data relate the predominant use of proximal prosthetic grafts for short, carotid-subclavian bypass and resultant patencies of 90% to 100%.[1,3,4,8–12] The one recent series by Kretschmer et al[11] reported only 78% 5-year patency rate by Life Table analysis for 19 carotid-subclavian bypasses but included four vein grafts. In patients with subclavian aneurysm, who are generally young and require graft placement in an anatomic position, vein is the recommended conduit.

Acknowledgments
This work was supported in part by the Alyce F. Salerno Fund and the Gaylord Freeman Aneurysm Research Fund.

REFERENCES

1. Welling RE, Cranley JJ, Krause RJ, et al. Obliterative arterial disease of the upper extremity. Arch Surg. 1981;116:1593–1596.
2. Bergqvist D, Ericsson BF, Konrad P, et al. Arterial surgery of the upper extremity. World J Surg. 1983;7:786–791.
3. Harris RW, Andros G, Dulawa LB, et al. Large-vessel arterial occlusive disease in symptomatic upper extremity. Arch Surg. 1984;119:1277–1282.
4. Crawford ES, DeBakey ME, Morris GC, et al. Surgical treatment of occlusion of the innominate, common carotid, and subclavian arteries: a 10-year experience. Surgery. 1969; 65:17–31.
5. Bartlett ST, Olinde AJ, Flinn WR, et al. The reoperative potential of infrainguinal bypass: long-term limb and patient survival. J Vasc Surg. 1987;5:170–179.
6. Hertzer NR. Fatal myocardial infarction following lower extremity revascularization: two hundred sixty-three patients followed six to eleven postoperative years. Ann Surg. 1981;193:492–498.
7. McCarthy WJ, Flinn WR, Yao JST, et al. Results of bypass grafting for upper limb ischemia. J Vasc Surg. 1986;3:741–746.
8. Gerety RL, Andrus CH, May AG, et al. Surgical treatment of occlusive subclavian artery disease. Circulation. 1981;64(suppl II):228–230.
9. Maggisano R, Provan JL. Surgical management of chronic occlusive disease of the aortic arch vessels and vertebral arteries. Can Med Assoc J. 1981;124:972–977.
10. Moore WS, Malone JM, Goldstone J. Extrathoracic repair of branch occlusions of the aortic arch. Am J Surg. 1976;132:249–257.
11. Kretschmer G, Teleky B, Marosi L, et al. Obliterations of the proximal subclavian artery: to bypass or to anastomose? J Cardiovasc Surg. 1991;32:334–339.
12. Gross WS, Flanigan DP, Kraft RO, et al. Chronic upper extremity arterial insufficiency. Arch Surg. 1978;113:419–423.
13. Veith FJ, Gupta SK, Ascer E, et al. Six-year prospective multicenter randomized comparison of autologous saphenous vein and expanded polytetrafluoroethylene grafts in infrainguinal arterial reconstructions. J Vasc Surg. 1986;3:104–114.

14. Davis JB, Grove WJ, Julian OC. Thrombotic occlusion of the aortic arch, Martorell's syndrome: report of a case treated surgically. *Ann Surg.* 1956;144:124–126.

15. Garrett HE, Morris GC, Howell JF, et al. Revascularization of upper extremity with autologous vein bypass graft. *Arch Surg.* 1965;91:751–757.

16. Whitehouse WH, Zelenock GB, Wakefield TW, et al. Arterial bypass grafts for upper extremity ischemia. *J Vasc Surg.* 1986;3:569–573.

17. Rapp JH, Reilly LM, Goldstone J, et al. Ischemia of the upper extremity: significance of proximal occlusive disease. *Am J Surg.* 1986;152:122–126.

18. Wood PB. Vein-graft bypass in axillary and brachial artery occlusions causing claudication. *Br J Surg.* 1973;60:29–30.

19. Holleman JH, Hardy JD, Williamson JW, et al. Arterial surgery for arm ischemia: a survey of 136 patients. *Ann Surg.* 1980;191:727–737.

20. Coleman SS, Anson BJ. Arterial patterns in the hand based upon a study of 650 specimens. *Surg Gynecol Obstet.* 1961;113:409.

21. Bundin JA, Casarella WJ, Harisiabis L. Subclavian artery occlusion following radiotherapy for carcinoma of the breast. *Radiology.* 1976;118:169.

22. Pearce WH, Yao JST. Overview of upper extremity ischemia. *Semin Vasc Surg.* 1990;3:207–210.

23. Ricotta JJ, Scudder PA, McAndrew JA, et al. Management of acute ischemia of the upper extremity. *Am J Surg.* 1983;145:661–666.

24. James EC, Khuri NT, Gardner RJ, et al. Upper limb ischemia resulting from arterial thromboembolism. *Am J Surg.* 1979;137:739–744.

25. Rob CG, Standeven A. Arterial occlusion complicating thoracic outlet compression syndrome. *Br J Med.* 1958;2:709–712.

26. Brown SCW, Charlesworth D. Results of excision of a cervical rib in patients with thoracic outlet syndrome. *Br J Surg.* 1988;75:431–433.

27. Cormier JM, Amrane M, Ward A, et al. Arterial complications of the thoracic outlet syndrome: fifty-five operative cases. *J Vasc Surg.* 1989;9:778–787.

28. Orcutt MB, Levine BA, Gaskill HV, et al. Civilian vascular trauma of the upper extremity. *J Trauma.* 1986;26:63–67.

29. McCollum CH, Mavor E. Brachial artery injury after cardiac catheterization. *J Vasc Surg.* 1986;4:355–359.

30. Close ME, Ahmed R, Ryan RB, et al. Complications of long-term transbrachial hepatic arterial infusion chemotherapy. *Am J Roentgenol.* 1977;129:797–803.

31. Kempczinski R, Penn I. Upper extremity complications of axillofemoral grafts. *Am J Surg.* 1978;136:209–211.

32. McCarthy WJ, Yao JST, Schafer MF, et al. Upper extremity arterial injury in athletes. *J Vasc Surg.* 1989;9:317–327.

33. Abbott WM, Darling RC. Axillary artery aneurysms secondary to crutch trauma. *Am J Surg.* 1973;125:515–520.

34. McNamara MF, Takaki HS, Yao JST, et al. A systematic approach to severe hand ischemia. *Surgery.* 1978;83:1–11.

35. Erlandson EE, Forrest ME, Shields JJ, et al. Discriminant arteriographic criteria in the management of forearm and hand ischemia. *Surgery.* 1981;90:1025–1036.

36. Sumner DE, Barkmeier LD. Noninvasive evaluation of upper extremity ischemia. *Semin Vasc Surg.* 1990;3:211–218.

37. Yao JST, Pearce WH. Reconstructive surgery for chronic upper extremity ischemia. *Semin Vasc Surg.* 1990;3:258–266.

38. Norem RF, Short DH, Kerstein MD. Role of intraoperative fibrinolysis therapy in acute arterial occlusion. *Surg Gynecol Obstet.* 1988;167:87–91.

39. Ziomek S, Quinones-Baldrich WJ, Busuttil RW, et al. The superiority of synthetic arterial grafts over autologous veins in carotid-subclavian bypass. *J Vasc Surg.* 1986;3:140–145.

40. Cohen ES, Holtzman RB, Johnson GW. Axillobrachial artery bypass grafting with *in-situ* cephalic vein for axillary artery occlusion: a case report. *J Vasc Surg.* 1989;10:683–687.

41. Guzman-Stein G, Schubert W, Najarian DW, et al. Composite *in-situ* vein bypass for upper extremity revascularization. *Plast Reconstr Surg.* 1989;3:533–536.
42. Scher LA, Veith FJ, Haimovici H, et al. Staging of arterial complications of cervical rib: guidelines for surgical management. *Surgery.* 1984;95:644–649.
43. Flinn WR, Rohrer MJ, Yao JST, et al. Improved long-term patency of infragenicular polytetrafluoroethylene grafts. *J Vasc Surg.* 1988;7:685–690.
44. Kretschmer G, Wenzl E, Piza F, et al. The influence of anticoagulant treatment on the probability of function in femoropopliteal bypass surgery: analysis of a clinical series (1970–1985) and interim evaluation of a controlled clinical trial. *Surgery.* 1987;102:453–459.
45. Diethrich EB, Garrett EH, Amersio J, et al. Occlusive disease of the common carotid and subclavian arteries treated by carotid-subclavian bypass. *Am J Surg.* 1967;114:800–808.
46. Vogt DP, Hertzer NR, O'Hara PJ, et al. Brachiocephalic arterial reconstruction. *Ann Surg.* 1982;196:541–552.

32

Long-Term Results After Operation for Thoracic Outlet Syndrome:

Factors Affecting Results

Richard M. Green, MD, Jere W. Lord, Jr., MD,
Kenneth Ouriel, MD, and James A. DeWeese, MD

The thoracic outlet syndrome (TOS) describes a variety of conditions caused by compression of one or a combination of neurovascular structures traversing the thoracic outlet.[1] There are those who believe that TOS is overdiagnosed and those who believe it is underdiagnosed.[2] The "overdiagnosed" group would divide TOS into four distinct categories: arterial, venous, neurologic, and disputed neurologic.[3] The former three share many common features. They each have characteristic symptoms, physical findings, definitive diagnostic tests, and a low incidence (e.g., the neurologic condition has an incidence of one per 1,000,000).[4] In the latter and most common category (the disputed neurologic), the diagnosis is uncertain, the severity of symptoms cannot be objectively quantitated, the natural history is unknown, the result of treatment is unpredictable, and the analysis of the result is subjective. It is a problem no surgical specialty seeks to treat and an unlikely one for the vascular surgeon because no blood vessel is involved. Long-term results after treatment of the disputed neurologic syndrome are difficult to obtain and analyze for all the reasons cited above. The "underdiagnosed" group feels that TOS represents a continuum of compression syndromes that initially were recognized as purely vascular. The entity is now evolving into a mainly neurologic condition related to cervical trauma superimposed on a congenital predisposition for compression. Existing data do not settle this controversy. The intent of this review is to study the combined experiences at the University of Rochester (JAD, RMG), at New York University (JL), and in selected large series reported in the literature to provide guidelines in management focusing on long-term results.

HISTORIC DEVELOPMENTS

Bony cervical ribs have been associated with neurovascular compression syndromes since the 18th century.[5,6] The first resection was performed by Coote in 1861, and as the roentgenogram became universally available, the diagnosis of cervical rib became more common. Halsted[7] reviewed the literature in 1916 and found that one-third of the 715 documented cases presented with vascular symptoms caused by aneurysm or thrombosis. Removal of a normal first rib for the "cervical rib syndrome" was first reported in 1910 in Australia by Murphy.[8]

The concept that downward shoulder migration could cause neurovascular compression implicated the clavicle in the pathogenesis of TOS around this same period.[9] Total resection of the clavicle was advocated to treat the entity now referred to as the "costoclavicular syndrome."[10] Concerns about the appearance of the incision and potential shoulder instability reduced the appeal of this procedure.

Nonosseous structures were implicated in TOS when Murphy[11] successfully relieved a patient of upper extremity arterial symptoms by dividing the anterior scalene muscle in 1905. A cervical rib was present but not removed. Many others, including Adson and Coffey,[12,13] postulated that the anterior scalene muscle alone could cause compression and thus the term *scalenus anticus syndrome* was coined, and this operation was performed for almost 35 years. This syndrome lost credibility because of a high failure rate (60%) after operation.[14] Muscle operations through the neck were rejuvenated by Sanders, who felt that the failures with division of the anterior scalene muscle were due to an inadequate removal of muscle rather than a conceptual error.[15]

Compression caused by fibrous bands was recognized by Bonney[16] when he reported the association of a sharp fibrous band extending from the tip of the C7 transverse process to the first rib over which the C8 and T1 nerve roots were angulated. Roos[17] described a variety of fibrous bands each of which may impinge on the brachial plexus and predispose to the development of neurologic symptoms. Identification of these bands is important because it provides concrete evidence of a congenital predisposition to the neurologic syndrome.

In a presidential address to the American Association for Thoracic Surgery in 1962, Clagett[18] attempted to provide a unifying concept for the variety of compression syndromes already described and named. He postulated that the common denominator of all the entities was the first rib and recommended that all the variants of TOS be treated by resection of the rib through a posterior approach.[18] Roos[19] described the technique of transaxillary first-rib resection (FRR) in 1966, and because of its cosmetic appeal, simplicity, and alleged safety, it generated a wave of enthusiasm and nearly 5,000 cases had been reported by 1984.[20]

Despite all claims to the contrary, the most appropriate treatment for TOS, with the exception of those cases with subclavian artery aneurysms or thrombosis, is in dispute. The dispute not only involves whether operative or nonoperative therapy is superior but also which operation is performed when that option is chosen.

LONG-TERM RESULTS: ARTERIAL THORACIC OUTLET SYNDROME

The incidence of cervical rib is 0.4% in the general population with a 1:2 male/female ratio.[21] Cervical ribs cause neurologic symptoms more often than arterial, but most arterial symptoms are due to these anomalous structures. Supraclavicular nonosseous structures rarely cause fixed arterial pathology. Treatment must focus on both arterial reconstruction *and* removal of the inciting cause. Long-term results are in large part a function of the degree of ischemia at the time of presentation but also the adequacy of the arterial repair and the removal of the compressive structure. The patient's initial complaint may be severe digital ischemia caused by thromboembolism from a subclavian artery aneurysm, requiring digital amputation.

The method of arterial reconstruction is dictated by the presentation. The subclavian artery is often elongated in the setting of a cervical rib, so that mobilization allows primary repair after resection of the involved segment. When a primary repair is not feasible, aneurysms of the subclavian artery should be resected and reconstructed with an autogenous vein graft. Dilated subclavian arteries can be left alone, providing that no thromboembolic events have occurred and the offending compressive structures are resected.[22,23] Although this does leave the potential for future embolic episodes, this late phenomenon has not been reported. The arteriogram in Figure 32–1 shows a dilated subclavian artery in a patient with a large bony cervical rib. This patient did present with digital artery emboli, and therefore the artery was opened. An ulcerated plaque was identified, which prompted arterial reconstruction with a saphenous vein graft. Subclavian artery stenosis or occlusion differs from the typical atherosclerotic occlusion because it occurs distal to the thyrocervical trunk and is treated with resection and either primary anastomosis or a bypass. The site of arterial compression is seen in the angiogram shown in Figure 32–2.

We have preferred resection of the medial half of the clavicle for these procedures and have not seen any disability from this approach. In our experience the cervical ribs associated with arterial pathology are short, broad, and complete, whereas the ribs associated with the neurologic compression syndromes tend to be long, thin, and often incomplete. A supraclavicular incision is adequate for removal of a cervical rib but may not allow sufficient room distally if an arterial reconstruction with a vein graft is necessary. An infraclavicular incision is inadequate both for the arterial aspect and the bony resection. The transaxillary approach is ideal for an FRR but inadequate, in our experience, for arterial repair. This incision also has limits when the cervical rib is broad. Cormier et al[24,25] reviewed their large experience and recommended a

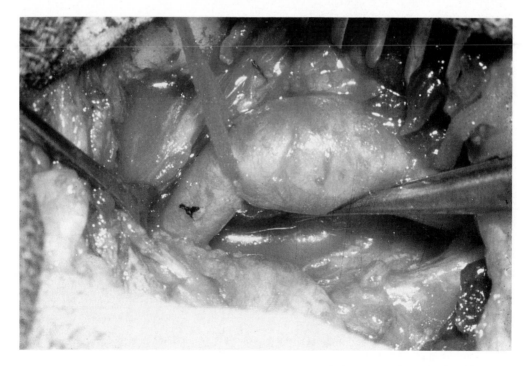

Figure 32–1. Aneurysm of the subclavian artery distal to compression from a bony cervical rib. Patient presented with atheroemboli to his fingers. Aneurysm was excised and replaced with a saphenous vein graft.

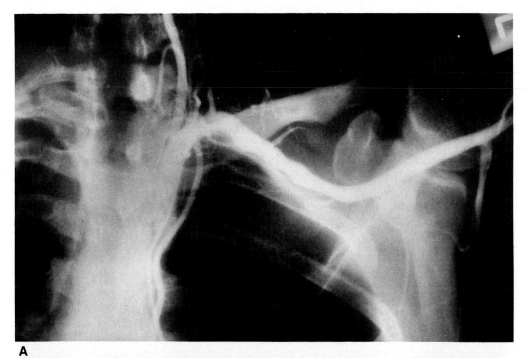

A

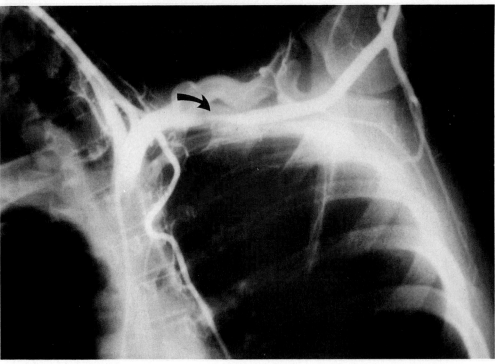

B

Figure 32–2. (A) Arteriogram in a housepainter with "tired" arms when used over his head. In the resting position, there is no obvious abnormality. **(B)** This same patient with his shoulder abducted, showing compression at site of a cervical rib (*arrow*).

combination supra- and infraclavicular approach. This approach allows for resection of cervical ribs, the first or second rib, a complete neurolysis, and arterial repair.

A variety of thromboembolic complications may occur that require additional procedures. The angiograms shown in Figure 32–3 are from a patient with a cervical

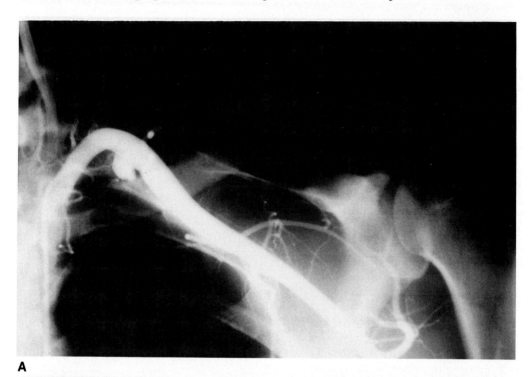

A

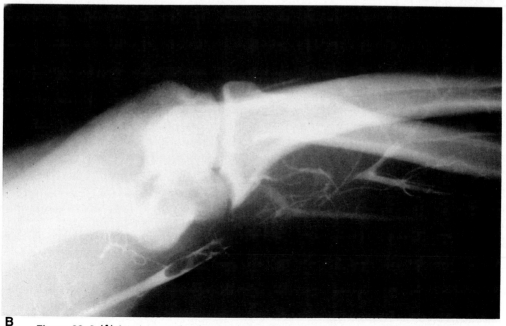

B

Figure 32–3. (A) Arteriogram showing a subclavian artery aneurysm associated with a broad cervical rib. This was resected and repaired primarily. **(B)** This patient presented with a brachial artery occlusion. A separate incision was made and the embolus was removed with a Fogarty catheter.

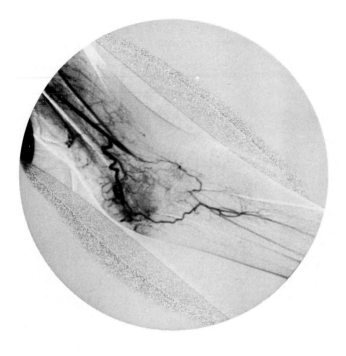

Figure 32–4. Arteriogram showing a chronically occluded brachial artery in a patient with a subclavian artery aneurysm. A venous bypass was required for arterial reconstruction.

rib and subclavian artery aneurysm who presented with an acute brachial artery occlusion. An embolectomy was performed through the brachial artery in the antecubital space, flow was re-established, and then the aneurysm and rib were removed. This patient has been asymptomatic for 15 years. The angiogram in Figure 32–4 shows a chronically occluded brachial artery caused by an embolus from a subclavian artery aneurysm. This patient was successfully treated with a venous bypass graft. The goal of reperfusion is to provide flow to the level of the elbow. When digital ischemia occurs in the setting of palpable radial and ulnar pulses, a cervical sympathectomy is performed. A nonoperative approach should be taken when arterial disease extends below the elbow. Cormier et al[24] reported on the late results in 46 of 55 patients with arterial problems related to the thoracic outlet syndrome. Patients were followed for an average of 5 years after operation. There were only four patients with residual arterial symptoms, and only one patient required a distal digital amputation. Symptoms were the result of thromboembolism to the arteries of the forearm and hand that was inoperable at the time of initial diagnosis. These excellent results support an aggressive approach to patients with arterial symptoms based on removal of compression sites, reconstruction of the subclavian artery, and reperfusion of the arm proximal to the elbow.

LONG-TERM RESULTS: VENOUS THORACIC OUTLET SYNDROME

Venous compression at the thoracic outlet produces symptoms in one of three ways: (a) intermittent obstruction related to arm position, (b) acute thrombotic obstruction (Paget-Schroetter syndrome) or (c) chronic post-thrombotic obstruction with intermittent obstruction of large collateral veins. Compression of the subclavian vein in the costoclavicular space is exacerbated with hyperabduction and external rotation of the arm and when a patient in the erect position braces his or her shoulders, as in the military position. Venous complications occur in only 5% of the patients with TOS.

Because the number of reported cases is small, long-term results of treatment for each of these entities are mostly anecdotal.

Intermittent Venous Obstruction

This syndrome is characterized by signs and symptoms of venous hypertension in certain positions of the arm. It is diagnosed by venous pressure measurements taken in the median antecubital vein first in the resting position and then with the arm elevated. At rest, the pressure will be slightly elevated but will increase two or three times in the symptomatic arm in the stressed position. Phlebograms performed in similar positions show a beak deformity of the subclavian vein at the junction of the first rib and clavicle.

Treatment of this problem by division of the anterior scalene, pectoralis minor, and/or subclavius muscles gives poor results.[26] A phlebogram in a patient with massive arm swelling shows an abrupt venous cutoff at the level of the pectoralis minor tendon in Figure 32–5. Division of the tendon provided no relief. Results after either resection of the medial half of the clavicle or the first rib are better.[27] Follow-up phlebograms at 5 years show patent veins even in the stressed position after bony decompression.

Acute Thrombotic Obstruction: Paget-Schroetter or "Effort" Thrombosis Syndrome

The natural history of this condition was first described by Sir James Paget in 1875[28] and by Von Schroetter in 1884 in a previously healthy man who was painting at the

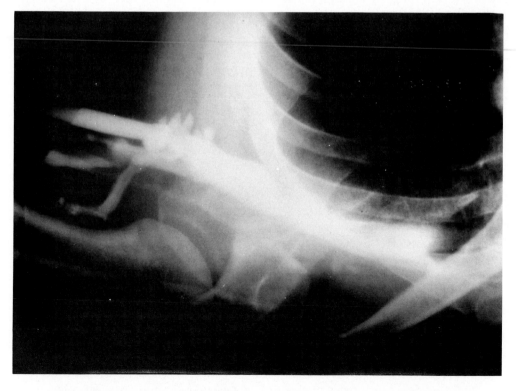

Figure 32–5. Phlebogram showing compression of axillary vein by pectoralis minor tendon. At operation the finding was confirmed, but division of the tendon did not provide any relief from arm swelling. Transaxillary first-rib resection was eventually performed with a good result.

time the thrombosis occurred.[29] Despite the spontaneous nature of the acute event, there is usually an underlying anatomic point of venous compression at the thoracic outlet. Residual symptoms have been reported in 40% to 85% of patients[30,31] with the standard treatment of elevation and anticoagulation.

Immediate thrombectomy of the occluded vein is no longer recommended but is of historic interest. A number of series with good follow-up demonstrated that when thrombectomy was accomplished through a medial claviculectomy or an FRR, the patient had a good symptomatic result.[32-34] It is not clear whether the thrombectomy or the bone removal is the most important element in treatment, however.

Thrombolytic therapy has now replaced thrombectomy and anticoagulation as the initial treatment of choice for this condition, but when used alone, recurrences are common.[35] Clot lysis is best achieved with local infusion of urokinase directly into the clot, initially at doses of 4,000 U/min for 2 hours and then reduced to 1,000 U/min for 20 hours.[36] The catheter used is a coaxial one that allows for the simultaneous administration of heparin at a dose of 800 IU/h. Systemic heparinization is maintained until anticoagulation with Coumadin is established.

Once the vein has been opened, a search for the underlying compressive anatomic lesion must be made. Stenotic lesions have been treated by balloon angioplasty, but this has resulted in thrombotic reocclusion and is not recommended.[37] Instead, either an FRR or a medial claviculectomy should be performed. Sykes[38] used this staged approach to patients with effort thrombosis and reported excellent results with an average follow-up of 30 months.

Chronic Post-thrombotic Occlusions

When a patient develops symptoms of venous hypertension caused by a chronically occluded subclavian vein, a variety of procedures can provide relief. Phlebograms (Fig. 32–6) in these patients typically reveal large collateral veins passing around the

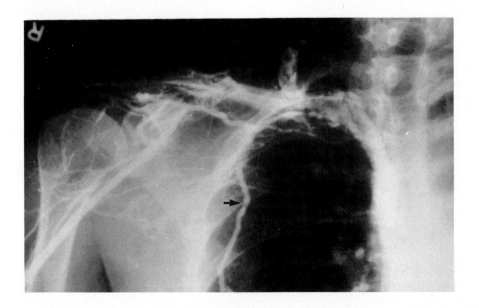

Figure 32–6. Phlebogram in a patient with a chronically occluded subclavian vein. A large collateral vein can be seen draining through chest wall. Elevation of the arm produced symptoms of swelling and pain, which were relieved by first-rib resection.

shoulder girdle that become compressed with elevation of the arm. An FRR or a medial claviculectomy will eliminate the compression of these collaterals.

There have been several reports of venous reconstruction in this setting.[32,39] The operation is performed with a supraclavicular incision, removing the medial half of the clavicle, dividing the internal jugular vein and anastomosing it into the distal subclavian vein proximal to the occlusion. Critics of this operation claim that the medial claviculectomy would accomplish the same goal. Nevertheless, personal follow-up of three cases for up to 7 years has demonstrated the efficacy of this approach. The phlebogram in Figure 32–7 shows the result of an internal jugular to distal subclavian vein bypass at 5 years. This patient had severe swelling and pain after an acute subclavian vein thrombosis. Collateral venous development was inadequate for this patient, and operation was recommended. The patient has since returned to normal activities and is asymptomatic.

LONG-TERM RESULTS: NEUROLOGIC THORACIC OUTLET SYNDROME

The Debate

The "classic" neurologic syndrome is quite rare (incidence estimated at one per 1,000,000) and some neurologists[3,40] would argue that operation be limited to those patients with weakness and wasting of the small muscles of the hand (partial thenar atrophy, Fig. 32–8) in the setting of either a cervical rib or a congenital fibrous band extending from an elongated transverse process of C7. The hard neurologic signs are often preceded by several years of arm pain. Sectioning the fibrous band or removing the cervical rib stops the sensory symptoms and the progression of the motor abnormalities. Although no one would question the operative indication in these cases, the long-term results after operation for the classic syndrome with definite muscle wasting are poor. In our own series, the neurologic deficit persisted in five of eight patients, and only three of the eight patients would undergo operation again if

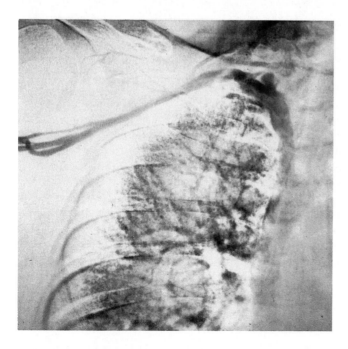

Figure 32–7. Phlebogram taken 5 years after an internal jugular to subclavian vein bypass. Anastomosis is patent with no evidence of collateralization.

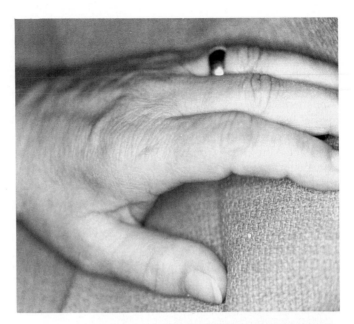

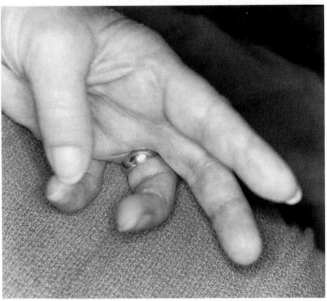

Figure 32–8. Patient with a cervical rib band and a severe ulnar neuropathy. There is atrophy of ulnar innervated muscles and an inability to flex fingers fully.

the result were the same.[41] Earlier operation before the development of muscle wasting would have given better results. It is our preference to decompress patients before the development of muscle wasting of the hand and not to limit operation to only those patients with measurable neurologic deficits.

It is estimated that 8% of the United States population has symptoms consistent with this syndrome. Critics claim that the syndrome lacks definable characteristics, the diagnosis is subjective, and it owes its popularity to overdiagnosis by "non-neurologically trained surgeons."[2] The critics further maintain that the lack of consensus among the entity's advocates relative to the clinical presentation, method of diagnosis, and proper operative approach further questions the existence of this as a discrete problem. The reasons for their concern are the potential for large numbers of inappropriate operations and mislabeling "true" neurologic conditions such as carpal tunnel syndrome.

Advocates of the "disputed" neurologic TOS syndrome state that this condition is an evolutionary precursor of the "classic" syndrome. The congenital anomalies of musculoskeletal tissue that predispose this patient population to develop neurologic symptoms after trauma are analogous to a cervical rib or fibrous band in the "classic" variant.[17] Cadaveric dissections have supported this "susceptibility" theory, finding a 33% incidence of anatomic abnormalities capable of producing compression at the thoracic outlet. Sophisticated tests such as computed tomography, magnetic resonance imaging, electrodiagnostics, and the vascular laboratory fail to demonstrate compression that can only be determined by the surgeon at operation. The responsible physician therefore must rely on careful physical examination, history, and clinical experience to evaluate prospective operative candidates.

Whatever one calls this syndrome, a rational approach to treatment is necessary given its overall prevalence. Physical therapy programs have been successful in 75% of the patients with this problem.[1,42] Initially the program should be concerned with pain relief using heat or ice, ultrasound, transcutaneous electrical nerve stimulator, and biofeedback. Exercises are directed at widening the thoracic outlet, improving posture, and strengthening the shoulder girdle suspensory muscles. Occasionally these exercises aggravate the muscle spasm and must be discontinued. When no other pathologic condition can be demonstrated or treatment of another condition fails to relieve symptoms, patients can be offered thoracic outlet decompression if (a) symptoms prevent the patient from working or performing normal activities and (b) physical examination reproduces the symptoms by abducting the shoulder to 90 degrees.

Operations for Neurologic Thoracic Outlet Syndrome

If the patients could be categorized preoperatively by objective standards and the results could be similarly analyzed, there would be no debate about the proper operative approach. This unfortunately is not the case and there are proponents for a variety of decompressive procedures. The following data summarize the experiences with 147 transaxillary FRRs were performed on 136 patients with neurologic TOS by Dr. Green between 1977 and 1989 at the University of Rochester Medical Center Rochester[43] and 115 decompression operations performed at New York University by Dr. Lord between 1950 and 1983, plus several large series reported in the literature.

The subjective nature of the symptoms and the lack of objective diagnostic criteria make patient selection difficult. We have been unimpressed by the variety of screening tests proposed to identify those patients who will benefit from FRR[43-47] and feel that the role of these tests is to exclude other neurologic disorders. The elevated arm stress test procedure described by Roos[17] as a predictor of success after FRR is positive in 92% of patients with carpal tunnel syndrome.[48] We do not believe that obliteration of the radial pulse has any diagnostic or prognostic value in evaluating these patients. This had been confirmed by Wright,[49] who found that 92.6% of normal subjects had obliteration of the radial pulse in at least one extremity test in an elevated position. The most helpful physical finding in our series was the reproduction of symptoms with the shoulder abducted less than 90 degrees.

Results were analyzed differently at the various institutions. In Rochester, success was measured by the patients' ability to return to preillness activities and whether they would undergo operation again if the same result could be assured. The New York cases were all personally reviewed by Dr. Lord and Dr. Wright and were categorized as excellent, good, fair, or poor. Follow-up ranged from 2 months to 34 years. Sanders and Pearce[15] used this same grading system for 668 operations and then grouped the excellent, good, and fair results into "successes" and the poor results into "failures." Regardless of the operative approach and method of follow-up, each of these series has a long-term success rate of greater than 70%. Most of the 30% of patients who fail do well initially but develop recurrent symptoms often after another trauma, and those who have a poor result from operation are usually because of improper patient selection.

Role of Trauma

Trauma has become an integral part of TOS as it has evolved from a purely vascular condition to a neurologic one over the past 100 years. Neurologic symptoms are produced by a combination of injury to the scalene muscles and a predisposition to plexus compression. Injury to the scalenes produces muscle fibrosis. This has been confirmed in microscopic studies of scalene muscles removed from patients with trauma that show an abnormal fiber-type change plus an increase in connective tissue compared with normal skeletal muscle.[50] A history of trauma can be obtained in most patients with anomalous ribs and neurologic symptoms. Sanders reported a history of neck trauma in 87% of his cases. In the Rochester series, there were 61 operations (41%) performed on 53 patients with a specific history of trauma.

In addition to being an etiologic factor in the development of neurologic symptoms, trauma also had a significant negative influence over the Rochester results in women when a workmen's compensation claim was filed. This type of trauma was usually in patients who had assembly line or keyboard jobs. This agrees with the larger series from Denver, where work-related injuries were associated with a 43% failure rate as compared with only 18% failure for nonspecific trauma (RJ Sanders, personal communication).

Table 32–1 shows the effects of the type of trauma on return to activities in each gender in the Rochester series. The 25 patients with injuries covered under a workmen's compensation policy fared poorly after FRR. Nine of these patients (36%) were able to return to normal activities compared with 16 of 28 patients who had a noncompensation incident. These differences did not reach statistical significance ($P = .10$) until the sex of the patient was considered. Whereas men did not demonstrate any differences in return to activities, only three of 16 women (19%) were able to return after a compensation injury compared with 14 of 26 after a noncompensation injury.

Anatomic Abnormalities

Anatomic abnormalities were documented in 48 (33%) patients in the Rochester series. There were 26 complete cervical ribs, 19 incomplete cervical ribs with taut fibrous bands attaching to the first rib, two clavicular exostoses, and one fusion of the first and second ribs. Symptoms were precipitated by a traumatic event in seven of these patients with anatomic anomalies. Symptoms began insidiously in the remain-

TABLE 32–1. IMPACT OF TYPE OF TRAUMA AND GENDER ON RETURN TO PRE-ILLNESS FUNCTION

Status	Nonspecific Injury (%)	Work-related Injury (%)	Men Nonspecific/ Work-related (%)	Women Nonspecific/ Work-related (%)
Return to activity	16 (57)	9 (36)	6/7 vs. 2/4 (86 vs. 50)	14/26 vs. 3/16 (54 vs. 19)
No return to activity	12 (43)	16 (72)	1/7 vs. 2/4 (14 vs. 50)	7/26 vs. 13/16 (27 vs. 81)
Total	28 (100)	25 (100)	11 (100%)	42 (100)

Comparisons: Compensation vs. noncompensation injury: $P < .02$; men, compensation vs. noncompensation injuries: $P = $ NS; women, compensation vs. noncompensation injuries: $P < .05$.

ing 41 cases. Sanders reported a 4.5% incidence of bony abnormalities and a high but unspecified incidence of congenital bands and variations in the anatomic relationships between the cords of the brachial plexus and the scalene muscles. Roos[17] documented a 7.5% incidence of cervical ribs and a 34% incidence of congenital bands in 980 operations for TOS. Finally, a current review reported on 9 cervical ribs and 10 pathologic clavicles that were removed for a bony anomaly incidence of 13%. Dale[51] and Lord[52] stated that the presence of a cervical rib was associated with a better postoperative result. Although there is no question that the presence of a bony abnormality supports the diagnosis and makes the decision to operate easier, other factors affect long-term results more than the mere presence of such an anomaly.

Impact of Other Factors

The role of preoperative neurologic or musculoskeletal deficits, anatomic abnormalities, and the need to return to a job requiring repetitive activities from this series is analyzed in Table 32–2. Anatomic abnormalities had no effect on return to activities or satisfaction. The presence of a preoperative neurologic deficit had an adverse effect on patient satisfaction. We therefore disagree with Wilbourn and Gilliatt,[4] who feel that operation should only be offered those patients with classical neurologic TOS and fixed neurologic symptoms because earlier operation might have prevented the neurologic disability. The same anatomic abnormality responsible for neurologic damage in the classic group, namely, a complete or incomplete cervical rib, was present in the disputed group as well. Fixed neurologic impairment was not seen in this group. This gives some credence to those who claim that the neurologic condition is indeed a continuum and that decompression in appropriate patients without a fixed neurologic deficit is indicated.

"Best" Operation for Neurologic Thoracic Outlet Syndrome

The extensive experience with a wide variety of decompressive procedures performed well in properly selected patients demonstrates that either FRR or scalenectomy combined with division of any anomalous bands provides significant relief of symptoms in most patients. Concern about the risks of transaxillary FRR followed a survey sent to the members of the International Society for Cardiovascular Surgery in 1981, which revealed that partial or complete postoperative paralysis was observed in 273 cases. Actually, the incidence of brachial plexus injuries after FRR reported in the neurologic literature is considerable and antedates the concerns raised by Dr. Dale. Nonetheless, this report to the society led to a recommendation that the "lesser" procedure of scalectomy should be the preferred initial procedure.[51]

TABLE 32–2. IMPACT OF OTHER FACTORS ON RESULTS

Status[a]	Preoperative Neurologic Deficit			Bony Anatomic Anomaly			Repetitive Job Activity		
	Yes	No	P	Yes	No	P	Yes	No	P
Returned (90)	8	82		19	71		14	76	
Not returned (46)	3	43	ns	9	35	ns	23	23	.01
Satisfied (107)	4	103		22	85		28	79	
Not satisfied (29)	7	22	.01	6	23	ns	9	20	ns

[a] "Returned" means back to preillness life style; "satisfied" means willing to undergo operation again if same result could be assured.

Brachial plexus injuries were an acknowledged complication of cervical rib resections as early as 1907, observed in 17% of the first 42 operative cases.[53] We did not experience any sensory or motor brachial plexus injuries but did have three patients who developed painful vasospasm after FRR. Others have observed this same phenomenon.[54] The rarity of plexus injuries in our series and in Roos'[55] much larger experience suggests that transaxillary FRR can be a safe and effective method of removing the first rib. It is interesting that Sanders, the original proponent of scalenectomy, now recommends rib resection in certain situations.

When we analyzed a group of patients who had initial supraclavicular procedures, we found a recurrence rate of five times the incidence after rib resection. Roos[55] described a similar difference, 5% after rib resection and 19% after scalenectomy. Because our experience with scalectomy has not been as positive as reports in the literature, we recommend FRR as the initial procedure in virtually all cases of the neurologic syndrome. There are no randomized data comparing the two procedures, however, and the choice remains one of operator preference.

There are conflicting reports about the long-term effects of claviculectomy. Some are reluctant to use it because of alleged cosmetic dissatisfaction and others because of shoulder instability. This series of 37 claviculectomies has been followed for up to 34 years, and the results are comparable with the other procedures. It remains a useful approach when the bone is pathologic or access to the vessels is required. No cases of shoulder instability were noted.

Treatment of Recurrences

The incidence of recurrent neurologic TOS depends on whether one is referring to a return in symptoms or the need for a reoperation. Roos[55] reported a long-term operative recurrence rate of 2.2%, but others have reported a range more consistent with our own experience of somewhere between 15% to 20%. This large difference in reported series is most likely due to the difficulties in quantifying the symptoms in these patients and perhaps in the intensity of the follow-up. That is why we opted for a functional analysis of results. Although most of our patients had some persistent symptoms, only 20 (15%) required reoperation. In 19 of these secondary operations, abundant scarring from the previously divided anterior and middle scalene muscles was identified rather than anomalous fibrous bands. The formation of this scar tissue around the plexus is an inevitable consequence of any operation in this area. Sanders and co-workers[56] reviewed their experience with 134 operations for recurrence and found that results were better if the return of symptoms was precipitated by a trauma rather than spontaneous event.

RECOMMENDATIONS

The keys to long-term success are proper patient selection, complete removal of compressive structures, and repair of fixed vascular lesions. Table 32–3 outlines the authors' recommendations for the variety of conditions. Adherence to these principles can result in excellent results and very grateful patients.

TABLE 32-3. RECOMMENDATIONS FOR TREATMENT

Condition	Diagnosis	"Preferred" TOS Approach	Adjuncts
Venous **Intermittent** **Acute thrombosis** **Chronic thrombosis**	Phlebogram via median antecubital vein, pressures in relaxed and stress position	Medial claviculectomy or first-rib resection Venous reconstruction for incapacitating symptoms	Thrombolytic Rx for acute thrombosis
Arterial **Dilatation w/emboli** **Aneurysm or** **thrombosis**	Vascular studies with digital plethysmography, arteriogram	Medial claviculectomy Primary arterial reconstruction or saphenous vein graft	Embolectomy or autogenous reconstruction to level of elbow Sympathectomy for digital emboli
Neurologic	Neurology consult, electromyelogram, cervical spine films, magnetic resonance imaging or myelogram	First-rib resection via axilla unless broad cervical rib requires neck approach	Avoid patients with work-related injuries because failure rate high

REFERENCES

1. Peet RM, Henriksen MD, Anderson TP. Thoracic outlet syndrome: evaluation of a therapeutic exercise program. *Mayo Clin Proc.* 1956;31:281–287.
2. Roos DB. Thoracic outlet syndrome is underrated. *Arch Neurol.* 1990;47:327.
3. Wilbourn AJ. The thoracic outlet syndrome is overdiagnosed. *Arch Neurol.* 1990;47:328–330.
4. Gilliatt RW. Thoracic outlet syndromes. In: Dyck PJ, Thomas PK, Lambert EH, Bunge R, eds. *Peripheral Neuropathy.* 2nd ed. Philadelphia, Pa: WB Saunders; 1984:1409–1424.
5. Willshire WH. Supernumeray first rib. *Lancet.* 1860;2:633.
6. Schein CJH, Haimovici H, Young H. Arterial thrombosis associated with cervical ribs: surgical considerations. *Surgery.* 1956;40:428.
7. Halsted WS. An experimental study of circumscribed dilatation of an artery immediately distal to a partially occluding band, and its bearing on the dilatation of the subclavian artery observed in certain cases of cervical rib. *J Exp Med.* 1916;24:271.
8. Murphy T. Brachial neuritis from pressure of the first rib. *Aust Med J.* 1910;15:582.
9. Todd TW. The descent of the shoulder after birth. *Anat Anz.* 1912;41:385.
10. Falconer MA, Weddell G. Costoclavicular compression of the subclavian artery and vein. *Lancet.* 1943;245:539.
11. Murphy JB. Case of cervical rib with symptoms resembling subclavian aneurysm. *Ann Surg.* 1905;41:399.
12. Adson AW, Coffey JR. Cervical rib. *Ann Surg.* 1927;85:839.
13. Ochsner A, Gage M, DeBakey M. Scalenus anticus (Naffzinger) syndrome. *Am J Surg.* 1935;28:669.
14. Wilbourn AJ, Porter JM. Thoracic outlet syndromes. In: Weiner MA, ed. *Spine: State of the Art Reviews.* Philadelphia, Pa: Hanley and Belfus; 1988;2:597–626.
15. Sanders RJ, Pearce WH. The treatment of thoracic outlet syndrome: a comparison of different operations. *J Vasc Surg.* 1989;10:626.
16. Bonney G. Scalenus medius band. *J Bone Joint Surg.* 1965;47B:268.
17. Roos DB. Congenital anomalies associated with thoracic outlet syndrome: anatomy, diagnosis and treatment. *Am J Surg.* 1976;132:771.
18. Clagett OT. Research and prosearch. *J Cardiovasc Surg.* 1962;44:153.

19. Roos DB. Thoracic outlet syndromes: symptoms, diagnosis, anatomy and surgical treatment. *Med Probl Perfor Art.* 1986;1:90.

20. Fernandez NE, Lopex S. Thoracic outlet syndrome: diagnosis and management with a new techinque. *Herz.* 1984;9:52.

21. Kerley P, Twinning EW, Dow J, et al. The cardiovascular and respiratory systems. In: Shanks SC, Kerley P, eds. *A Textbook of X-ray Diagnosis by British Authors.* London: Lewis; 1962;2:376.

22. Scher LA, Veith FJ, Haimovici H, et al. Staging of arterial complications of cervical rib: guidelines for surgical management. *Surgery.* 1984;95:757.

23. Rob CG, Standeven A. Arterial occlusion complicating thoracic outlet compression syndrome. *Br Med J.* 1958;2:709.

24. Cormier JM, Amrane M, Ward A, et al. Arterial complications of the thoracic outlet syndrome: fifty-five operative cases. *J Vasc Surg.* 1989;9:778.

25. Ward AS, Cormier JM. *Operative Techniques in Arterial Surgery.* Lancaster, UK: MTP Press; 1986:283.

26. Adams JT, DeWeese JA, Mahoney EB, et al. Intermittent subclavian vein obstruction. *Surgery.* 1968;63:147.

27. Urschel HC Jr, Razzuck MA. *N Engl J Med.* 1972;287:567. Letter.

28. Paget J. *Clinical Lectures and Essays.* London: Longmans, Green & Co; 1875.

29. Hughes ESR. Venous obstruction in the upper extremity (Paget-Schroetter's syndrome): a review of 320 cases. *Int Abstr Surg.* 1949;88:89.

30. Adams JT, DeWeese JA. "Effort" thrombosis of the axillary and subclavian veins. *J Trauma.* 1971;11:923.

31. Crowell LL. Effort thrombosis of the subclavian and axillary veins: review of the literature and case report with two year follow-up and venography. *Ann Intern Med.* 1960; 52:1337.

32. Blebea J, DeWeese JA, Ouriel K, et al. Long-term results of surgical therapy for axillary-subclavian vein thrombosis. Submitted for publication.

33. Aziz S, Straehley CJ, Whelan TJ. Effort-related axillo-subclavian vein thrombosis. *Am J Surg.* 1986;152:57.

34. Roos DB. Experience with first rib resection for thoracic outlet syndrome. *Ann Surg.* 1971;173:429.

35. Strange-Vognsen HH, Hauch O, Anderson J, et al. Resection of the first rib following deep arm vein thrombolysis in patients with thoracic outlet syndrome. *J Cardiovasc Surg.* 1989;30:430.

36. Kunkel JM, Machleder HI. Treatment of Paget-Schroetter syndrome. *Arch Surg.* 1989;124:1153.

37. Machleder HI. Effort thrombosis of the axillosubclavian vein: a disabling vascular disorder. *Comp Ther.* 1991;17:18.

38. Sykes MT. Effort thrombosis of the subclavian vein: Paget-Schroetter syndrome. In: Veith FJ, ed. *Current Critical Problems in Vascular Surgery.* St. Louis, Mo: Quality Medical Publishing; 1990;2:359.

39. Witte CL, Smithy R. Single anastomosis vein bypass for subclavian vein obstruction. *Arch Surg.* 1966;93:664.

40. Gilliatt RW. Thoracic outlet compression syndrome. *Br Med J.* 1976;1274. Letter.

41. Green RM, McNamara J, Ouriel K. Long-term results after thoracic outlet decompression: an analysis of factors determining outcome. *J Vasc Surg.* 1991;6:739.

42. Britt LP. Nonoperative treatment of the thoracic outlet syndrome symptoms. *Clin Orthop.* 1967;51:45.

43. Urschel HC, Razzuk MA. Management of thoracic outlet syndrome. *N Engl J Med.* 1972;286:1140–1143.

44. Glover JL, Worth RM, Bendick PJ, et al. Evoked responses in the diagnosis of thoracic outlet syndrome. *Surgery.* 1981;89:86–93.

45. Cherington M. Ulnar nerve conduction velocity in thoracic outlet syndrome. *N Engl J Med.* 1979;77:169–173.

46. Machleder HI, Moll F, Nuwer **M, et al.** Somatosensory evoked potentials in the assessment of thoracic outlet syndrome. *J Vasc Surg.* 1987;6:177–184.
47. Lord JW Jr. Critical reappraisal of diagnostic and therapeutic modalities for thoracic outlet syndromes. *Surg Gynecol Obstet.* 1989;168:337–340.
48. Costigan DA, Wilbourn AJ. The elevated arm stress test: specificity in the diagnosis of the thoracic outlet syndrome. *Neurology.* 1985;35(suppl 1):74–75.
49. Wright IS. The neurovascular syndrome produced by hyperabduction of the arms. *Am Heart J.* 1945;157:1.
50. Sanders RJ, Jackson CGR, Banchero N, et al. Scalene muscle pathology in traumatic thoracic outlet syndrome. *Am J Surg.* 1990;159:231–236.
51. Dale WA. Thoracic outlet compression syndrome: critique in 1982. *Arch Surg.* 1982;117:1437.
52. Lord JW. Thoracic outlet syndrome. Real or imaginary? *NY State J Med.* 1981;81:1488–1489.
53. Keen WW. The symptomatology, diagnosis and surgical treatment of cervical ribs. *Am J Med Sci.* 1907;133:173–218.
54. Horowitz SH. Brachial plexus injuries with causalgia resulting from transaxillary rib resection. *Arch Surg.* 1985;120:1189–1191.
55. Roos DB. The place for scalenectomy and first-rib resection in thoracic outlet syndrome. *Surgery.* 1982;92:1077–1085.
56. Sanders RJ, Haug CE, Pearce WH. Recurrent thoracic outlet syndrome. *J Vasc Surg.* 1990;12:390.

VII

The Extra-Anatomical Bypass

33

Femorofemoral Bypass:

A Twenty-Five-Year Experience

Bruce J. Brener, MD, Donald K. Brief, MD,
Joseph Alpert, MD, Robert J. Goldenkranz, MD,
David E. Eisenbud, MD, Jan Huston, MD,
Victor Parsonnet, MD, Debra Creighton, B A , and
Frances Cross, MD

It is generally acknowledged that the aortofemoral bypass is the most predictable, consistent, and durable procedure to treat aortoiliac occlusive disease.[1-3] Because of the magnitude of that procedure, however, alternative strategies have been developed over the past two decades. These include transluminal angioplasty, axillofemoral bypass, ileofemoral bypass, and femorofemoral bypass (FFB). The latter, introduced by Oudot and Beaconfield[4] and Freeman and Leeds[5] in the 1950s and popularized by Vetto[6,7] in the 1960s, has been used by our group during the past 25 years to alleviate the ischemia resulting from unilateral iliac occlusive disease. We originally used this procedure in high-risk patients[8]; because of acceptable patency rates, we extended the indications to include good-risk patients as well.[9] Subsequently, continued success prompted us to apply this procedure to patients with compromised donor inflow vessels, sometimes using balloon angioplasty, iliac endarterectomy, and iliac bypass grafting to improve inflow.

Adhering to the standards of the Society for Vascular Surgery and the North American Chapter of the International Society for Cardiovascular Surgery,[10] we recently reported the long-term success of FFB in 196 patients.[11] Primary patency rates at 5, 10, and 15 years were 63%, 56%, and 40%, respectively; secondary patency rates were 77%, 71%, and 43%, respectively. Early failures were usually a result of inability to establish adequate flow through the recipient profunda femoris artery. Late failures were a result of progressive outflow, donor iliac artery inflow stenosis, or infection. This chapter updates that report, documenting results with 228 femorofemoral grafts implanted and followed since 1967. Results with FFB have been poorer during the past decade compared with our early experience, but these data are not strictly comparable because more strict criteria for patency are now being used. Perhaps more important, during the past 10 to 15 years patients with compromised inflow vessels have been accepted as candidates for FFB. Since 1978 we have entered data in a prospective fashion into a registry. We focus more closely on this group because the follow-up is more complete and the data are more accurate.

MATERIALS AND METHODS

During the 25-year period from 1967 through 1991, 228 FFBs were performed for aortoiliac occlusive disease by a single surgical group. Patients with aneurysmal disease and those with ischemia as a result of intra-aortic balloon insertion were excluded, but patients who underwent previous aortoiliac and infrainguinal reconstructions were included. The extent and distribution of aortoiliac disease were evaluated by arteriography and measurement of femoral artery pressures. The status of the superficial femoral artery was noted on angiography and noninvasive testing. Segmental limb pressures were determined pre- and postoperatively.

Graft patency was determined during the follow-up period (0 to 260 months; mean, 46 months) by physical examination, noninvasive testing, pulse volume recording, segmental limb pressures, and duplex scans. Failing grafts were examined by angiography. Primary and secondary patencies, early and late morbidity, and mortality were defined according to the criteria established by the committee on standards of reporting as noted above.[10] In contrast to some of our earlier reports,[9] grafts revised within 48 hours of surgery were considered to have failed. Procedures designed to prevent thrombosis of the graft such as balloon angioplasty or endarterectomy signified the end of primary patency of the graft, even though the graft was still functioning. Patent grafts removed because of infection were considered to have failed. Grafts were considered to be secondarily patent independent of the number of revisions if the major portion of the original graft remained.

Statistical differences between groups were determined by a two-tailed test for continuous variables and Pearson χ^2 test for discrete variables. Long-term patency data were analyzed using the Kaplan-Meier technique. Differences between patency curves were compared using the Log Rank test.

RESULTS

Patient Characteristics

Demographic information for 110 patients treated since 1978 is outlined in Table 33–1. Fifty-seven percent of patients undergoing FFB were men, a lower figure than expected in patients with atherosclerosis. Women were not older than the men. Only 46% had documented coronary disease, a lower figure than expected.

TABLE 33–1. PATIENT DEMOGRAPHICS

Age (mean, years)	63
Male gender (%)	57
Diabetes (%)	29
Smoking (%)	61
Hypertension (%)	54
Coronary artery disease (%)	46
Cerebrovascular disease (%)	24

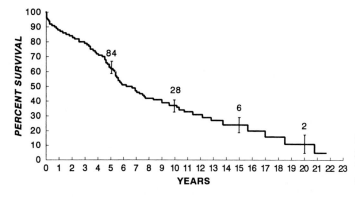

Figure 33–5. Actuarial survival of 228 patients who underwent FFB 1967 to 1991. Sixty-three percent survived 5 years.

DISCUSSION

The 5- and 10-year primary patencies for 228 FFBs placed during the past 25 years were 55% and 46%. This is lower than we had expected for several reasons. The first relates to the definition of primary patency. In 1980,[9] we reported a 5-year primary patency of FFB of 73%. At that time, early occlusions that were revised were not considered to be graft failures; furthermore, patients who had undergone previous operations were excluded. In our report in 1989,[11] we followed the criteria recommended by the two vascular societies. In addition, we segregated out those patients who had undergone previous attempts to revascularize the ileofemoral system from those who had not had surgery. Five-year primary patency was 53% after a previous reconstruction and 67% when no prior surgery had been carried out. In that 1989 study, grafts that required revision but remained patent were still considered patent. In the current study, however, patients who had undergone previous infrainguinal bypass were not segregated from those who had no such surgery. Only previous aortoiliac surgery was considered a risk factor. In the current study, all revisions were considered to signify failure of the graft, even if the graft remained patent at the time of revision. Grafts that required iliac angioplasty, anastomotic revisions, or removal because of infection were considered to have failed. As a result, the current 5-year primary patency rates for FFB of 55% overall, 63% with no previous aortoiliac reconstruction or adjunctive treatment of donor iliac artery disease, and 41% with previous aortoiliac surgery are the most conservative figures that could be calculated.

Few recent papers have stringently followed the criteria for patency established by the Society for Vascular Surgery and the North American Chapter of the International Society for Cardiovascular Surgery. Therefore it is difficult to compare the results in this report with previous studies. Rutherford et al,[12] Kalman et al,[13] and Piotrowski et al[14] recently reviewed results of FFB using these new definitions of patency. The first study[12] reported 5-year patencies of 74% for FFB when no inflow attempts had been made and 39% when a previous aortoiliac procedure had been carried out. Kalman et al[13] have shown 3-year patencies to be 90% and 47%, respectively, in these two groups.

Probably the most important reason for the low overall patency was the inclusion of two groups at high risk for failure. Fifty-one patients had undergone previous aortofemoral, ileofemoral, or femorofemoral grafting. One might expect the disease that prompted the first operation to progress after the second procedure. In fact, 18 of the 28 failures in this group were caused by outflow lesions, either incompletely corrected at surgery or progressing after bypass. Similar findings have been noted by others.[12,13] Interestingly, three patients developed inflow lesions despite previous inflow operations. Two patients had an aortofemoral bypass: one developed proximal aortic stenosis, and one developed donor iliac thrombosis. One patient had recurrent iliac stenoses at a site of angioplasty. (This patient could have also been classified with the group who had donor iliac artery disease—see below.)

A second group of 27 patients with donor iliac disease were at high risk for recurrent or progressive disease. In reviewing all cases of failure, we found rather unexpectedly that disease in the segment of iliac artery just proximal to the proximal anastomosis occasionally became involved in a stenotic process. In six patients, this was the cause of graft failure. One patient had an ileofemoral endarterectomy, two had interposition, and one had iliac artery dilatation. In the 12 patients who underwent donor iliac angioplasty, as noted above, only one graft failed because of recurrent disease at the angioplasty site. Brewster et al[15] noted good results with FFB after iliac angioplasty. Nevertheless, one can expect restenosis in at least 20% to 30% of these patients with time, depending on the location and extent of the iliac lesion.

During the 25-year period 1967 through 1991, 150 of the 228 grafts were placed in patients who had neither disease in the donor iliac artery or had undergone a previous inflow procedure that failed. During the first 11 years (series A), 104 of 118 (87%) of grafts fell into this category. During the last 13 years, with increasing expansion of the indications for FFB, only 47 of 110 (43%) grafts were placed in this most favorable environment. Despite these conditions, the 5- and 10-year patencies were only 63% and 54%. Some of the early failures were preventable. Recipient iliac endarterectomy, the cause of four earlier graft failures, was abandoned more than 15 years ago because it eliminates the disease for which the bypass was intended. Inflow disease, which accounted for 12 graft failures, may have been avoided by better selection and persistent surveillance. Attention to details of tunneling and curvature of the graft probably would have prevented a few more occlusions. Thus most of the failures occurred within the first year, some of which may have been avoided.

A final speculation to account for the diminished patency of the FFB was the willingness to use diseased profunda vessels. Unfortunately, this practice would be difficult to evaluate because no reliable method of quantitating profunda runoff has been tested. However, it is clear that some grafts were anastomosed to severely diseased vessels because (a) the risk of a procedure limited to the groin was low and failure could be more easily accepted than an abdominal operation or (b) the procedure could be easily combined with an infrainguinal bypass.

Through a variety of techniques, secondary patency at 5 years was extended to 69% in FFB. The method used depended on the cause of failure. Iliac angioplasty, endarterectomy, or bypass grafting were useful for repairing an inflow problem. Endarterectomy or interposition grafting was used at the donor common femoral level. The usual methods of endarterectomy, interposition grafting, and infrainguinal reconstruction were used at the recipient outflow tract. As a result of an aggressive approach to the occluded or failing FFB, secondary patency reached 75% in those grafts that were not complicated by simultaneous donor artery inflow procedures or preliminary attempts at aortoiliac reconstruction.

It is unrealistic to expect that FFB will have the same patency as aortofemoral bypass. Inflow through the FFB depends on the quality of iliac and common femoral vessels, whereas aortofemoral bypass depends solely on the quality of the infrarenal aorta. In this study, 22 of 92 failures of FFB were caused by progressive disease in the aorta, donor iliac, or proximal donor femoral artery. The aortofemoral bypass is not exposed to these influences. Furthermore, the aortofemoral graft is used in patients with adequate profunda vessels. In our practice, aortic procedures are reserved for good-risk patients with significant bilateral aortoiliac disease. FFB is preferred for patients with unilateral iliac occlusions, particularly occlusions of the common iliac artery. Therefore, it is not valid to use the current study to compare the two procedures.

Nevertheless, when a good-risk patient with a unilateral iliac occlusion needs surgery, a decision between the two procedures must be made. This decision weighs the relative risks and long-term patency of each. Does the better long-term success justify the slightly higher risk of death and serious morbidity of the aortofemoral graft? What is the incidence of interference with sexual function, embolization into the normal ileofemoral system, and life-threatening graft infection in one's experience with aortic surgery? Will repeat operations on the FFB put a patient at increased risk? Performing aortofemoral bypass in *all* patients with unilateral iliac disease may subject certain patients to unacceptable risks. Denying good-risk patients with dubious donor arteries a longer-lasting procedure by avoiding aortic surgery may represent poor judgment as well. We continue to recommend aortofemoral grafts for good-risk patients with bilateral aortoiliac disease and use FFB for both good- and poor-risk patients with unilateral iliac occlusion. Even though FFB will require surgical revision in about half the patients, secondary patency will remain lower than the primary patency of the aortic procedure.

REFERENCES

1. Brewster DC, Darling RC. Optimal methods of aortoiliac reconstruction. *Surgery.* 1978;84:739–747.
2. Crawford ES, Bomberger RA, Glaeser **DH, et al.** Aortoiliac occlusive disease: factors influencing survival and function following reconstructive operation over a twenty-five-year period. *Surgery.* 1981;90:1055–1066.
3. Szilagyi DE, Elliott JP Jr, Smith RF et al. A thirty-year survey of the reconstructive surgical treatment of aortoiliac occlusive disease. *J Vasc Surg.* 1986;3:421–436.
4. Oudot J, Beaconfield P. Thrombosis of the aortic bifurcation treated by resection and homograft replacement. *Arch Surg.* 1953;66:365–374.
5. Freeman NE, Leeds FH. Operations on large arteries: application of recent advances. *Calif Med.* 1952;77:229–233.
6. Vetto RM. The treatment of unilateral iliac artery obstruction with a trans-abdominal, subcutaneous, femorofemoral graft. *Surgery.* 1962;52:345.
7. Vetto RM. The femoro-femoral shunt: an appraisal. *Am J Surg.* 1966;112:162–165.
8. Parsonnet V, Alpert J, Brief DK. Femoro-femoral and axillofemoral grafts: compromise or preference. *Surgery.* 1970;67:26–32.
9. Dick LS, Brief DK, Alpert J et al. A 12-year experience with femorofemoral crossover grafts. *Arch Surg.* 1980;115:1359–1365.
10. Rutherford RB, Flanigan DP, Gupta SK, et al. Suggested standards for reports dealing with lower extremity ischemia. *J Vasc Surg.* 1986;4:80–94.
11. Brener B, Eisenbud DE, Brief DK, et al. Utility of femorofemoral crossover grafts. In: Bergan JJ, Yao JST, eds. *Aortic Surgery.* Philadelphia: WB Saunders; 1989:423–428.
12. Rutherford RB, Patt A, Pierce WH. Extra-anatomic bypass: a closer view. *J Vasc Surg.* 1987;6:437–446.
13. Kalman PG, Hoserg M, Johnston KW et al. The current role for femorofemoral bypass. *J Vasc Surg.* 1987;6:71–76.
14. Piotrowski JJ, Pearce WH, Jones DN, et al. Aortobifemoral bypass: the operation of choice for unilateral iliac occlusion? *J Vasc Surg.* 1988;8:211–218.
15. Brewster DC, Cambria RP, Darling RC, et al. Long-term results of combined iliac balloon angioplasty and distal surgical revascularization. *Ann Surg.* 1989;210:324–330.

34

Axillofemoral Bypass:

Long-Term Results

F. William Blaisdell, MD

Since its inception in 1962, the use of axillofemoral bypass for elective revascularization of aortoiliac occlusive disease has been controversial when it is used as an alternative to conventional anatomic operations.[1] However, recent technical advances have resulted in outcomes for axillofemoral grafts nearly as good as conventional procedures when used in comparable good-risk cases.

There are a number of problems that make comparison between the two procedures difficult. First, no randomized studies have been performed comparing the two operations, and second, the inclination, including our own, is to use the normal anatomic route when the patients are good risks and to use axillofemoral bypass in patients who are not good risks or who have complications such as infection that preclude conventional procedures. There is also the theoretic possibility that the inflow provided by the subclavian axillary arteries may not be comparable with that provided by the abdominal aorta. Nonetheless, unless there is proximal disease in the inflow vessels, the axillary artery is capable of supplying normal flow to the lower limb, and it is the distal resistance in the outflow vessels that determines the degree of blood flow in the bypass. Another factor that might theoretically be disadvantageous is the relatively exposed position of the axillofemoral graft, which makes it vulnerable to compression and kinking.

Although there is great variability in the reported results from axillofemoral bypass, it is of interest that the large series that have been followed for 5 years or more generally demonstrate excellent long-term patency, whereas smaller series followed for modest periods of time have usually reported high risk for early thrombosis. This is undoubtedly because technical factors influence outcome more often than standard bypass operations.

RESULTS

In Table 34–1,[2–19] we have listed all the axillofemoral graft series that we are aware of in the English literature that report follow-up of 5 or more years. The table classifies the grafts by whether they were axillounifemoral (AF) or axillobifemoral (AFF). AF

TABLE 34–1. AXILLOFEMORAL GRAFTS

		Mortality			Graft Patency			
Date	Reference	No.	30-Days (%)	5-yr (%)	Type	No.	1-yr (%)	5-yr (%)
1971	Moore et al[2]	52	8	70	AF(F)	52	62	9
1977	Eugene et al[3]	59	8	73	AF	35	62	30
					AFF	24	62	30
1977	LoGerfo et al[4]	130	8	23	AF	64	64	37
					AFF	66	89	74
1977	Johnson et al[5]	56	2	37	AFF	56	82	76
1978	Sheiner[6]	45	2	32	AF	25	60	51
1979	Ray et al[7]	84	3.7	32	AF	33	75	67
					AFF	21	90	77
1982	Kenny et al[8]	92	—	—	AF	58	85	66
1982	Courbier et al[9]	220	3.6	24	AF	220	87	64
1985	Ascer et al[10]	56	5.3	57	AF	34	68	44
1985	Allison et al[11]	109	6.4	44	AF	87	48	16
					AFF	25	58	45
1986	Chang[12]	88	2	47	AF	47	—	33
1986	Christenson et al[13]	85	3.6	45	AF(F)	85	74	67.6
1986	Foster[14]	52	12	60	AF(F)	52	60	32
1986	Donaldson et al[15]	100	8	31	AF(F)	72	78	48
1986	Savrin et al[16]	33	18	59	AF(F)	96	91	75
1986	Schulz et al[17]	41	—	—	AF(?)	41	95	80
1987	Rutherford et al[18]	42	12	50	AF	15	48	19
					AFF	27	78	62
1988	Hepp et al[19]	124	4.9	40	AF	102	60	46
					AFF	22	83	80

AF, Axillounifemoral graft; AFF, axillobifemoral graft; AF(F), combined AF and AFF; AF(?), AF or AFF not specified.

grafts on the whole had a 1-year patency of 48% to 87% and a 5-year patency of 19% to 67%; the AFF grafts had a 1-year patency of 58% to 90% and a 5-year patency rate of 30% to 80%.

In reviewing these reports, there does not appear to be any significant difference between those series using polytetrafluoroethylene grafts and those using Dacron grafts,[20] although one report suggested that polytetrafluoroethylene was superior.[13] In addition, there did not seem to be any difference whether 8- or 10-mm Dacron grafts were used,[3] although we found a difference in long-term patency between woven and knitted Dacron grafts that markedly favored the latter.[3]

As previously alluded, technical factors also influence the immediate and long-term patency of axillofemoral grafts. The factors that I believe are important are listed in Table 34–2. They are proximal placing of the axillary anastomosis, directing the graft laterally so that it lies in the axis of flexion of the body, using externally

TABLE 34–2. TECHNICAL FACTORS THAT IMPROVE PATENCY

Proximal anastomosis on axillary artery

Graft placed in axis of flexion of the trunk

Externally supported graft

Double outflow from distal graft

Avoid parallel flow in native arteries

supported grafts, maximizing outflow by using AFF grafts whenever possible, and avoiding parallel flow in native arteries.

The importance of proximal placement of the anastomosis on the axillary artery cannot be overemphasized. In those series that report poor results, in many instances these appear to result from placing the anastomosis distally on the second or third portion of the axillary artery.[21,22] I believe that the optimal location for the axillofemoral graft is between the clavicle and pectoralis minor tendon. To ensure the proximal placement of the graft, the pectoralis minor should not be cut, and the dissection should mobilize the entire segment between the clavicle and the pectoralis minor muscle. This segment contains only one branch, the highest thoracic, which is a 1-mm vessel. The collateral potential for this segment is excellent, and should this segment thrombose, viability of the arm is not threatened. When the anastomosis is placed in this region, there is minimal movement of the anastomotic area when the shoulder is elevated, whereas the more distal the anastomosis is placed, the greater the potential for stress of the graft and false aneurysm formation.

Because of the potential possibility for kinking the graft with flexion of the trunk, it is optimal to curve the tunnel for the graft laterally into the posterior axillary line so that it lies in the axis of flexion of the trunk. This requires a counter incision, as no tunneler has been devised that will ensure adequate lateral curvature of the graft tunnel. Therefore, we routinely make a small counter incision in the mid or posterior axillary line and tunnel in both directions toward this incision. We then pull an umbilical tape the entire length of the dissected tunnel. The tunnel, incidentally, is placed under pectoralis major muscle by dissection from above and under the external oblique fascia by dissection from below. The areolar plane under the fascia and muscle results in less trauma during the dissection, less bleeding, and less cosmetic deformity.

Cavallaro et al[23] studied ankle pressure index and pulse/volume wave amplitude changes after 5 and 10 minutes of external compression by body weight on the side of the reconstruction. Eight patients with axillofemoral bypasses were evaluated, and the external body weight compression caused important changes in graft hemodynamics. These included both a decrease in ankle pressure index and in pulse/volume recorder wave amplitude at 5 and 10 minutes. The use of an externally supported graft, with support rings the entire length of the graft, is important to protect the graft from compression trauma when the patient is lying on his or her side. We agree with Sauvage's group[8,17] that support rings have constituted a major technical advance in decreasing thrombosis in these superficially placed grafts.

Ray et al[7] believed that the patency rate of axillofemoral grafts is directly related to flow. This is our position as well. LoGerfo et al[4] did studies of blood flow in patients and found that AFF grafts had an average flow rate of 621 cc/min versus the average flow rate of AF grafts of less than 300 cc/min. In their series, there was a 75% 5-year patency rate of AFF grafts as opposed to a 32% 5-year patency with AF grafts. Ray et al[7] demonstrated a higher 5-year patency rate for axillofemoral grafts in limbs with a patent superficial femoral artery than for those with an occluded superficial femoral artery. This is consistent with our experience. Thus, when the nature of the operation permits, we use AFF rather than AF grafts. We prefer the double outflow technique that involves dividing the common femoral artery at the inguinal ligament, doing an end-to-end anastomosis of the proximal femorofemoral graft to the distal end of the divided femoral artery, and placing the axillofemoral graft anastomosis on a distal part of the common femoral artery, often overlapping onto the superficial artery or the profunda femoral artery (Fig. 34–1). This means that, should the outflow to the right or left limb become obstructed, there is still outflow provided to the

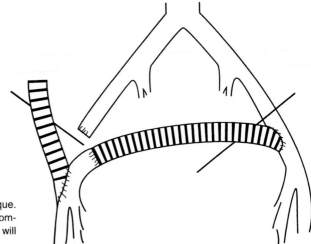

Figure 34–1. Double outflow technique. Should one extremity's blood flow be compromised, flow to the opposite limb will maintain axillofemoral graft patency.

opposite leg. This technique improves patency and ensures maximal outflow through the entire length of the graft. An alternative when the ipsilateral common femoral artery is diseased is to resect this vessel, bring the graft through the external oblique fascia more laterally than usual, and do a side-to-end anastomosis to the graft. The distal end is then tunneled across the lower abdomen for anastomosis to the contralateral groin (Fig. 34–2).

The final principle that is important to ensure maximal flow through the graft is avoiding parallel flow. If the common iliac arteries are completely occluded, then end-to-side anastomosis of one of the femoral limbs is appropriate to provide retrograde pelvic perfusion. However, should an iliac artery still have prograde flow, then interruption of the common femoral artery should be performed and an end-to-end anastomosis to the distal common femoral artery carried out.

In summary, there are widely different reports concerning the results of axillofemoral grafting. If the technical factors outlined in this chapter are used, the long-term outcome of these grafts should parallel those of the best-reported series.

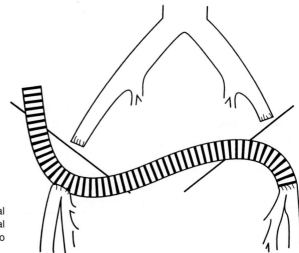

Figure 34–2. When dealing with aneurysmal disease that requires resection, ipsilateral femoral anastomosis can be side-to-end to the common femoral bifurcation.

REFERENCES

1. Blaisdell FW, Hall AD. Axillary-femoral artery bypass for lower extremity ischemia. *Surgery*. 1963;54:563.
2. Moore WS, Hall AD, Blaisdell FW. Late results of axillary-femoral bypass grafting. *Am J Surg*. 1971;122:148.
3. Eugene J, Goldstone J, Moore WS. Fifteen-year experience with subcutaneous bypass grafts for lower extremity ischemia. *Ann Surg*. 1977;186:177.
4. LoGerfo FW, Johnson WC, Corson JD, et al. A comparison of the late patency rates of axillobilateral femoral and axillounilateral femoral grafts. *Surgery*. 1977;81:33.
5. Johnson WC, LoGerfo FW, Vollman RW, et al. Is axillo-bilateral femoral grafts an effective substitute for aortic-bilateral iliac-femoral graft? *Ann Surg*. 1977;186:123.
6. Sheiner NM. Peripheral vascular surgery: alternate anatomical pathways and the use of allograft veins as arterial substitutes. In: Wilson SE, Van Wagener P, Passaro E Jr, eds. *Current Problems in Surgery: Arterial Infection*. Chicago, Ill: Year Book Medical; 1978:2–76.
7. Ray LI, O'Connor JB, Davis CC, et al. Axillofemoral bypass: a critical reappraisal of its role in the management of aortoiliac occlusive disease. *Am J Surg*. 1979;138:117.
8. Kenny DA, Sauvage LR, Wood SJ, et al. Comparison of noncrimped, externally supported (EXS) and crimped, nonsupported Dacron prostheses for axillofemoral and above knee femoropopliteal bypass. *Surgery*. 1982;92:931.
9. Courbier R, Jausseran JM, Bergeron P. Axillo-femoral bypass material of choice. In: Greenhalgh RM, ed. *Extra-anatomic Secondary Arterial Reconstruction*. Bath, England: Pitman Press; 1982:122–130.
10. Ascer E, Veith FJ, Gupta SK, et al. Comparison of axillounifemoral and axillobifemoral bypass operations. *Surgery*. 1985;97:169.
11. Allison HF, Terblanche J, Immelman EJ. Axillofemoral bypass: a 2-decade experience. *S Afr Med J*. 1985;68:559.
12. Chang JB. Current state of extra-anatomic bypasses. *Am J Surg*. 1986;152:202.
13. Christenson JT, Broome A, Norgren L, et al. The late results after axillo-femoral bypass grafts in patients with leg ischaemia. *J Cardiovasc Surg (Torino)*. 1986;27:131.
14. Foster MC. A review of 155 extra-anatomic bypass grafts. *Ann R Coll Surg Engl*. 1986;68:1.
15. Donaldson MC, Louras JC, Buckham CA. Axillofemoral bypass: a tool with a limited role. *J Vasc Surg*. 1986;3:757.
16. Savrin RA, Record GT, McDowell DE. Axillofemoral bypass: expectations and results. *Arch Surg*. 1986;121:1016.
17. Schulz GA, Sauvage LR, Mathisen SR. A five to seven year experience with externally supported Dacron prostheses in axillofemoral and femoropopliteal bypass. *Ann Vasc Surg*. 1986;1:214.
18. Rutherford RB, Patt A, Pearce WH. Extra-anatomic bypass: a closer view. *J Vasc Surg*. 1987;6:437.
19. Hepp W, deJonge K, Pallua N. Late results following extra-anatomic bypass procedures for chronic aortoiliac occlusive disease. *J Cardiovasc Surg*. 1988;29:181.
20. Burrell MJ, Wheeler JR, Gregory RT. Axillofemoral bypass: a ten-year review. *Ann Surg*. 1982;195:796.
21. Gorman JF, Douglass FM. Axillary-femoral artery bypass. *Arch Surg*. 1965;91:509.
22. White GH, Donayre CE, Williams RA. Exertional disruption of axillofemoral graft anastomosis. *Arch Surg*. 1990;125:625.
23. Cavallaro A, Sciacca V, deMarzo L, et al. The effect of body weight compression on axillo-femoral bypass patency. *J Cardiovasc Surg*. 1988;29:476.

VIII

Late Results in the Management of Venous Problems

35

Arteriovenous Malformation:

Long-Term Follow-Up

Elizabeth Scott, MD, William H. Pearce, MD,
Walter J. McCarthy, MD, William R. Flinn, MD,
and James S.T. Yao, MD, PhD

No other vascular disorder enjoys a history as rich in imagination and folklore as vascular malformations. At the center of this history is the concept of maternal impression—that a mother could alter the phenotype of her offspring through experience, emotion, or craving during her pregnancy. Because midwifery was essentially women's work, little was known about female reproductive anatomy and childbirth. *Imaginatio gravidarum* was used to explain not only phenotypic variation but also the birth of malformed children.[1-3] Women were urged to guard against emotional disturbances of any sort, but particularly grotesque or frightening scenes. Because 30% of hemangiomas are located on the head and neck, maternal fear could mark a child by a mother's tendency to touch the face and neck in a gesture of fright.[1] Also, the inability to satisfy cravings for various fruits during pregnancy (i.e., strawberries, cherries, raspberries) could leave a child with a cutaneous stain. Early theories regarding treatment included rubbing the lesion with the placenta or the hand of a corpse, which was thought to induce regression.[2] Also mothers of infants born with vascular birthmarks believed that licking the lesion for nine consecutive mornings postpartum would bring a cure. Because most hemangiomas (~80%) involute spontaneously, it is easy to understand how such theories would go unchallenged. During the first half of the 18th century, Dr. James Augustus Blondel published the earliest criticisms of the teratogenic potential of maternal thought.[1] Although he was supported by a number of prominent physicians, the debate continued for almost another two centuries.

The long history of folklore and superstition has left the legacy of ambiguous nomenclature and misunderstanding, often resulting in the mismanagement of vascular malformations. The etiology of terms such as *strawberry hemangioma* and *port wine stain* are obvious. Rudolf Virchow reclassified this lesion into *agioma simplex, racemosum,* and *cavernosum,* terms that are used today. In 1982 Mulliken and Glowacki[4] proposed a classification system based both on the clinical behavior and the histopathologic features of these lesions. Previous classification systems that were merely descriptive or embryologic lacked clinical usefulness. In this system there are two major categories of vascular birthmarks, hemangiomas and malformations (Table 35–1).[1]

Clinically there are profound differences between the hemangiomas and malformations. Hemangiomas, the most common tumors of infancy, are dynamic lesions. They are generally not present at birth but may be preceded by the "herald spot," a small, blanched, or telangiectatic patch. They proliferate rapidly during the first weeks of life and then gradually involute over the next 5 to 7 years. There is a slight female-to-male predominance of 2 to 3:1.

Vascular malformations, however, are true inborn errors in the embryologic maturation of the vascular system. Vascular malformations are, by definition, present at birth, although they may not be evident until adolescence or pregnancy. Malformations occur with equal frequency in both boys and girls and tend to grow with the child.

On a cellular level, proliferating hemangiomas demonstrate significant endothelial cell hyperplasia as demonstrated by tritiated thymidine incorporation and a more than 30% increase in the mast cell population.[4] It seems logical that endothelial cells retain their proliferative potential throughout their lifetime and respond to some, as yet unidentified angiogenic signal after injury. Folkman et al[5] proposed that the angiogenic stimulus also induces "helper" cells (i.e., mast cells) to secrete growth factors, thereby setting up a self-perpetuating cycle.

However, malformations are characterized by normal appearing, flat endothelial cells, with normal turnover (doubling time = years) and normal mast cell numbers.[6] Normal development of the peripheral vascular system is dependent on a number of forces acting in concert during the critical period of remodeling that follows formation of the plexus. Mechanical tension, hormones, the chemical microenvironment, and metabolic demands may all play a role in determining the formation of mature vessels. Blood flow through the plexus exerts physical forces causing portions of the plexus to grow in calibre, wall thickness, and size of the capillary bed.[1] Conversely, a diminution of flow and pressure will cause other parts of the plexus to decrease their calibre and wall thickness or cause the capillary bed to resorb completely. The final stage is the formation of mature vessels. As the limb bud develops, one axial artery and two axial veins, a pre- and postaxial vein, reaches the distal retiform plexus. Further remodeling may occur in the third stage with resorption of the axial arteries of the upper extremity and the postaxial veins in the legs. Preaxial veins are the precursors of the cephalic and long saphenous. The axial arteries in the lower

TABLE 35–1. SYSTEMS OF CLASSIFICATION

		Malformation	
	Old Terminology	**High-flow**	**Low-flow**
Hemangioma			
←————————Capillary hemangioma			
←————————Strawberry hemangioma			
←————————Capillary-cavernous hemangioma			
	Arteriovenous ————————————→Arteriovenous malformation		
	Port wine stain ————————————→ Capillary malformation		
	Cavernous hemangioma ————————→Venous malformation		
	Hemangio-lymphangioma ——————————→Lymphatic venous malformation		
	Lymphangioma ——————————————→Lymphatic malformation		

(Adapted with permission from Mulliken JB. Classification of vascular birthmarks. In: Mulliken JB, Young AE, eds. Vascular Birth Marks: Hemangiomas and Malformations. Philadelphia: WB Saunders: 1988:32.)

extremities persist and eventually form the femoral and popliteal vessels. Lymphatics develop after blood vessels, and although it has not been proven conclusively, it appears that the lymphatics sprout from veins. Nodes develop after fibrous septae divide the lymphatics, which are subsequently invaded by lymphocytes. No single putative injury has been identified in the formation of arteriovenous malformations. Vascular malformations may involve any one component of the vascular tree or may exist as mixed lesions, with or without lymphatic involvement.

DIAGNOSIS

Physical examination is helpful in differentiating hemangiomas from malformations. On palpation, hemangiomas are rubbery and cannot be completely emptied of blood. On angiography, hemangiomas are homogeneous and well circumscribed and supplied by several large branches of adjacent normal vessels, equatorial vessels. Capillary malformations yield the typical port wine stain and should alert the observer to the possibility of other lesions. In contrast, malformations are compressible, can be completely emptied of blood, and often have palpable thrombi within. High-flow malformations are notorious for extensively involving adjacent structures such as bone and muscle. Vascular malformations may be extensive penetrating skin, subcutaneous tissue, muscle, tendon, and bone, often excluding complete primary resection, short of amputation. Because of propensity to involve many tissues, presentation may vary tremendously. Magnetic resonance imaging is helpful in defining location and extent.[7] If the fistulous connections are large, significant shunting of blood from the distal arterial bed will occur and patients will exhibit ischemic symptoms as well as primary venous stasis. Other secondary effects of vascular malformations increase limb length discrepancy, hypertrophy, and venous tortuosities.

TREATMENT

The treatment of vascular malformations has undergone an evolution paralleling technologic advances and a better understanding of their pathogenesis. A number of therapies have been applied including proximal ligation, radical excision, electrocautery, sclerotherapy, and radiation[8,9] with varying results. However, treatment that may be appropriate for hemangiomas is not necessarily appropriate for arteriovenous malformations and the misidentification of these lesions may confuse the reported results.[10]

HEMANGIOMAS

It was not until the middle of this century that observation alone became the accepted standard of care for hemangiomas. William Lister[11] followed a cohort of more than 70 patients with rapidly proliferative hemangiomas from birth through their seventh birthdays and reported that 100% of the patients exhibited spontaneous regression of their lesions, on the average, in 5 years.

In 1965 Margileth and Museles[12] compared a group of patients with hemangiomas managed with either radiation or surgery with a group managed by observation alone. More than half of the treated patients experienced either no improvement, recurrence of the lesions, or complications including skin necrosis, scar tissue formation requiring grafting, bleeding, and secondary sepsis. The complication rate in the untreated group was 5%. Margileth and Museles recommended conservative therapy in most patients, with observation, serial measurements, and frequent color photographs of the lesion to reassure parents of the natural tendency of hemangiomas to involute. Using "before and after" photos of patients whose lesions had undergone repression was especially useful. Indications for more aggressive therapy in this group of patients (i.e., surgery or radiation) included rapidly expanding hemangiomas, giant hemangiomas complicated by platelet trapping (Kasabach-Merritt syndrome), and rarely lack of regression.

Moroz[13] at Children's Hospital in Montreal compiled treatment data on the largest cohort of patients with hemangiomas to date (Table 35–2).

Eight hundred and three patients were followed by observation for 7 years. Forty-six percent had complete resolution of their lesions; 36% had minimal telangiectasias that were cosmetically acceptable; 18% had either atrophy, scarring, or residual hemangiomas.

Follow-up was also obtained on 94 patients who had undergone radiation therapy, surgery, or a combination of the two. Of the patients receiving radiation alone, 21% had complete resolution and 10% had minimal telangiectasias. The remaining 69% had atrophy, scarring, or residual hemangioma. All the patients treated by surgery alone or radiation plus surgery had either atrophy, scarring, or residual hemangioma.

For large disfiguring hemangiomas with bleeding, a variety of therapies has been recommended. Steroid suppression of the rapidly proliferative phase, palliative embolization for ulceration and hemorrhage, antifibrinolytic therapy for thrombocytopenia, and occasionally surgery. Steroid therapy is based on the finding that hemangiomas demonstrate an abnormally high level of estrogen receptors and that high-dose corticosteroids may suppress the stimulatory effects of endogenous proliferative hormones.[14] Compression therapy with elastic garments is marginally effective in hastening the involution phase, but compliance is a major problem for most children.

Surgical intervention is indicated where the lesion is life-threatening: bleeding visceral hemangiomas or refractory congestive heart failure secondary to an hepatic hemangioma. Other indications for surgical treatment include respiratory compromise, feeding difficulties, and eyelid lesions because they lead to astigmatism, proptosis, and visual or eye loss. Nasal tip, labial lesions, and bulky head and neck masses are sometimes treated by subtotal excision, revision, and grafting for cosmetic reasons before involution.

TABLE 35–2.

Modality	No.	Lost to Follow-up	Results Resolved	Telangiectastic	Residual Hemangioma/Scar
Observation	803	0	369 (46%)	289 (36%)	145 (18%)
Excision	49	10 (20%)	0	0	24/15 (49%)[a]
Radiation	91	40 (44%)	11 (12%)	5 (6%)	35 (38%)
Surgery and radiation	7	3 (43%)	0	0	4 (57%)
Cryotherapy	12	0	1 (8%)	0	11 (92%)
Electrodessication	2	1 (50%)	0	0	1 (50%)
Steroids	10	0	0	1 (10%)	9 (90%)

From ref. 13, with permission.

[a] Because surgery always leaves some scar, this result refers only to patients with residual hemangioma after resection.

VASCULAR MALFORMATION

Vascular malformations are notoriously difficult to treat because of their variable extension into adjacent structures. One of the few treatment successes involves laser therapy for port wine stains or capillary malformations of the dermis. Port wine stains may appear on any part of the body, either randomly or in association with a number of vascular syndromes or developmental defects of the central nervous system. When they occur on the face, they frequently follow the distribution of one of the branches of the fifth cranial nerve, producing a flat pink to purple patch. Port wine stains are stable lesions that do not involute as hemangiomas do. Frequently, however, port wine stains tend to darken with age, and the previously smooth overlying skin becomes increasingly nodular. Because of the natural tendency of port wine stains to progress, numerous treatments have been described, again paralleling industrial progress. The most notable have been scarification, electrocoagulation, ultraviolet and ionizing radiation, tattooing, excision, and grafting.[15,16] Unfortunately, the treatment often failed. Cosmetics and excision with skin grafting or tissue expanders for large lesions continue to be options. More recently, laser therapy has been developed that results in a much more aesthetic result.

The principle underlying argon laser therapy is that light energy is selectively absorbed by oxyhemoglobin in ectatic vessels causing thrombosis with conversion of that light energy to heat.[17] Initially, it was thought that injury to the epidermis with the argon laser was negligible, but it quickly became evident that younger patients were especially prone to hypertrophic scar formation after argon laser therapy.[18,19]

The CO_2 laser causes a nonspecific thermal burn of exposed tissue by vaporization of water-containing cells. CO_2 lasers are presently used to treat adults with verrucous hypertrophic lesions refractory to argon lasers. Lanigan and Cotterill[20] reported in 1990 "good" results in 53% of 22 children with nonresponding "pink" lesions using CO_2 laser therapy. Because the international standards for acceptable results are a good response in 60% to 70% of adult patients treated with argon laser therapy,[21] no less was expected of laser therapy used to treat children, and this led to the development of the tunable-dye laser. The tunable-dye laser not only targets oxyhemoglobin but, by virtue of its longer wavelength, decreases absorption by epidermal melanocytes and spares the epidermis.[21] Nelson et al reported good results in children treated for port wine stains with the pulsed-dye laser "without the adverse complications of hypertrophic scarring, permanent pigmentation abnormality, or textural changes . . . often seen with conventional laser systems."[15]

Unfortunately, treatment strategies for malformations of larger vessels have not been as satisfying as laser therapy has been for capillary malformations. However, even treatment failures have merit in defining guidelines. The axiom to be gained from the past 30 years of experience is that treatment of arteriovenous malformations should be individualized to each patient. To tailor therapy to a particular patient's problem, a thorough investigation of the location, extent, and hemodynamic significance of the lesion must be made. In the event of a planned surgical intervention, preoperative studies should include Doppler, magnetic resonance imaging, and arteriography. Often venography is needed to define the lesion completely.

Tables 35–3, 35–4, and 35–5 compare locations of arteriovenous malformations for a number of investigators, including our experience at Northwestern. These data are included because location and severity portend final treatment outcome (i.e., end artery lesions tend to do poorly over time).

In the series reviewed, patients with upper extremity lesions presented with swelling and pain, and those with lower extremity lesions complained of varicosities

TABLE 35–3. ARTERIOVENOUS MALFORMATION LOCATION

Investigator	Date	No.	Upper Extremity[a]	Lower Extremity[b]	Head/Neck (%)	Pelvis/Trunk (%)
Szilagyi et al[27]	1976	82	18	82		
Vercellio et al[31] (Halliday & Mansfield) (1989)	1988	32	47	53		
Kromhout et al[23]	1990	81	40	60		
Flye et al[24]	1983	25	12	24	44	20
Trout et al[22]	1984	9	11	44	33	11
Widlus et al[26]	1988	27	44	26	0	30
Northwestern	1992	35	23	57	14	6

[a] Mean follow-up from initial presentation for upper extremity lesions is 70 months (range, 12–240 months).
[b] Mean follow-up from initial presentation for lower extremity lesions is 154 months (range, 60–240 months).

and ulceration in addition to pain and swelling. Patients with lesions of the trunk and pelvis presented with pain, a palpable mass, and hematuria. Not surprisingly, patients with head and neck lesions most often sought treatment for disfigurement. For the cohort of patients at Northwestern, a poor prognosis is associated with recurrent ulceration and hemorrhage regardless of anatomy, upper extremity venous malformations, distal lesions, fingers fairing worse than hands, and enlarging cutaneous vascular stains or malformations.

A variety of treatment modalities for malformations from several different institutions is reviewed in Table 35–4. Trout et al[22] reviewed operative management and did not follow a cohort of patients by observation alone. The results for surgical excision by Kromhout et al[23] are reported as one figure, as they did not distinguish between patients who underwent complete versus staged resections.

Ten patients in studies by Flye et al[24] and Trout[22] were treated by ligation of a proximal artery. Five of the six patients in Flye's study required additional procedures to control their arteriovenous malformations. One progressed to amputation 1 month after ligation. In Trout's study only one patient of the four receiving ligation as part of their therapy received any benefit but only after multiple ligations. One patient progressed to amputation, and the remaining two recurred. Proximal ligation of vessels feeding malformations was an early surgical technique now recognized not only as ineffective in controlling the arteriovenous malformation but, in fact, as

TABLE 35–4. MANAGEMENT OF ARTERIOVENOUS MALFORMATIONS

	Investigator			
	Flye et al 1983[24]	Trout et al 1984[22]	Kromhout et al 1990[23]	Northwestern 1992
Treatment modality (n)	25	9	81	35
Complete excision	9 (36%)	3 (33%)	8 (23%)	21 (26%)
Partial excision	2 (8%)	0		6 (17%)
Embolization	1 (4%)	0	45 (56%)	3 (9%)
Ligation	1 (4%)	2 (22%)	0	0
Amputation	1 (4%)	2 (22%)	0	4 (11%)
Combined treatment	6 (24%)	2 (22%)	11 (14%)	5 (14%)
Observation	6 (24%)	N/A	4 (5%)	6 (17%)
Lost to follow-up	0	0	0	3 (9%)

TABLE 35–5. SURGERY VERSUS OBSERVATION IN ARTERIOVENOUS MALFORMATIONS[a]

Investigator	Date	Condition	Excision	Observation
Szilagyi et al[27]	1976		$n = 18$	n = 64
		Improved	10 (55%)	12 (19%)
		Unchanged	2 (11%)	· 42 (65%)
		Worse	6 (33%)	10 (17%)
Flye et al[24]	1983		$n = 16$	$n = 5$
		Improved	13 (81%)	1 (20%)
		Unchanged	1 (6%)	4 (80%)
		Worse	2 (13%)	0 (0%)
Northwestern	1992		$n = 15$	$n = 5$
		Improved	5 (33%)	0 (0%)
		Unchanged	2 (13%)	2 (40%)
		Worse	3 (20%)	1 (20%)
		Lost to follow-up	5 (33%)	2 (40%)

[a] These figures pertain to complete excision. Partial excisions or surgical procedures performed as an adjunct to conservative therapy are not included.

detrimental. One patient in the Northwestern University treatment group underwent ligation of her right facial artery 4 years before presenting for a vascular malformation of her ear. The malformation continued to grow after ligation, with ulceration requiring numerous transfusions. This patient subsequently underwent excision of the malformation. Proximal ligation of the arteriovenous malformation should be avoided because it precludes later embolization and it induces collateralization.

Promising results using transcatheter embolization have been published in recent years. The semiliquid Ethibloc is a mixture of amino acids, ethanol, and lipid contrast material that polymerizes under acidic conditions. Ethibloc produces thrombosis more distally than other agents in the capillary bed. Gel foam, coils, and particulate embolization often result in proximal occlusion and subsequent collateralization similar to proximal ligation. Gel foam, in addition, will recanalize over time. Yakes et al[25] obtained follow-up studies in 19 of 20 patients with arteriovenous malformations who were treated with ethanol embolization. All patients showed persistent occlusion of the malformation between 3 and 24 months postembolization. Cyano-acrylate compounds, or glue, have also been used to thrombose malformations. These compounds may be diluted and, like ethanol, embolize the nidus of the arteriovenous malformations. Widlus et al[26] treated 11 patients with isobutyl cyanoacrylate (IBCA). During a 40-month follow-up period, nine (82%) had complete resolution of their symptoms and the remaining two had partial resolution.

The most serious complication common to both Ethibloc and IBCA therapy is passage of the material into the venous circulation and pulmonary embolism. Ethibloc, because of its viscosity, must be injected under high pressure and can lead to inadvertent embolization. IBCA polymerizes so rapidly that it can glue the catheter itself to the vessel wall. Complications were few in the above studies, owing to superselective embolization. Superselective embolization is a technique that allows the angiographer to seat the catheter tip just proximal to the portion of the arteriovenous malformation to be embolized. Small catheters, often with coronary guide wires, are used for positioning. This maintains access to the arteriovenous malformation through open feeding vessels for repeat embolization and protects adjacent normal tissue from inadvertent embolization by catheter placement too far proximally.

Also of note are the three patients that were lost to follow-up in our study. There is probably also an attrition bias with respect to follow-up. Patients discharged for observation, second opinions, etc., may tend not to keep follow-up appointments. Two of these three patients were being followed by observation alone; the third was discharged for second opinion and never returned.

The results of excision are compared with observation in Table 35–5. Outcome categories are broad to encompass the wide range of patient responses. The unchanged category means either that surgery did little to alter the lesion or that symptoms rapidly reoccurred. There are few studies with complete long-term follow-up (Table 35–6).

The literature suggests that management of both upper and lower extremity arteriovenous malformations should be conservative.[27] Both venous and lymphatic malformations can cause significant deformity, swelling, and edema. In patients with pure venous malformations, pain tends to be the most common presenting symptom. Patients with lymphatic malformations, however, are limited because of large bulky lesions whose cystic spaces can spread into the adjacent chest wall. Rather than pain, these patients experience a loss of function. Although both venous and lymphatic malformations may benefit from compression therapy, pure venous disorders show the greatest decrease in volume with elastic garments. Extensive lymphatic malformations are associated with repeated bouts of ascending lymphangitis. Because complete excision is not usually functionally or cosmetically satisfactory, these patients often do better with amputations of affected limbs and prosthetics rather than staged excisions.[24]

Combined lymphatic-venous malformations in association with a cutaneous vascular stain where the lymphatics are profoundly hypoplastic is known as Klippel-Trenaunay syndrome. Presenting symptoms are similar to patients with pure lymphatic anomalies and are related to bulky deformities. Klippel-Trenaunay syndrome manifests itself with minor limb length discrepancies, soft tissue swelling, and curiously, large toes.[28] These patients have normal arterial architecture, extensive varicosities, and all the concomitant problems associated with arteriovenous malformations. Other than compression therapy, no other treatment is available. Surgery is rarely indicated.

High-flow arteriovenous malformations are a challenge both diagnostically and in terms of management. Arteriography is frequently inadequate in completely defining the malformation. After subtotal resection or skeletalization, rapid re-establishment of flow to the lesion occurs by opening up of adjacent vessels that were not visualized. Surgical indications include unremitting pain, distal ischemia, and functional loss. High-flow arteriovenous malformations are best treated by combined modalities including multiple embolizations and staged excisions with the cooperative efforts of interventional radiologists, vascular, orthopedic, and plastic surgeons.[29]

TABLE 35–6. FOLLOW-UP PERIOD

Investigator	Date	Mean Follow-up (mo)	Range (mo)
Szilagyi et al[27]	1976	120	<12–>240
Flye et al[24]	1983	a	10–120
Northwestern	1992	93	36–240
UE		70	12–240
LE		154	60–240

a Unable to calculate.

In assessing patients with recurrence, simple clinical and hand-held Doppler should be complemented by ascending and descending venography and varicography.[16-20] It is thus possible to divide most patients into one of three principal morphologic types.

Type 1

In these patients there is no evidence on Doppler insonnation of the distal varicosities of recurrence in saphenofemoral or saphenopopliteal junctions. A cough fails to register a propagated signal from the deep system. Varicography demonstratres in most that the source of new varicosities is through one or more incompetent thigh perforating veins and less frequently calf veins.

Type 2

In this form of "recurrence," the cause is attributable to persistence or evolution of varicosities derived from problems in a second saphenous system, either in the short saphenous after previous great saphenous surgery, the more common event, or less frequently in the opposite situation.

Type 3

In these patients, a positive sonic impulse is heard with hand-held Doppler on patient coughing when insonnation is carried out over a distal varicosity. This implies a system of incompetence from the femoral vein in the groin to the point of examination. In these patients, descending venography is of particular value in achieving precise definition as to the source of these recurrences, which can be further classified into three subgroups.

In type 3A, the recurrence is due to an incomplete or an inadequate previous ligation at the time of the initial surgery. It is illustrated in Figure 36–1. The appearance is typical and demonstrates an untied tributary proximal to the point of previous ligation of the saphenofemoral junction linking with the varicosity in the more distal limb.

Type 3B recurrence is shown in Figure 36–2. Here reflux is seen to occur down an incompetent superficial femoral vein and out through a midthigh perforator. Strictly speaking, this might be regarded as a variation of type 1, but on the basis of clinical and Doppler examination, it is indistinguishable. Occasionally this may be more complex. Figure 36–3 shows recurrence emanating from a distal tributary of an incompetent deep femoral vein.

Type 3C recurrence is due to reconstitution of the saphenofemoral or, less frequently, saphenopopliteal junction as shown in Figures 36–4 and 36–5, respectively. These show the typical appearance of bizarre and tortuous multichanneled trunks, which re-establish a connection between the common femoral vein and either a persistent and previously unremoved long saphenous trunk or less commonly varicosities in the thigh. This phenomenon was first described on venography by Starnes et al[17] and on histologic study by Sheppard.[10] In interesting recent reports in humans and animals, serial studies have documented the development. After initial saphenous ligation with retention of the main trunk, there is an organizing thrombus in which numerous small vessels grow. Over a period of months these coalesce, thus forming a single or a few major trunks. These develop muscle and elastin in the walls, resembling mature veins. It may become clinically significant within 6 months of surgery[18,20-23] (Fig. 36–6).

What is the relative incidence of these different forms of morphologic recurrence, and thus how important are they? Table 36–2 shows the results of a recent study by

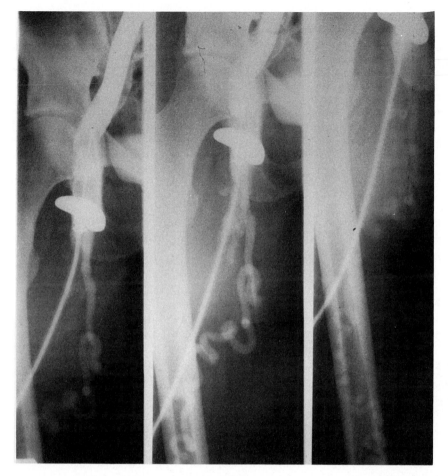

Figure 36–1. Descending venogram showing a single nontortuous trunk communicating with a distal varicosity. It is thought to represent an untied tributary.

the author,[15] evaluated during an 18-month period from a consecutive series of new patients referred for treatment of varicose veins. Of 444 patients seen during this period, 349 (79%) had no previous surgery. Ninety-five patients were documented by clinical history and by the presence of surgical scars to have had previous surgery directed toward one or another saphenous system. All patients had recurrences of sufficient severity to be seeking further treatment. The mean period since previous surgery was 20 years, and in seven limbs the recurrence had already been reoperated on twice before (re-recurrent).

It is seen from Table 36–2 that there were 29 with type 1 recurrence from thigh perforators and 10 patients in type 2, of which nine had emergence in the sapheno-popliteal junction. The largest single group was those with recurrent saphenofemoral incompetence. Table 36–3 defines the nature of this recurrence in 47 limbs that were fully evaluated. Only in a relative few was there an untied tributary (type 3A). Most recurrences appear to be due to reconstitution of this junction (type 3C).

For completeness, it is worthwhile mentioning that there were two further patients who had complex recurrence through pelvic veins, which is a rare form of the problem and indeed difficult to treat.

Other important and interesting aspects among these patients were the extent to

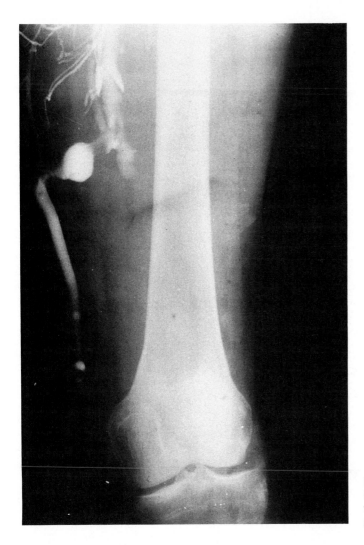

Figure 36–2. Reflux through an incompetent superficial femoral vein and thigh perforator into a persistent long saphenous trunk.

which a residual long saphenous trunk played a role in the pathogenesis. One of the advantages of venography is that it clearly demonstrates this feature. Twenty-three of the 29 patients with recurrence through a thigh perforator (type 1) had a persistent long saphenous trunk. This aspect is not relevant in type 2. Of the type 3 patients, there was an identifiable residual long saphenous trunk in 26 of the 47 limbs evaluated (55%). A further feature of type 3 patients was that 64% of them had primary deep incompetence, demonstrated on descending venography.

Minimizing the Recurrence Rate

These data demonstrate the importance of systematic and routine evaluation of saphenofemoral and saphenopopliteal junctions at the time of preliminary examination. Type 2 recurrence may indeed be a legitimate and unavoidable emergence of a new problem subsequent to the original surgery. However, it is not unreasonable to speculate as to whether this lesion may have been missed at this time. These therefore would not strictly constitute recurrences; they are persistences.

The second major issue is what role the retained long saphenous trunk might play in the evolution of recurrence. Two prospective randomized trials have shown a

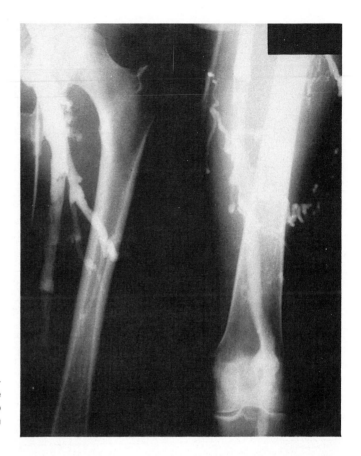

Figure 36–3. Descending venogram. Complex recurrence through an incompetent deep femoral vein communicating with a distal superficial varicosity.

statistically significant increase in recurrence rate in those treated by saphenofemoral ligation alone compared with ligation and synchronous stripping.[11,24] From the morphologic data presented above, it is not difficult to see why this might be so. We know that if the saphenous is simply ligated, the trunk remains patent. Indeed protagonists of this policy cite this because a viable potential conduit remains for future bypass surgery.[25] Furthermore, in most the trunk valves are incompetent and connected to a deep system by incompetent perforators, thus reflux is not controlled.[26,27] This surely constitutes an anatomic recipe for recurrence of type 1, those with incompetent thigh perforators, and type 3A, those with an incompetent femoral and perforator.

Finally, we come to the difficult problem of the reconstituted saphenofemoral junction. It seems likely a retained saphenous trunk if nothing else will potentiate this phenomenon. However, it must be conceded that this cannot reflect the problem in its entirety because type 3C recurrence occurred in some patients in the absence of a retained trunk.

On a more general note, it has been suggested that saphenous junction reconstitution (type 3C) can be minimized by applying a Dacron patch to the denuded femoral vein at the time of initial surgery.[28] Whether this is effective is difficult to say. No controlled study has been published. The whole question of recurrence is deserving of fuller study and research. There is clearly a major factor that is inherent within the patient's constitution over which there is potentially limited influence from a surgical standpoint. The re-recurrent rate in a proportion of patients bears testimony to this concept.

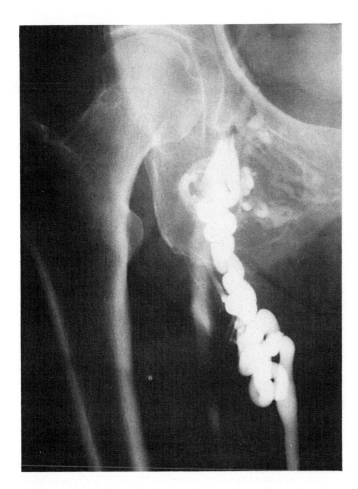

Figure 36–4. Descending venogram showing typical appearance of reconstituted saphenofemoral junction with multiple tortuous channels communicating with a persistent long saphenous trunk.

Recurrent Short Saphenous Incompetence

This area does pose special problems that are worthy of separate consideration. The application of morphologic types as used above for the great saphenous system are not as widely appropriate. Type 1 does not have a comparable pattern. This is essentially because the deep calf veins have a different anatomic system. Instead of a single major trunk, the superficial femoral vein in the thigh, there are multiple small veins. Although recurrence can be derived from these through incompetent calf and ankle perforator veins, this is not a function of the short saphenous system *per se*. Furthermore, the short saphenous trunk is usually deep to the calf fascia for most of its length. As such, therefore, it is rather more a vein of the deep system and thus less vulnerable to be the source of recurrence.

Type 2 recurrences have already been considered, and no more on this subject needs to be said.

The question of type 3 recurrence is important. The criteria for diagnosis are, of course, different. Reflux of the saphenopopliteal junction is characterized by hand-held Doppler signals on calf squeeze and then on release.[7]

This was seen in 10 patients (see Table 36–2), so it is not inconsiderable. Identification of the precise morphology poses special problems. The first of these is that it is not as easy to image venographically. A descending phase, so valuable for the saphenofemoral junction, cannot be obtained unless the femoral and popliteal systems happen to be incompetent as well (Fig. 36–5). The appearance and nature of

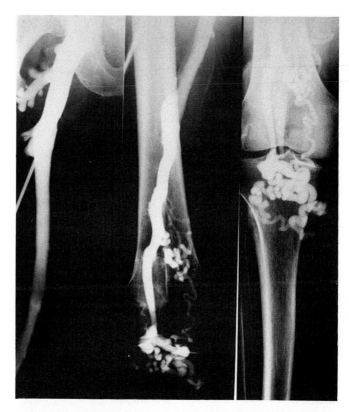

Figure 36–5. Descending venogram showing strikingly similar appearance to Figure 36–4, in a reconstituted saphenopopliteal junction. This is demonstrable because the saphenofemoral segment is fortuitously co-existently incompetent.

recurrence is thus more difficult to investigate. However, duplex scanning can be invaluable at this site. However, there seems no doubt that reconstitution caused by neovascularization can occur as at the saphenofemoral junction (type 3C). Figure 36–5 depicts that most clearly. But it is not always possible to obtain adequate imaging to be sure of this point for the reasons mentioned above. Furthermore, it is not necessarily possible to say from duplex studies or indeed operative findings either. The author's view is that type 3A is more common because of the variation of anatomy and potential sites of origin of varicosities that exist behind the knee. In more than 60% of patients, the popliteal vein is double.[29] The saphenopopliteal junction itself is in the popliteal fossa in only 80% of limbs. A number of veins other than the short saphenous itself may be the site of incompetence and the source of varicosities: the gastrocnemius veins—more usually the medial, the popliteal area vein, and other muscular veins.[30]

SAPHENOUS AND ANKLE PERFORATOR LIGATION FOR VENOUS ULCER

Venous ulcer is a clinical entity for which the indications for and benefits of surgery are more clearly defined and recognized. It represents only 20% of patients seeking treatment for superficial vein problems (see Table 36–1), and surgery will not be appropriate in all these (see below). Nonetheless because the global problem is so prevalent, the potential pool of patients for whom rewarding benefit can be achieved is considerable. It has to be conceded that the technical aspects of surgery of this nature are relatively prosaic and undemanding, particularly when compared with

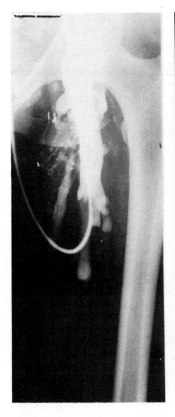 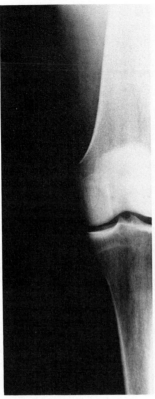

Figure 36–6. Descending venogram taken only 6 months after saphenous ligation without stripping at another institution. Already patient has developed recurrent incompetence on Doppler, and a myriad of venous channels have developed between femoral vein and persistent venous trunk.

TABLE 36–2. TYPE OF RECURRENCE

Type 1	Thigh perforator	29
Type 2	Emergence of saphenopopliteal incompetence	9
	Emergence of saphenofemoral incompetence	1
Type 3	Recurrent saphenofemoral incompetence	46
	Recurrent Saphenopopliteal incompetence	10
Total		95

reconstructive arterial surgery. This may be one reason why this area has received little attention in terms of research and published scientific literature. What little there is, is out of proportion to the considerable and durable benefits that can be offered to patients by simple procedures relatively devoid of operative morbidity and mortality. However, correct case selection is of crucial importance.

TABLE 36–3. NATURE OF RECURRENT SAPHENOFEMORAL INCOMPETENCE

3A	Untied tributary	4
3B	Incompetent **saphenofemoral** vein and thigh perforator	9
3C	Reconstituted junction	28
3B & 3C	Combined	4
Total limbs evaluated[a]		47

[a] In addition to those described here there were two limbs in whom the recurrent was found to be from incompetent pelvic veins.

Patient Selection

Taken that a confident diagnosis of venous ulceration has been made and that other causes have been excluded, it is in turn absurd to regard all such lesions as the consequence of a single underlying morphologic process. It may well be that ultimately venous hypertension targets ankle skin nutrition by a single pathway, be it leucocyte trapping[31] or fibrous deposition.[32] But the reasons for venous hypertension, although complex, vary. And thus, in turn, it is necessary when planning, and in due course evaluating the 5- to 10-year results of treatment, to do it in the context of this underlying pathology. Recognition of this concept has been growing over recent years.[18,33]

When evaluating a patient with venous ulcer, the first priority therefore is to identify those entities that may contribute to venous hypertension.

There may be primary incompetence of the great or short saphenous vein. For this, the simple unidirectional hand-held Doppler is invaluable.[4–7] There may be incompetence of the ankle perforating veins. Here the gold standard probably remains tourniquet-assisted ascending venography.[18] However, this gives no quantifiable information, and it is unlikely that more sophisticated duplex studies will replace radiology. Ankle perforators remain something of an enigma and, in the author's view, are overstated in importance. One problem is that a degree of "incompetence" can be demonstrated by a skilled venographist in most patients with venous ulcer. It is quite another matter to extrapolate this observation into citing these as the universal cause.[18] This will be discussed further below.

Next comes the question of primary deep incompetence. The credit for introducing this into contemporary thinking must go to Kistner,[34–36] which has stimulated the development of a variety of innovative procedures to restore valve function.[34–38] This form of reflux may be detected in the femoral system by descending venography[18,33–36] and, more recently, by duplex.[39] Quantified tests of venous function such as plethysmography are also used.[40] Popliteal incompetence can be detected from hand-held Doppler, although it may be difficult to distinguish from saphenopopliteal reflux, especially if they co-exist.[18] If there is doubt, duplex scanning is invaluable.

Finally comes the important question of postphlebitic damage, which leaves a combination of outflow obstruction and reflux caused by valvular destruction. Although it may be difficult to exclude the possibility with absolute confidence, the best method remains careful and comprehensive venograph.[18] To rely on a past history alone is certainly inadequate.[18]

Thus having completed this comprehensive evaluation, a number of abnormalities may be detected. In any one patient there may be a variety. However, it is possible to classify patients into one of four principal types. The author's experience in pursuing this policy is summarized in Table 36–4.

Type 1 is those in whom the only abnormality is ankle perforator incompetence. These patients are rare and represent less than 4% of the total.

Type 2 is the single biggest group (40%). In these patients, the principal abnormality is one of saphenous incompetence. In most of these patients, a degree of ankle perforator incompetence is also demonstrable.

Type 3 patients are in many ways the single most challenging and interesting. Their main feature is primary deep incompetence, but many have saphenous and perforator reflux as well. Clearly the proportion of patients in this group compared with those in type 2 depends on by what criteria you judge deep incompetence to be of clinical significance. Much work still needs to be performed on this important area. One problem is the difficulties experienced in trying to quantify this form of reflux

TABLE 36–4. DISTRIBUTION OF TYPES OF VENOUS MORPHOLOGY: CONSECUTIVE SERIES OF PATIENTS WITH 232 LIMBS WITH VENOUS ULCERATION

		No. Limbs	No. Female	%
Type 1	Calf perforator incompetence alone	9	6	3.9
Type 2	Calf perforator incompetence alone (saphenous incompetence)	91	54	39.2
Type 3	Primary deep venous incompetence (often with associated saphenous and perforator incompetence)	81	24	34.9
Type 4	Postphlebitic damage	51	24	22.0

and its hemodynamic consequences. In this series of patients, Kistner grade 2 reflux[34–36] (to knee level) was taken as significant, but this was arbitrary and may or may not be legitimate. Type 4 patients (22%) are those with a truly "postphlebitic" limb. There is a combination of valve and luminal destruction with incomplete recovery.

Outcome of Treatment

Type 1 patients are such a small group that the author is unable to present data on the outcome of treatment. However, protagonists of ankle perforator ligation would feel confident that subfascial ligation would be expected to give a durable result.[43]

Type 2 patients are the simplest and easiest to treat. The author has recently published the outcome of simple saphenous ligation and stripping to knee level in these patients.[41,42] A specific policy at the outset of this series was to reserve subfascial ligation should these simple measures fail. It proved to be unnecessary. The outcome after up to 8 years postoperatively was complete healing achieved in 49 of 54 limbs followed up for a mean period of 3 to 4 years. Most of these patients have worn no support stockings. Those that did, did so on their own discretion. In the five limbs with persistent ulceration, other factors found on further review were thought likely to account independently for this persistence. One had developed leukemia, one had diabetes, two had short saphenous incompetence, possibly previously missed, and the last patient had popliteal incompetence. These results suggest that in this group of patients, an excellent and durable outcome can be achieved in most if not all. Avoidance of subfascial ligation is of obvious benefit because this carries extra morbidity, particularly with wound healing.[43] The distribution of great and short saphenous incompetence in this and in other groups is shown in Table 36–5, and once more emphasizes the need to evaluate the saphenopopliteal junction with care, not only in primary varicose veins but also in those with ulceration.

TABLE 36–5. INCIDENCE OF SAPHENOUS INCOMPETENCE

		Type of Incompetence		
Morphology	Total No. of Limbs	Long Saphenous Vein Alone	Short Saphenous Vein Alone	Long Saphenous Vein + Short Saphenous Vein
1	9	—	—	—
2	91	82	2	7
3	81	49	7	9
4	51	16	1	2

Type 3 patients represent a more formidable challenge, and the results of surgery are certainly less predictable. Of the 81 limbs in this category, 25 had already undergone a saphenous ligation and thus represented a failure of this modality of treatment. Of this group of patients with previous surgery, recurrent saphenofemoral incompetence was found in 18 of the 25. Religation of the groin incompetence failed to achieve ulcer healing in five of seven limbs (see Table 36–5). It would appear therefore that once recurrent saphenous incompetence has occurred in the presence of ulceration, further measures are likely to be needed to achieve healing. There were, however, 65 limbs in this group (see Table 36–4) in which no previous surgery had been directed toward an incompetent saphenous system. Of these, durable healing has been achieved in 27 of 35, followed up for a mean period of 4.6 years and up to 8 years.

Of those that failed after previous or current ligation, 19 have been treated by subfascial ligation. Ten have remained healed for a mean period of 4 to 5 years. These results are summarized in Table 36–6.

Conclusions

What inference can be drawn from these results? It is apparent that with the co-existence of deep incompetence, the durability of simple ligation of an incompetent saphenous system is in doubt. Only about half have achieved maintained healing. This is in contrast to those in type 2. The addition of subfascial ligation of incompetent ankle perforators in patients with failed saphenous ligation seems to benefit a further proportion with a sustained result. But about one-quarter of the patients fail to achieve a durable result with these two procedures. It must be concluded that deep incompetence remains a critical factor. In these, deep valve repair might justifiably be considered, in some perhaps prospectively.

OVERALL CONCLUSIONS

Superficial Vein Problems and Venous Ulceration

What is the explanation for these observations in pathophysiologic terms? It would appear from these data that ankle perforator saphenous or deep incompetence may, independently, be of sufficient severity and duration to bring about ulceration. When they co-exist, which is more commonly the case, they probably have a synergistic effect. To correct one may be sufficient to achieve healing. But these are inherent and progressive problems, so the duration of benefit will depend on the severity and rate of progression in those areas of incompetence that remain. So a sequence can emerge in the severe patient: an initially successful saphenous ligation, which then fails; healing from subsequent perforator ligation in a proportion; and deep valve repair. What needs to be answered is whether it is preferable to correct all these sequentially

TABLE 36–6. OUTCOME OF SURGERY TYPE 3 PATIENTS

	No. of Limbs	Healed	Follow-up (yr)
Ligation saphenofemoral incompetence	35	27	4.6
Subfascial ligation for failed saphenoligation	19	10	4.5
Religation recurrent saphenofemoral incompetence	7	2	2.1

as and when clinical need arises, or whether they should be addressed synchronously and prospectively at the time of preliminary evaluation.

Type 4

It is perhaps fortunate that postphlebitic damage causing a combination of outflow obstruction and valve destruction accounts for less than one-quarter of patients (see Table 36–4). The potential for effective surgery is limited, as are the therapeutic options.

Although there may be incompetence of a saphenous system, surgery directed toward this finding is seldom beneficial and may be actively contraindicated. Either this finding is just one part of widespread and irremedial problems or the dilated saphenous is acting as an important superficial collateral to overcome the consequences of deep obstruction. Much information about the hemodynamics of the saphenous contribution to reflux and outflow can be obtained from a variety of plethysmographic techniques used with or without a superficial occlusive tourniquet. This simulates the effects of surgery. Details of these investigative procedures are outside the remit of this chapter.

But does subfascial ligation of incompetent ankle perforators play any role in the management of these difficult cases? For this we do have a conclusive answer. Burnand and colleagues[44] studied 41 patients with venous ulcer by ascending venography. Twenty-three patients were found to have evidence of deep vein damage on the initial venogram (i.e., type 4). Recurrent ulceration occurred within 5 years in every one of them after operative ligation of incompetent calf perforating veins. Of the remaining 17 patients with normal deep veins (i.e., types 1 to 3), all but one remained healed after a combination of saphenous and subfascial ligation. This finding is in line with the data described above.

So what can be done for these patients? Compression stockings and more recently drug therapy with oxypentifyline have been reported to give encouraging results, although the value in type 4 patients specifically was not addressed.[45] Reconstructive surgery in the author's experience has little to offer in most patients,[46] although some have reported encouraging results with brachial valve transplant.[47]

REFERENCES

1. Coon WW, Willis PW III, Keller JB. Venous thrombo-embolism and the venous disease in the Tecumseh Community Health Study. *Circulation.* 1973;48:839.
2. Widmer LK, Mall T, Martin H. Epidemiology and sociomedical importance of peripheral venous disease. In: Hobbs JT, ed. *The Treatment of Venous Disorders.* Lancaster, England: MPT Press; 1977:3–12.
3. Reagan B, Folse R. Lower limb haemodynamics in normal persons and children of patients with varicose veins. *Surg Gynecol Obstet.* 1971;152:15–22.
4. Chan A, Chisholm I, Royle JP. The use of directional Doppler ultrasound in the assessment of saphenofemoral incompetence. *Aust NZ J Surg.* 1984;53:399–402.
5. Hoare MC, Royle JP. Doppler ultrasound detection of sapheno-femoral and sapheno-popliteal incompetence and operative venography to ensure precise sapheno-femoral ligation. *Aust NZ J Surg.* 1984;54:49–52.
6. McIrvine AJ, Corbett CRR, Aston ND, et al. The demonstration of sapheno-femoral incompetence; Doppler ultrasound compared with standard clinical tests. *Br J Surg.* 1984;71:506–508.
7. Mitchell DC, Darke SG. The assessment of primary varicose veins by Doppler ultrasound—the role of sapheno popliteal incompetence and the short saphenous system in calf varicosities. *Eur J Vasc Surg.* 1987;1:113–116.

8. Hobbs JT. Surgery and sclerotherapy in the treatment of varicose veins. *Arch Surg.* 1974;104:793–796.

9. Doren FSA, White M. A clinical trial to discover if primary treatment of varicose veins should be by Fagan's method or by an operation. *Br J Surg.* 1975;62:72–76.

10. Sheppard M. A procedure for the prevention of recurrent sapheno femoral incompetence. *Aust NZ J Surg.* 1978;48:322–326.

11. Jakobsen BH. The value of different forms of treatment for varicose veins. *Br J Surg.* 1979;66:182–184.

12. Lofgren EP. Treatment of long saphenous varicosities and their recurrence: a long term follow up. In: Bergan JJ, Yao YST, eds. *Surgery of the Veins.* Orlando, FL: Grune & Stratton; 1985:285–299.

13. Royle JP. Recurrent varicose veins. *World J Surg.* 1986;10:944–953.

14. Berridge DC, Makin GS. Day case surgery; a viable alternative for surgical treatment of varicose veins. *Phlebology.* 1987;2:103–108.

15. Darke SG. The morphology of recurrent varicose veins. *Eur J Vasc Surg.* 1993;6:512–517.

16. Corbett CR, McIrivine AJ, Astor NO, et al. The use of varicography to identify the sources of incompetence in recurrent varicose veins. *Ann R Coll Surg.* 1982;66:412–415.

17. Starnes HF, Vallance R, Hamilton DNH. Recurrent varicose veins: a radiological approach to investigation. *Clin Radiol.* 1984;35:95–99.

18. Darke SG, Andress MR. The value of venography in the management of chronic venous disorders of the lower limb. In: Greenhalgh RM, ed. *Diagnostic Techniques and Assessment Procedures in Vascular Surgery.* Orlando, Fl: Grune & Stratton; 1985:421–446.

19. Darke SG. Recurrent varicose veins and short saphenous insufficiency. In: Bergan JJ, Yao JST, eds. *Venous Disorders.* Philadelphia: WB Saunders; 1991:217–232.

20. Darke SG. Chronic venous insufficiency—should the long saphenous vein be stripped? In: Barros D'SA AAB, Bell PRF, Darke SG, Harris PL, eds. *Vascular Surgery Current Questions.* Oxford: Butterworth-Heinemann; 1991:207–218.

21. Glass GM. Neovascularisation in recurrence varices of the great saphenous vein in the groin, phlebography. *Angiology.* 1988;39:577–582.

22. Glass GM. Neovascularisation in recurrence of the varicose great saphenous vein following transection. *Phlebology.* 1987;2:81–91.

23. Glass GM. Neovascularisation in restoration of continuity of the not femoral vein following surgical interruption. *Phlebology.* 1987;2:1–6.

24. Munn SR, Morton JB, MacBeth WAAG, et al. To strip or not to strip the long saphenous vein? A varicose vein trial. *Br J Surg.* 1981;68:426–428.

25. Hammersten J, Pedersen P, Claes-Goran C, et al. Long saphenous vein saving surgery for varicose veins. A long term follow up. *Eur J Vasc Surg.* 1990;4:361–364.

26. Sutton R, Darke SG. Stripping the long saphenous vein: preoperative retrograde saphenography in patients with and without ulceration. *Br J Surg.* 1986;73:305–307.

27. McMullin GM, Coleridge Smith PD, Scurr JH. Objective assessment of high ligation without stripping the long saphenous vein. *Br J Surg.* 1991;78:1139–1142.

28. Glass GM. Prevention of recurrent sapheno femoral incompetence after surgery for varicose veins. *Br J Surg.* 1989;76:1210.

29. Williams AF. The formation of the popliteal vein. *Surg Gnyecol Obstet.* 1953;97:769–772.

30. Dodd H. The varicose tributaries of the popliteal vein. *Br J Surg.* 1965;52:350–354.

31. Coleridge-Smith PD, Thomas PRS, Scurr JH, et al. Cause of venous ulceration: a new hypothesis. *Br Med J.* 1988;296:1726–1727.

32. Burnand KG, Whimster I, Naidoo A, et al. Pericapillary fibrin in the ulcer bearing skin of the leg: the cause of lipodermatosclerosis and venous ulceration. *Br Med J.* 1982;285:1071–1072.

33. McEnroe CS, O'Donnell TF, Mackey WC. Correlation of clinical findings with venous haemodynamics in 386 patients with chronic venous insufficiency. *Am J Surg.* 1988;156:148–152.

34. Kistner RL. Surgical repair of the incompetent femoral vein valve. *Arch Surg.* 1975;110:1336–1342.

35. Kistner RL. Primary venous valve incompetence of the leg. *Am J Surg.* 1980;140:218–224.
36. Kistner RL, Ferris EB. Technique of surgical reconstruction of femoral vein valves. In: Bergan JT, Yao JST, eds. *Operative Techniques in Vascular Surgery.* Orlando, FL: Grune & Stratton; 1980:291–300.
37. Jones JW, Elliott F, Kerstein MD. Triangular venous valvuloplasty. A new procedure for correction of venous incompetence. *Arch Surg.* 1982;117:1250–1251.
38. Raju S, Fredericks R. Valve reconstruction procedures for non obstructive venous insufficiency. *J Vasc Surg.* 1988;7:301–310.
39. Vasdekis B. Quantification of venous reflux by means of duplex scanning. *J Vasc Surg.* 1989;10:670–677.
40. Nicolaides AN, Miles CM. Photoplethysmography in the assessment of venous insufficiency. *J Vasc Surg.* 1987;5:405–412.
41. Sethia KK, Darke SG. Long saphenous incompetence as a cause of venous ulceration. *Br J Surg.* 1984;71:754–755.
42. Darke SG, Penfold C. Venous ulceration and saphenous ligation. *Eur J Vasc Surg.* 1992;6:4–9.
43. Negus D, Friedgood A. The effective management of venous ulceration. *Br J Surg.* 1983;70:623–627.
44. Burnand KG, O'Donnell TF, Lea Thomas M, et al. Relation between post phlebitic changes in the deep veins and results of surgical treatment of venous ulcers. *Lancet.* 1976;1:936–938.
45. Colgan MP, Dormandy JA, Jones PW, et al. Oxypentifylline treatment of venous ulcers of the leg. *Br Med J.* 1990;300:972–974.
46. Darke SG. Venous reconstruction. In: Bell PRF, Jamieson CW, Ruckley CV, eds. *Surgical Management of Vascular Disease.* London: WB Saunders; 1992:1221–1238.
47. O'Donnell TF, Mackey WC, Shepard AD, et al. Clinical phlebographic and haemodynamic assessment of popliteal vein valve transplant. *Proceedings of 2nd International Vascular Symposium.* London. September 1986. Abstract S22.6.

37

Fate of the Greenfield Filter:

Ten-Year Follow-Up

Lazar J. Greenfield, MD, and Mary C. Proctor, MS

The importance of establishing well-defined criteria to evaluate the Greenfield stainless steel vena caval filter and the need to document the course of thromboembolic disease were recognized early in the development of the Greenfield filter. Long before the current evaluation programs were mandated by federal regulation, long-term patient follow-up was considered essential to comprehensive care. The results from these evaluations provide a wealth of information available for this device and its relationship to the underlying disorder.

The efficacy and safety of the Greenfield filter was initially studied in an animal model. Cavagrams, lung scans, and careful autopsy studies revealed that all experimental thrombi were successfully trapped, caval patency was maintained, there was no proximal extension of the thrombus, there was no evidence of retroperitoneal bleeding, and at 16 weeks, there was evidence of resolution of the thrombi.[1] The animal studies also demonstrated that the filter was safely implanted and that the curved hooks assured fixation without penetration of the inferior vena cava. In addition, the relationship between the volume of thrombus trapped and the cross-sectional area of the filter available for flow was demonstrated to allow 70% to 80% filling without a pressure gradient.[2] (Fig. 37–1). This finding was significant in light of the high rate of caval occlusion reported with earlier devices.[3]

Publications introducing the Greenfield vena cava filter identified the performance standards, which included effective filtration of emboli, continued patency after capture of an embolus, lack of thrombogenicity, and a low risk for the insertion procedure.[1,2] (Fig. 37–2).

Comprehensive patient data files have been maintained in a computerized relational database containing records of more than 800 patients since 1972. This database allows longitudinal assessment of patient outcomes obtained from prospective routine evaluation.

VENA CAVA FILTER FOLLOW-UP

During animal examinations, the stability and patency of the filter are assessed, the status of the underlying venous disease is determined, and patients are provided with

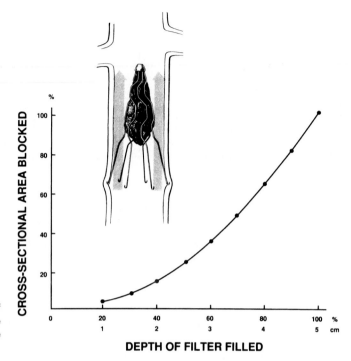

Figure 37–1. Conical shape of Greenfield filter allows it to be filled to 80% of its length before flow and pressure are affected.

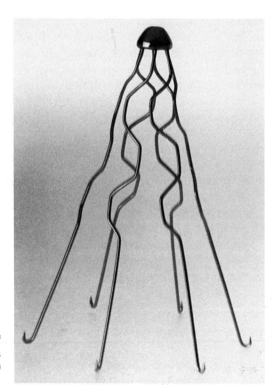

Figure 37–2. Original Greenfield filter is made of stainless steel and held in position within the vena cava by curved hooks that provide secure fixation without caval penetration.

an opportunity for ongoing education concerning their disease and the role of the filter in their care.

Secondary objectives of the assessment include evaluation of the safety and efficacy of this permanent device and increased knowledge of the natural history of venous thromboembolic disease. Finally, it enables characterization of the population of patients who have received vena caval filters and allows estimation of survival.

Stability of the filter within the vena cava is measured in terms of proximal or distal movement as well as change in filter base diameter. Plain abdominal radiographs taken in the anteroposterior projection are compared with prior studies. If the position of the filter is difficult to interpret, lateral and angled views can be used to determine limb position. After correcting for radiographic magnification, the relative position of the filter can be determined and gross changes can be identified. From these same films, any change in filter base diameter can be detected. Significant change in base diameter may be indicative of caval penetration and requires clinical correlation. If clinical findings suggest penetration, an abdominal computed tomography may be obtained to confirm the suspicion.[4] Reports such as published by Redhead et al[5] are indicative of information obtained from these studies.

Clinical information is obtained regarding hospitalization since the last follow-up as well as any patient complaints that suggest possible recurrent pulmonary embolism (PE). Patients who present with clinical symptoms of recurrent PE should always undergo pulmonary angiography or ventilation/perfusion scanning. If embolism has occurred, vena cavography is indicated to determine whether there is thrombus in the filter. If it is found to contain thrombus with proximal extension, an additional filter may be placed proximal to the first to ensure continued protection. If thrombus is present without proximal extension, thrombolytic therapy may also be used.

Maintenance of long-term patency of the vena cava is an important characteristic of the Greenfield filter. If caval occlusion occurs, there is significant risk of proximal propagation with possible PE as well as lower extremity venous hypertension. Initially, caval patency was determined by contrast or isotope vena cavography. Currently, duplex scanning is routinely used because it is a sensitive, specific, noninvasive method of evaluation. The examination may be precluded by body habitus in the obese patient, but limitations related to large amounts of bowel gas may be minimized through the use of an antiflatulent before the study. In addition to determining patency, some authors have suggested that duplex scanning may be useful for determining device migration or structural deformities, but plain radiographs appear to be more reliable for these parameters.[4,6]

The natural history of the patient's underlying venous disease is monitored by venous duplex studies of the lower extremities. Patients are also questioned regarding the presence of edema, ulceration, or other signs of venous insufficiency. Special attention is given to the filter insertion site to determine patency. Information is obtained regarding the use of oral anticoagulants or elastic compression stockings. Changes occurring over time are documented.

In addition to the standard modes of evaluation, more advanced technologies may be used when there is a need for more detailed information. Liebman et al[7] studied the safety and efficacy of magnetic resonance imaging in evaluating vena caval filters and in the diagnostic imaging of patients who coincidentally have filters. They concluded that magnetic resonance imaging can be safely and effectively performed in most patients with vena caval filters.[7] Teitelbaum et al[8] explored the use of gradient-echo imaging in addition to spin-echo imaging and found that it was well suited for determining filter position and caval patency, as well as the patency of side branch vessels. Gradient-echo imaging also demonstrated the presence and extent of intraluminal thrombus, as well as the compressive effects on the vena cava caused by tumor masses and hepatomegaly.[8]

The use of intravascular ultrasound has recently been reported by Marx et al,[9] who used an animal model to compare the use of IVUS with cavography and concluded that the roles were complementary. McCowan et al[10] used intravascular ultrasound in evaluation of 24 patients with vena caval filters and found it superior to cavography in detecting inferior vena cava thrombus in six cases and superior to external duplex in all cases available for comparison.

RESULTS OF LONG-TERM PATIENT FOLLOW-UP

At various times, summary findings from the Filter Registry have been reported. Some reports were comprehensive in nature, but others were focused on a specific patient population or aspect of the evaluation.

1977

The study published in 1977 reported results for the initial 76 patients treated during a 4-year period with follow-up to 53 months. The methods of evaluation included physical examination with careful attention to the condition of the lower extremities, vena cavography, and if clinically warranted, peripheral venography, pulmonary angiography, or V/Q scanning. Detailed postmorten examinations were performed when permitted. The rate of recurrent PE was 2% to 3%, with an operative mortality rate of 4%. In addition to establishing the efficacy and safety of the device, the benefit of preserving flow around a trapped embolus was demonstrated including the lysis of trapped emboli on successive cavography.[11]

1981

The 1981 review extended the experience to 156 patients with up to 63 months of evaluation. The results indicated a recurrent PE rate of 2%, no migration or deaths from recurrent PE, and a long-term patency rate of 95%. Recurrent thrombophlebitis was noted in 4% of the patients. Trapped emboli were observed in 25% of the patients, with lysis occurring in 8% at a subsequent evaluation. The most important development from this report was the recommendation for suprarenal position as an alternative location in clinically warranted cases. The excellent long-term outcomes for patients who had suprarenal filters provided the basis for this recommendation.[12]

1984

By 1984, 260 patients had been entered into the Filter Registry and the follow-up experience was extended to 100 months. The purpose of the study was to explore current indications for filter insertion. This was prompted by the increased number of requests for prophylactic filter placement. Despite 8 years of experience indicating no decrease in vena caval patency or damage to the cava or adjacent structures, the indication for prophylactic filter placement remained limited to patients with life-threatening deep vein thrombosis or those high-risk patients with a proved deep vein thrombosis who could not tolerate even a small recurrent embolism. The rate of recurrent PE was 5%, with a long-term filter patency rate of 98%. There was one death possibly related to recurrent PE. The data also suggested that long-term anticoagulation might not be necessary to maintain filter patency.[13]

1988

The most recent analysis of the Registry data was published in 1988 and contained the experience of 469 patients with follow-up to 138 months. The methods of follow-up were extended to include plain radiographs of the abdomen, duplex evaluation of the inferior vena cava, which replaced the isotope or contrast venacaograms, and noninvasive measurements of venous insufficiency. Pulmonary angiography was the preferred diagnostic method of detecting clinically suspected PE. The standard location for filter placement remained the third lumbar vertebra except when clinical conditions warranted more proximal placement. Results of this review indicated a recurrent PE rate of 4% diagnosed by angiography, V/Q scan, or change in clinical condition. The short-term vena caval patency rate was 93%, but subsequent studies indicated recanalization in a number of cases, resulting in a long-term patency rate of 96%.[14]

Four important findings were reported. The problem of filter misplacement was significantly reduced from 7% to 4% by the standard use of a guide wire during the insertion procedure. The lack of clinical sequelae in patients with misplaced filters who had been followed over several years led to a reduction in the number of attempted removals. It was recommended that unless the filter was in the tricuspid valve or was causing a disturbance of cardiac rhythm, it did not warrant removal.[14]

The question of correlation between filter tilt and recurrent pulmonary embolism was addressed by studying the radiographs of patients who experienced recurrent PE. All these filters were well positioned within the vena cava, and patients with angled filters remained symptom-free. Recurrent pulmonary embolism did not appear to be a function of filter angulation. Finally, the experience in 32 patients who had filters positioned above the renal vein revealed no caval occlusion, no renal impairment, and no difference in the incidence of recurrent PE. Inserting the filter in the suprarenal position in young women of childbearing age as well as in those patients with thrombus extending into the vena cava to the level of the renal veins became accepted practice based on the available follow-up information.

In these reports, certain issues had priority: indications for filter placement, efficacy of the device and long-term sequelae, ease and safety of insertion, and the natural history of the venous disease. Analysis of data from the Filter Registry has provided information on all these issues, in addition to documenting the effects of technologic changes. Tables 37–1 to 37–4 compare and contrast patterns over the four major analyses.

Patient demographics remained constant throughout the period, with a mean age of 53 to 57 years and a male/female ratio of approximately 3:2. The mean length of follow-up increased from 23 to 43 months from 1977 to 1988. The percentage of the total registry added at each time point changed significantly, reflecting the increased

TABLE 37–1. DEMOGRAPHIC INFORMATION FOR PATIENTS WITH GREENFIELD VENA CAVAL FILTERS

Demographics	Year of Publication			
	1977	1981	1984	1988
Number of patients	76	156	260	469
Female	28	57	105	185
Male	48	99	155	284
Age (yr)	54	53	57	56
Mean follow-up (mo)	—	23	34	43
Length of follow-up (mo)	53	63	100	138

TABLE 37–2. SUMMARY OF PLACEMENT AND OUTCOME EVENTS

	Year of Publication			
	1977	*1981*	*1984*	*1988*
Recurrent pulmonary embolism	2[a]	2	5	4
Patency	97	95	98	96
Jugular insertion	61	72	80	83
Femoral insertion	39	36	19	16
Location	Below renal vein	L-3	L-3 or suprarenal	L-3 or suprarenal
Alterations	Jugular inserter	Heparin infus. port	Guide wire	
Misplacement	7	7	3	4

[a] All values presented as % of those available for evaluation.

level of confidence in the efficacy and safety of the Greenfield filter. Approximately 20% of the patients were added at each of the first three reports, but more than 50% enrolled between the third and fourth (Table 37–1).

The rate of recurrent pulmonary embolism (2% to 5%) and vena caval patency (95% to 98%) is consistent over time, indicating that the impressive, early findings were not artifactual but were highly reproducible. The misplacement rate of 7% in the earliest reports decreased with time as operator experience increased and the use of a guide wire became standard procedure. The one parameter that demonstrated the most variation was the choice of insertion site. The earliest filters could only be placed through the femoral vein because of carrier design. When a jugular device became available, the use of this route increased by 22%, indicating the preference of surgeons for this approach. Since 1988 femoral placement has become more dominant, as it is preferred by radiologists who place a large number of filters percutaneously. Our Registry experience currently indicates that insertions from the femoral vein account for 32% of all placements (Table 37–2).

TABLE 37–3. COEXISTING DIAGNOSES IN PATIENTS WITH GREENFIELD VENA CAVAL FILTERS

	Year of Publication			
Disease	*1977*	*1981*	*1984*	*1988*
Venous disease	32[a]	52	NR	58
Acute	—	33		73
Chronic	—	19		15
Postoperative or postpartum	14	31		37
Trauma	13	6		9
Malignancy	14	19		17
Cardiac disease	12	23		24
Obesity	11	17		17
Arterial disease	9	8		9
Gastrointestinal disease	9	17		16
Psychological/alcoholism	5	16		5
Central nervous system disease	5	14		19
Pulmonary hypertension	4	13		13
Hypercoagulable state	3	3		4
Pulmonary disease	NR	7		9
Other	NR	19	NR	33

[a] All values presented as % of those available for evaluation.

TABLE 37–4. INDICATIONS FOR PLACEMENT OF GREENFIELD VENA CAVAL FILTERS

Indication	Year of Publication			
	1977	*1981*	*1984*	*1988*
Contraindication to anticoagulation	23[a]	30	35	38
Complication of anticoagulation	16	16	18	17
Prophylaxis	11	17	18	17
Failure of anticoagulation	38	30	31	27
Pulmonary embolectomy	8	10	9	8
Other	4	0	1	2

[a] All values presented as % of those available for evaluation.

The greatest change in coexisting disorders was in patients who received filters between the report in 1977 and the subsequent report in 1981. The incidence of reported venous disease increased by 20%, which probably reflects the inclusion of patients with chronic venous disease. Use of the filter in postoperative and postpartum patients also increased by more than 50%, reflecting the increased level of confidence in the use of the device in younger patients. Between 1981 and 1988, the number of patients with acute venous disease increased significantly as did the number of "other diseases." This is most likely related to extended use of the filter in patients with life-threatening deep vein thrombosis as indicated in the 1981 report[13] (Table 37–3).

The relative importance of a contraindication to anticoagulation and failure of anticoagulants as indications for filter placement reversed position from 1977 to 1988 as the others remained constant. As confidence in the device and ease of insertion have increased since the last review, the number of prophylactic insertions has most likely increased (Table 37–4).

BENEFITS OF EXTENDED FOLLOW-UP

The primary goal of long-term follow-up is to provide appropriate care to patients with vena caval filters whose underlying disorder is not affected by filter placement. In addition, a large body of experience has been obtained, which has resulted in modifications of the technique for placement and the design of the filter.

Modification of the Greenfield Filter

Improvement of the Greenfield filter has been an ongoing process since its introduction. Several adaptations of the filter resulted from concerns that arose from analysis of the follow-up data. The initial insertion carrier system was designed for femoral venous access but was soon adapted to allow internal jugular vein placement as well. Problems with incomplete opening and development of thrombus within the carrier were corrected with the addition of a port for heparin infusion during the insertion procedure. The use of a guide wire was shown to decrease significantly the rate of misplacement that was observed in the earlier summaries.

As radiologists became more active in placing vena caval filters during the late 1980s, interest in applying percutaneous techniques increased.[15–17] While insertion was simplified, an unacceptably high rate of insertion site venous thrombosis was observed because of the necessary dilation of the track required by the 24 F insertion

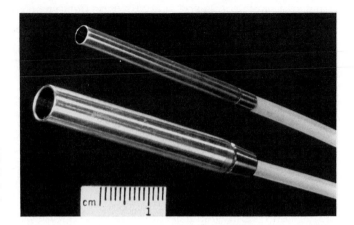

Figure 37–3. Development of a titanium Greenfield filter allowed the carrier system to be reduced in diameter from 24 FR (*below*) to 12 FR (*above*), facilitating percutaneous insertion.

system and the requirement for prolonged compression for hemostasis.[18] Attempts at reducing the size of the delivery system resulted in the development of a titanium version of the original filter, which used a 12 F insertion system[19] (Fig. 37–3). The early results of the multicenter clinical trial of the titanium Greenfield filter indicate it to be comparable with the original filter, both with respect to efficacy and safety.[20]

UNDERSTANDING COMPLICATIONS

More than 100,000 filters have been placed in patients during the past 20 years, and because the Greenfield filter has become the standard against which other devices are compared, a number of articles have appeared in the literature detailing both the benefits and the problems experienced by the authors. In many cases these findings have extended our understanding of the function of the filter in unique situations.

Bach et al[21] reported a case of misplacement of a filter into the right atrium and subsequent cardiac arrhythmias in a quadriplegic patient. This situation differs from the deformity of the filter in quadriplegics who are vulnerable to increased abdominal trauma from routine administration of the "quad cough."[3] Gelbfish and Ascer[22] followed a small series of patients with misplaced intracardiac or intrapulmonary filters who experienced no clinical sequelae. Both articles support the position taken as a result of data based on the Registry experience.

Fracture of a filter strut is a rare event, which is detailed in the literature.[23–26] Although there have been a small number of cases requiring surgical intervention, patients usually are unaware of this change and only rarely develop clinical conditions requiring intervention. Complications such as penetration of adjacent organs, movement of the filter, intraoperative disruption, and misplacement into tributary vessels have been detailed.[26–31] Many of these reports provide valuable insights into dealing with complications and, more importantly, avoiding them.

EXTENDING THE INDICATIONS

As the body of evidence documenting the safety and efficacy of the Greenfield filter continues to grow, there is an increasing demand to extend the indications for placement. Hux et al[32] and Banfield et al[33] have written about the use of the filter during pregnancy. Brenner et al[34] investigated placement of a suprarenal filter in patients with vena caval tumor thrombi with favorable outcomes. Several authors have reported the use of the Greenfield filter in transplant patients who develop deep vein thrombosis.[35,36] Pomper and Lutchman[37] studied the use of the filter in patients with deep vein thrombosis and chronic obstructive pulmonary disease. Fink and Jones[38] recommended the Greenfield filter as primary therapy for patients with venous thromboembolic disease who are more than 65 years old with a correspondingly higher risk from anticoagulation. Many orthopedic surgeons have suggested the use of a Greenfield filter as prophylaxis in high-risk patients who are to undergo total hip or knee arthroplasty.[39-44]

In each of these reports, a relatively small sample of patients has been studied, and although the information is often encouraging, it is certainly not sufficient to alter the indications that have withstood 20 years of evaluation. The currently available information on the Greenfield filter is based on a particular patient population who share a level of risk of developing thromboembolic disease on which the risk/benefit assessments have been based. By increasing prophylactic placements, the population characteristics are altered. It remains for interested investigators to complete more extensive evaluations of patients who receive filters for these indications and report their findings.

REFERENCES

1. Greenfield L, McCurdy J, Brown P. A new intracaval filter permitting continued flow and resolution of emboli. *Surgery.* 1973;73:599–606.
2. Elkins R, McCurdy J, Brown P, et al. Clinical results with an extracaval prosthesis and description of a new intracaval filter. *Okla State Med Assoc.* 1973;53–59.
3. Greenfield L. Use and abuse of intracaval devices. *Surgery.* 1986;99:383–384.
4. Guglielmo FF, Kurtz AB, Wechsler RJ. Prospective comparison of computed tomography and duplex sonography in the evaluation of recently inserted Kimray-Greenfield filters into the inferior vena cava. *Clin Imaging.* 1990;14(3):216–220.
5. Redhead D, Adam R, Allan P, et al. Radiological evaluation of caval patency and filter migration in patients with caval interruption/filtration. *J Int Radiol.* 1989;4:42–45.
6. Sandager G, Simmer S, Silba M, et al. Ultrasonographic characteristics of transvenous vena caval interruption devices. *DVU Conference Abstract.* 1991.
7. Liebman C, Messersmith R, Levin D, et al. MR imaging of inferior vena caval filters: safety and artifacts. *ARJ.* 1988;150(5):1174–1176.
8. Teitelbaum G, Ortega H, Vinitski S, et al. Optimization of gradient-Echo imaging parameters for intracaval filters and trapped thromboemboli. *Radiology.* 1990;174(3):1013–1019.
9. Marx V, Tauscher J, Williams D, et al. Evaluation of the inferior vena cava with intravascular US after Greenfield filter placement. *JVIR.* 1991;2:261–268.
10. McCowan T, Ferris EJ, Carver DK. Inferior vena caval filter thrombi: evaluation with intravascular US. *Radiology.* 1990;177(3):783–788.
11. Greenfield L, Zocco J, Wilk J, et al. Clinical experience with the Kim-Ray Greenfield vena caval filter. *Ann Surg.* 1977;185(6):692–698.
12. Greenfield L, Peyton R, Crute S, et al. Greenfield vena caval filter experience: late results in 156 patients. *Arch Surg.* 1981;116:1451–1456.
13. Greenfield L. Current indications for and results of Greenfield filter placement. *J Vasc Surg.* 1984;1(3):502–504.
14. Greenfield L, Michna B. Twelve-year clinical experience with the Greenfield vena caval filter. *Surgery.* 1988;104(4):706–712.
15. Kantor A, Glanz S, Gordon DH, et al. Percutaneous insertion of the Kimray-Greenfield filter: incidence of femoral vein thrombosis. *AJR.* 1987;149(4):1065–1066.

16. Hye R, Mitchell A, Dory C, et al. Analysis of the transition to percutaneous placement of Greenfield filters. *Arch Surg.* 1990;125(12):1550–1553.
17. Rose B, Simon D, Hess M, et al. Percutaneous transfemoral placement of the Kimray-Greenfield vena cava filter. *Radiology.* 1987;165:373–376.
18. Feinman L, Meltzer A. Phlegmasia cerulea dolens as a complication of percutaneous insertion of a vena caval filter. *J Am Osteopath Assoc.* 1989;89(1):63–68.
19. Greenfield L, Cho KJ. Progress in vena caval devices: the titanium Greenfield vena caval filter. In: Veith FJ, ed. *Current Critical Problems in Vascular Surgery.* St. Louis, Mo: Quality Medical Publishing; 1989:151–153.
20. Greenfield L, Cho KJ, Proctor M, et al. Results of a multicenter study of the modified hook titanium Greenfield filter. *J Vasc Surg.* 1991;14:253–257.
21. Bach JR, Zaneuski R, Lee H. Cardiac arrhythmias from a malpositioned Greenfield filter in a traumatic quadriplegic. *Am J Phys Med Rehabil.* 1990;69(5):251–253.
22. Gelbfish GA, Ascer E. Intracardiac and intrapulmonary Greenfield filters—a long-term follow-up. *J Vasc Surg.* 1991;14:614–617.
23. Plaus W, Hermann G. Structural failure of a Greenfield filter. *Surgery.* 1988;103(6):662–664.
24. Dufretay X, Pagny J, Relland J, et al. Intracaval breakage of a Kimray-Greenfield filter. *AJR.* 1990;154(6):1349–1350.
25. Bury T, Barman A. Strut fracture after Greenfield filter placement. *J Cardiovasc Surg.* 1991;32:384–386.
26. Balshi J, Cantelmo N, Menzoian J. Complications of caval interruption by Greenfield filter in quadriplegics. *J Vasc Surg.* 1989;9:558–562.
27. Howerton R, Watking M, Feldman L. Late arterial hemorrhage secondary to a Greenfield filter requiring late arterial hemorrhage secondary to a Greenfield filter requiring operative intervention. *Surgery.* 1991;109(3):265–268.
28. Adye BA, Rabbe RD, Zobell RL. Errant percutaneous Greenfield filter placement into the retroperitoneum. *J Vasc Surg.* 1990;12(1):60–61.
29. Patterson R, Fowl RJ, Lubbers DJ, et al. Repositioning of partially dislodged Greenfield filters from the right atrium by use of a tip deflection wire. *J Vasc Surg.* 1990;12(1):70–72.
30. Alexander J, Gewertz B, Zarins C. Intraoperative disruption of a Greenfield vena cava filter. *J Cardiovasc Surg.* 1989;30(1):130–132.
31. Appleberg M, Crozier JA. Duodenal penetration by a Greenfield caval filter. *Aust NZ J Surg.* 1991;61:957–960.
32. Hux C, Wapner R, Chayen B, et al. Use of the Greenfield filter for thromboembolic disease in pregnancy. *Am J Obstet Gynecol.* 1986;155:734–737.
33. Banfield PJ, Ptiiam M, Marwood R. Recurrent pulmonary embolism in pregnancy managed with the Greenfield vena caval filter. *Int J Gynaecol Obstet.* 1990;33(3):275–278.
34. Brenner D, Brenner C, Scott J, et al. Suprarenal Greenfield filter placement to prevent pulmonary embolus in patients with vena caval tumor thrombi. *J Urol.* 1992;147:19–23.
35. Walker H, Pennington D. Inferior vena caval filters in heart transplant recipients with perioperative deep vein thromboses. *J Heart Transplant.* 1990;9(5):579–580.
36. Jarrell B, Szentpetery S, Mendez-Picon G, et al. Greenfield filter in renal transplant patients. *Arch Surg.* 1981;116:930–932.
37. Pomper SR, Lutchman G. The role of intracaval filters in patients with COPD and DVT. *Angiology.* 1991;42:85–89.
38. Fink J, Jones B. The Greenfield filter as the primary means of therapy in venous thromboembolic disease. *Dr Chos.* 1991;172(4):253–256.
39. Emerson RH Jr, Cross R, Head WC. Prophylactic and early therapeutic use of the Greenfield filter in hip and knee joint arthroplasty. *J Arthroplasty.* 1991;6:129–135.
40. Barnes C, Collins D, Nelson C, et al. Vena caval filter use in orthopaedic patients with recognized preoperative deep venous thrombosis. *Orthop Trauma Assoc.* Paper presented November 7, 1990; Toronto, Canada.
41. Brooks R, Winslow M, Kenmore P. The week-old hip fracture: indication for prophylactic use of a vena cava filter? Report of two cases. *Orthopedics.* 1987;10(9):1287–1288.

42. Woolson S, Harris W. Greenfield vena caval filter for management of selected cases of venous thromboembolic disease following hip surgery. A report of five cases. *Clin Orthop.* 1986;204:201–206.
43. Golueke P, Garrett W, Thompson J, et al. Interruption of the vena cava by means of the Greenfield filter: expanding the indications. *Surgery.* 1988;103(1):111–117.
44. Vaughn B, Knezevich S, Lombardi A, et al. Use of the Greenfield filter to prevent fatal pulmonary embolism associated with total hip and knee arthroplasty. *J Bone Joint Surg.* 1989;71(10):1542–1548.

38

Fifteen Years' Experience with Spiral Vein Graft for Superior Vena Cava Syndrome

Donald B. Doty, MD

William Hunter[1] described the first case of superior vena cava syndrome in 1757. The symptoms and signs of obstruction of the superior vena cava have since come to be recognized as unmistakable syndrome. A recent review of the clinical problem of obstruction of the superior vena cava was presented by Nieto and Doty.[2] Data from more than 90 publications including 1,980 cases of superior vena cava syndrome reported in the literature since 1934 were reviewed by Ahmann.[3] These papers are good starting points for gaining a more complete overview of the problem of the syndrome caused by obstruction of the superior vena cava.

ANATOMY

The superior vena cava is located in the middle mediastinum, surrounded by relative rigid structures including the trachea, right bronchus, aorta, pulmonary artery, and perihilar and paratracheal lymph nodes. Disease in any of the adjacent structures may contribute to the pathogenesis of superior vena cava syndrome. The superior vena cava is a thin-walled vein that is compliant and easily compressible. Pressure within this great vein is low. The vena cava originates as the confluence of the right and left brachiocephalic (innominate) veins and extends for a distance of 6 to 8 cm to the right atrium. It is inside the pericardial sac for the distal 2 cm of its course. There is only one major venous channel entering the superior vena cava, the azygous vein, which enters posteriorly just above the pericardial reflection and is a very important venous collateral pathway.

Obstruction of the superior vena cava stimulates the formation of extensive venous collateral circulation. The azygous venous system in the chest wall is the most important collateral pathway. When the obstruction of the superior vena cava is located distal to a patent azygous vein, there is retrograde flow through the azygous-hemiazygous veins to the lumbar veins below the diaphragm and to the inferior vena cava. When the obstruction is proximal to the patent azygous vein, collateral veins in the neck allow blood flow to enter the azygous system and continue directly into the distal vena cava below the obstruction. When the azygous connection to the superior vena cava is included in the obstruction, more complex and varied pathways must develop to drain the upper compartment. One prominent system is the internal mammary veins, which connect to the superior and inferior epigastric veins and subsequently to the inferior vena cava by way of the external iliac veins. The lateral thoracic veins drain to the thoraco-epigastric veins, and eventually blood flow may enter the femoral veins. Paraspinous veins form a collateral network, which connects to the inferior vena cava through lumbar veins. The esophageal venous network also can decompress the thorax through the left gastric vein to the portal system. This pathway is not very important unless esophageal varicose veins develop, which are associated with bleeding into the gastrointestinal tract (rare). Subcutaneous veins are particularly important means of bringing blood flow from the upper compartment below the diaphragm to the inferior vena cava. Despite extensive collateral circulation that may develop, venous pressure in superior vena cava obstruction has been recorded as high as 200 to 500 cm of water in severe superior vena cava syndrome.

Cerebral venous decompression may be provided through a single internal jugular vein because the veins of the right and left sides of the brain are in continuity through midline venous sinuses.[4] The superior and inferior sagittal sinuses drain the cerebral hemispheres to the confluence of sinuses that communicate through the transverse and sigmoid sinuses to either internal jugular vein. The cavernous venous sinuses also communicate both sides of the brain to either internal jugular vein. The cerebral venous drainage, therefore, may be adequate through either one of the internal jugular veins to the right atrium.

PATHOGENESIS

Superior vena cava syndrome is the result of obstruction of the superior vena cava. This may be due to extrinsic compression, direct invasion by disease process, or thrombosis. Extrinsic compression usually produces obstruction that gradually and progressively worsens. Collateral circulation has time to develop so that obstruction is usually well tolerated and the patient may have few if any signs and symptoms of superior vena cava syndrome. When the obstruction develops more rapidly, as in cases of invasion of the vena cava by some disease process such as a malignant tumor, collateral circulation may not have time to develop to decompress the upper compartment veins adequately. The superior vena cava syndrome is more obvious in these cases.

The most severe syndrome develops in cases of thrombosis of the superior vena cava in which the obstruction occurs suddenly without time for any collateral venous channels to develop. Thrombosis may spread to involve the major caval tributaries and thus eliminate major collateral pathways. Thrombosis is often associated with superior vena cava obstruction from any cause and compounds the problem because subsequent organization of the clot with fibrosis results in a permanent closure of vena cava. Thrombosis will not respond to treatment directed at the primary disease process that caused obstruction of the superior vena cava.

Lymphatic drainage should be considered as well as venous hypertension in superior vena cava syndrome. The thoracic lymphatic ducts drain to the subclavian veins and are affected by venous hypertension associated with obstruction of the superior vena cava. The lymphatics of the lung may also be secondarily affected with occurrence of increased lung water and associated dyspnea. Respiratory insufficiency is frequently associated with acute obstruction of the superior vena cava and may be difficult to manage. Pleural effusion of chylous nature may be present and associated with thoracic lymphatic obstruction.

DESCRIPTION OF DISEASE

Obstruction of the superior vena cava may be caused by a wide spectrum of disease. There has been a change in the common causes of caval obstruction during the past 40 years. McIntire and Sykes[5] found the most common causes of caval obstruction were thoracic malignancy (33%), aortic aneurysm (30%), and chronic granulomatous mediastinitis (19%) before 1949. By 1962, only 25% of cases of superior vena cava obstruction were due to benign causes in a review reported by Effler and Groves.[6] In cases reviewed between 1969 and 1979, Lochridge and associates[4] found only 3% of caval obstruction caused by benign cause; all the rest were malignant causes. Contemporary studies of superior vena cava obstruction show that malignant etiologies account for more than 90% of cases.

Benign

The Mayo Clinic review[7] and the Cleveland Clinic review[8] reported mediastinal granulomatous disease resulting in fibrosing mediastinitis as a prominent cause of benign superior vena cava obstruction. The most common specific etiologic agent is histoplasmosis, which causes a caseating granulomatous process in mediastinal lymph nodes which compress, fibrose, and contract around the superior vena cava and may result in secondary thrombosis. Fibrosing mediastinitis secondary to radiation therapy may be progressive and involve the superior vena cava years after the radiation treatment has been completed.

Iatrogenic causes have been increasing in importance because of increase in use of invasive intravenous procedures such as cardiac pacemaker electrodes, central venous–pulmonary artery catheters, and hyperalimentation–chemotherapy catheters. Thrombosis of the superior vena cava around these catheters is especially troublesome when the prosthetic device is required as a permanent life support for the patient and cannot be conveniently removed.

Other benign causes include benign tumor, vascular aneurysm, a variety of cardiac causes, pulmonary causes, and mediastinal hematomas.

Malignant

Thoracic malignancy accounts for most of the causes of obstruction of the superior vena cava in current practice. More than 90% of superior vena cava syndromes will be associated with intrathoracic malignancy. Bronchogenic carcinoma is responsible for 67% to 82% of all cases of superior vena cava obstruction.[2] It is estimated that 3% to 15% of patients with bronchogenic carcinoma will develop superior vena cava syndrome. The cell type of bronchogenic carcinoma causing superior vena cava obstruction appears to be somewhat variable and may be related to individual series classifications. Squamous (epidermoid) carcinoma accounts for 22% to 27% of cases and appears to be relatively constant in most reports. Small cell carcinoma is the most variable (18% to 46%), perhaps related to variation in interpretation of small cell pathology, but there seems to be a real increase in frequency of small cell carcinoma as a cause of superior vena cava syndrome. Lymphoma is the second most frequent cause of superior vena cava obstruction, accounting for 5% to 15% of cases. These malignancies are located in the anterior mediastinum and produce caval obstruction by external compression from the front. Thoracic metastasis from extrathoracic malignancies account for a smaller number of vena cava obstructions, with breast and testicular malignancy particularly important.

SIGNS AND SYMPTOMS

Patients with superior vena cava obstruction usually present with a well-established syndrome, which is easily recognized and unmistakable. Rarely, complete obstruction of the superior vena cava may take place without noticeable signs or symptoms developing. The typical syndrome consists of symptoms of swelling of face, neck, and arms; shortness of breath; orthopnea; and cough. These patients may notice that a shirt collar is tight and that the face looks swollen especially around the eyes. The skin of the face appears flushed. Other symptoms include hoarseness, stridor, tongue swelling, nasal congestion, epistaxis, dysphagia, headaches, dizziness, syncope, lethargy, or chest pain. The symptoms are all aggravated by bending forward, stooping, or by lying down. Many patients become dyspneic when recumbent and must sleep in a chair.

The most common signs are dilation and tortuosity of the veins of the upper body; swelling of the face, neck, or arms; and plethora or cyanosis of the face. Other signs include proptosis, glossal edema, rhinorrhea, laryngeal edema, mentation changes, and elevation of the venous and cerebrospinal fluid pressure. Some patients may have pleural effusion that may be chylous.

Signs and symptoms suggesting cerebral and/or laryngeal edema are of prognostic importance.[4] Headache, vertigo, visual disturbances, decreased mentation, stupor, somnolence, and convulsions indicate cerebral edema, whereas hoarseness and stridor suggest upper airway obstruction. These symptoms have been associated with decreased survival time and should prompt more rapid workup and treatment.

DIAGNOSIS

Clinical diagnosis of superior vena cava obstruction is usually obvious in cases associated with superior vena cava syndrome. Specific characterization of the location, degree, and specific cause of the caval obstruction should be established in every case. There is some controversy regarding how specific this characterization should be inasmuch as more than 90% of cases are due to malignancy. Some physicians think that treatment directed at palliating intrathoracic malignancy should proceed without delay, but others argue that superior vena cava syndrome is seldom a medical emergency and that the condition should be characterized as completely as possible in an orderly fashion so that treatment may be specific. Specific etiology by tissue diagnosis can usually be obtained, but in some cases it may be difficult and even hazardous to the patient. All diagnostic methods should be used with judgment and consideration for patient safety and comfort. It should be remembered that patients with superior vena cava syndrome seek relief of the symptoms of the syndrome and seldom complain of symptoms relating to the actual etiologic cause of the caval obstruction. Treatment of the caval syndrome should always accompany treatment and diagnostic measures directed at the causative primary disease.

The chest radiograph is very helpful although not specific in the diagnosis of superior vena cava obstruction. Because bronchogenic carcinoma is the most common cause of superior vena cava syndrome, the chest radiograph will often show a right-sided hilar mass. Anterior mediastinal mass suggests lymphoma.

The most useful diagnostic procedure for patients with superior vena cava syndrome is the bilateral arm contrast venogram.[9,10] This procedure will establish the location and degree of obstruction of the vena cava, the degree of involvement of caval tributaries, and the extent of collateral venous pathways. It will establish whether the vena cava is completely obstructed or remains patent and is extrinsically compressed. Identification of thrombus on venography, especially retrograde propagation of thrombosis to involve the caval tributaries, may be a sign that caval obstructive symptoms are not as likely to respond to nonoperative therapy.

Computerized axial tomography provides an effective and noninvasive means of analysis of the superior vena cava and its tributaries. The advantages of this diagnostic measure have been outlined by Moncada and associates.[11] The caval anatomy can be clearly related to surrounding mediastinal structures. Mediastinal masses or lymph node pathology relative to the superior vena cava can be outlined. As this diagnostic technique is refined, it has assumed increasing importance in the workup of superior vena cava syndrome. It can also be of great assistance in obtaining directed needle biopsy of mediastinal masses. Patency of the internal jugular veins in the neck can also be assessed by axial tomography when there is extensive occlusion of the tributaries of the superior vena cava. Magnetic resonance imaging has also been shown to be useful in assessing graft patency after operation for superior vena cava syndrome.[12]

Other diagnostic methods including cytology, isotope venography, ultrasound, bronchoscopy, lymph node biopsy, mediastinal biopsy, and exploratory thoracotomy may have indications for individual cases. In each case, the risks of intervention in terms of patient comfort, bleeding, interruption of venous collateral, and the like should be carefully weighed against the chance of success in establishing the diagnosis. The more invasive diagnostic tests may actually worsen the caval syndrome and may best be avoided in favor of a more direct approach in which the vena cava obstruction is treated along with establishing the etiologic diagnosis.

THERAPY

Three basic treatment modalities for superior vena cava syndrome are (a) radiation therapy; (b) medical measures; and (c) operation. Radiation therapy is the most important primary therapeutic modality because most cases of superior vena cava syndrome are caused by malignancy, which is not resectable at operation. Medical measures may provide relief of some of the symptoms of the syndrome but are usually not curative interventions. Surgical intervention to provide definitive relief of superior vena cava obstruction by means of caval bypass or replacement is the most effective means of relief of symptoms of the syndrome but the least used and most controversial method of treatment. There is debate as to which treatment modality should be used, when therapy should be instituted, and even which patients should receive treatment. The spectrum of etiologies and patient presentation makes uniform treatment impossible, so that the therapeutic regimen must be tailored to individual patient needs.

INDICATIONS FOR OPERATION AND PATIENT MATERIAL

Indications for operation in patients with superior vena cava obstruction caused by malignant disease remains debatable, but operation may be indicated in those patients in whom superior vena cava syndrome itself is severe and life-threatening.[2,4,13] The malignancy, however, ultimately prevails so that long-term effectiveness of bypass grafts cannot be determined in these patients. Operation in patients with benign causes of superior vena cava obstruction provides the opportunity to observe the function of bypass conduits over a long time course.[14] It is the purpose of this paper to report the late follow-up of patients having superior vena cava bypass using a composite spiral saphenous vein graft as the conduit to relieve superior vena cava obstruction.

Nine patients had operations for obstruction of the superior vena cava with superior vena cava syndrome caused by benign disease. Three patients had fibrosing mediastinitis, four had fibrosing mediastinitis with caseous necrosis, one had thrombosis of the superior vena cava around a pacemaker electrode, and one had spontaneous thrombosis of superior vena cava. Patients ranged in age from 25 to 68 years. All the patients reported symptoms of superior vena cava syndrome that had not improved or gradually worsened over time. Two patients reported marked worsening of superior vena cava syndrome during observation before operation that was associated with progressing thrombosis of the superior vena cava and its tributaries. All bypass operations were performed using a composite spiral vein graft constructed from the patient's own saphenous vein, split longitudinally and wrapped around a stent in spiral fashion. The edges of the vein were sutured together to form a large conduit, ranging in diameter from 9.5 to 15.0 mm. Six grafts were from the left innominate vein and three grafts were from the internal jugular vein. The grafts were placed into the right atrial appendage in all except one, which was to the distal superior vena cava. Follow-up extends from 1 to 15 years.

OPERATIVE PROCEDURE

The operation is performed through a midline sternotomy[15] (Fig. 38–1A). The left brachiocephalic (innominate) vein is mobilized to the internal jugular vein and the subclavian vein junction. The innominate vein may be thrombosed in some patients. In these cases it is necessary to mobilize the internal jugular vein on the left or right side as the outflow point from the upper venous compartment. The operation is the same in these cases except that the thoracic inlet must be opened up by excision of strap muscles to provide an unrestricted passageway for the bypass conduit. Abnormal tissues surrounding the superior vena cava are biopsied. The diameter of the innominate or jugular vein is determined and distance from the vein to the right atrial appendage measured (Fig. 38–1B).

A simultaneous incision is made over the saphenous vein. The average diameter of the vein is measured. The length of saphenous vein to be removed is determined according to the ratio of the diameter innominate vein (desired conduit diameter) to the diameter of the saphenous vein multiplied by the length of conduit needed to reach to the right atrial appendage. For example, if the innominate vein measured 12 mm in diameter, the saphenous vein was 4 mm in diameter, and length to the right atrial appendage is 10 cm, then 30 cm of saphenous vein is required ($10 \times 12/4 = 30$). A thoracostomy catheter, which has the same diameter as the innominate vein, is selected as a stent on which to form the bypass graft.

The required length of saphenous vein is removed and incised longitudinally through its entire length. The opened vein graft is flattened out and wrapped in spiral fashion around the stent (Fig. 38–1C). A continuous suture of 7-0 polypropylene is used to join the edges of the graft to form a large conduit. Optical magnification ensures that no loose tissue is pulled into the suture line.

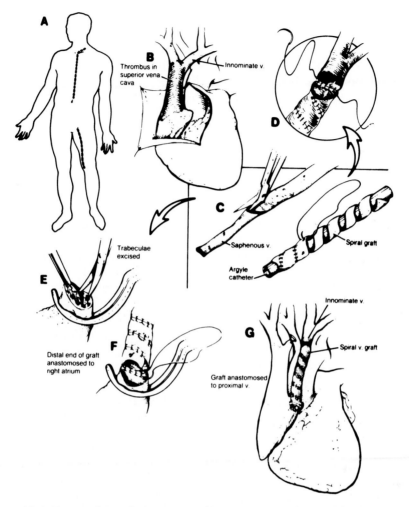

Figure 38–1. Bypass of superior vena cava with composite spiral vein graft. (**A**) Midsternal incision is made, which may be extended into the neck to obtain access to internal jugular vein if necessary. Incision is made in the leg directly over saphenous vein. (**B**) Upper portion of the pericardium is opened to expose right atrial appendage. Biopsy of obstructing process in superior vena cava may be taken. Innominate vein is completely mobilized. (**C**) Saphenous vein graft is distended and its branches ligated. It is opened longitudinally through its entire length. A stent catheter exactly the same size as the vein to which the graft will be anastomosed is selected. Opened saphenous vein is wrapped around the stent catheter in spiral fashion with intimal surface against the stent. Edges of vein graft are joined by continuous suture of 7/0 polypropylene, forming a spiral anastomosis the length of the graft. (**D**) Innominate vein is divided. End-to-end anastomosis of the graft to innominate vein is constructed with continuous stitches of 7/10 polypropylene suture. (**E**) Entire right atrial appendage is excluded by vascular clamp. Tip of appendage is removed, and all trabeculae within the appendage are removed. (**F**) End of vein graft is anastomosed to right atrial appendage with 5/0 polypropylene suture. (**G**) Completed graft lies anterior to aorta. (*From ref. 15, with permission.*)

Heparin 200 to 300 U/kg is administered intravenously. The innominate vein is ligated as close as possible to the superior vena cava. A soft jaw vascular clamp (Fogarty) is applied at the internal jugular-subclavian junction, and the innominate vein is divided, retaining as much length as possible. Thrombus or any abnormality of the intima or vessel wall is removed.

The graft is pushed slightly off the end of the stent catheter, and an end-to-end anastomosis to the innominate vein is constructed using 7-0 polypropylene continuous suture (Fig. 38–1D). The stent is removed from the graft. The tip of the right atrial appendage is excised, and the opening is cleared of trabeculae to ensure unrestricted blood flow into the atrium (Fig. 38–1E). The graft is anastomosed to the right atrium using 5-0 polypropylene suture (Fig. 38–1F). The graft should be precisely the right length; extra length serves no advantage as the graft may kink and impede blood flow.

RESULTS

At the time of report, seven of the patients are asymptomatic and relieved of superior vena cava syndrome.[14] Graft longevity ranges from 1 year to nearly 15 years. Five of the patients experienced no complications and have returned to normal life-styles and are able to sleep flat and enjoy such activities as tennis, swimming, and skiing. One patient recently passed the Iowa State Highway Patrol physical conditioning requirement at the highest level. One of the patients had survived for more than 11 years and was perfectly fine until the graft was divided during coronary artery bypass surgery at another institution. The graft was destroyed, and massive hemorrhage resulted from this surgical accident. The graft was replaced with a saphenous vein graft (not spiral). This patient now has some venous obstruction symptoms. Another patient developed thrombosis at the proximal graft anastomosis. Reoperation was performed 4 days after the original operation. The anastomosis was taken down, and the innominate vein was resected further back to remove abnormal intima. A new graft was reanastomosed, which remained patent, and the patient is asymptomatic.

Two patients experienced difficulty with the procedure because of thrombosis of the spiral vein bypass graft during the first year after operation. Both patients had anastomosis of the bypass graft to the internal jugular vein and crossing the thoracic inlet. One patient had aggressive sclerosing mediastinitis, which progressed after operation to obliterate in both internal jugular veins and the bypass graft. The inferior vena cava also thrombosed. This patient underwent reoperation at 1 year, and two saphenous vein grafts (not spiral) were taken from the right and left external jugular veins to the right atrium. These grafts have remained patent for more than 7 years and provided partial relief of superior vena cava syndrome. Ultimately, it was necessary to bypass from the remnant of the left internal jugular vein at the angle of the mandible to the right atrium, using an externally reinforced polytetrafluoroethylene (PTFE) graft. This graft is currently patent, and symptoms of superior vena cava syndrome are relieved. The other patient had reoccurrence of the superior vena cava syndrome 5 months after the operation. No further operative treatment has been given. Computerized axial tomography with contrast showed the graft had occluded apparently because of reoccurrence of spontaneous thrombosis in the venous system. This graft not only originated from the right internal jugular vein and crossed the thoracic inlet but also was the only graft placed directly to the superior vena cava, which could have exposed it to the pre-existing abnormalities in the intima of the superior vena cava. Anticoagulants had not been used after operation.

DISCUSSION

Haimovici and associates[16] reviewed grafts used in the venous system and concluded that autogenous veins are preferred for venous replacement. Experimental and clinical experience with vena cava replacement or bypass was reviewed by Scherck and associates.[17] Many types of conduits have been tried, including autogenous, homologous, or heterologous vein and aorta as well as various synthetic grafts. It was concluded that autogenous vein grafts of nearly the same size as the superior vena cava are most likely to remain patent. It is necessary to sacrifice another large vein from elsewhere in the body to obtain a large venous conduit. Hanlon and Danis[18] used the femoral, subclavian, or jugular veins to replace or bypass the superior vena cava. Gladstone and associates[19] used the femoral vein as a bypass conduit, and Marshall and Kouchoukos[20] combined the use of the femoral vein within a PTFE sleeve to provide resistance to external compression of the graft. Venous drainage problems are uncommon but remain a possible complication attending removal of these large veins for use as a bypass graft in another part of the body. The alternative to sacrifice of a large vein is to obtain a smaller autogenous vein and construct a larger composite conduit.

Synthetic grafts are attractive because of convenience. Graft thrombosis has limited the usefulness of prosthetic devices. Reconstruction of the superior vena cava using a PTFE graft was performed by Dartevelle and associates.[21] Graft patency in the short term was quite promising in 13 cases followed an average of 24 months in their series. Garcia-Rinaldi and associates[22] reported a case in which two 10-mm PTFE grafts were used to replace the resected superior vena cava and left innominate vein. These grafts remained patent for more than 4 years, but significant intimal irregularity and stenoses had developed. Although there is much to recommend the use of PTFE grafts, it is known that the inside lining of the healed graft consists of collagen matrix rather than living endothelium and therefore subject to thrombosis. Moore and associates[23] suggested that the use of a distal arteriovenous fistula into an external reinforced PTFE graft will result in patency rates comparable with spiral vein grafts, but I have no experience with this technique.

Composite vein grafts constructed from the saphenous or other small vein have the advantage of autogenous vascular tissue, which may be fashioned into a conduit of any diameter. Large composite vein grafts have been constructed in panel or longitudinal fashion and used clinically to bypass or replace the superior vena cava.[24,25] Chiu and associates[26] reported construction of a composite spiral vein graft that was used to replace the superior vena cava. Doty and Baker[27] successfully applied this technique in a man who had fibrosing granulomatous mediastinitis. This patient is the first patient reported in this series and is free of symptoms of superior vena cava syndrome nearly 15 years after operation. Results in this series suggest that once a spiral vein graft is established, it can be expected to function indefinitely unless the basic disease process causing caval thrombosis affects the graft. Progressive fibrosing mediastinitis closed not only the bypass graft but also the inferior vena cava in one patient in this series, whereas another patient apparently had recurrence of spontaneous thrombosis of the vena cava, which closed the graft. Perhaps long-term anticoagulation would have prevented this complication in the latter patient.

Critics of the composite spiral vein graft technique have argued that the operation is complex and that the construction of the bypass conduit is tedious and time-consuming. Time for construction of the bypass graft is about 20 to 30 minutes. Disadvantages of time for construction are offset by the advantage of being able to form a conduit to precisely the desired diameter. Critics have pointed out that the long suture line is a source for thrombosis of the graft. The potential problem of suture line as a foreign body stimulus for thrombosis is effectively reduced by the spiral suture technique, because flowing blood is only exposed to a single suture line at any cross-sectional level of the graft.

Fowl and associates[28] reported good results in three cases in which a spiral vein graft was used in heavily contaminated locations. This experience suggests use of this type of graft may be especially useful for vascular reconstruction in the presence of fungal or bacterial infection.

The results in this series of patients indicates that the most favorable situation is that where the bypass graft is constructed end-to-end to a large vein in the thorax. A graft of exactly the same size as the vein to which it is connected is preferred, so that there will be slight outflow resistance to ensure adequate venous distending pressure, along with obligatory flow into the graft.[2] End-to-end anastomosis of the graft to the vein, while technically easier to perform, is not as desirable. End-to-side anastomosis of a conduit to the internal jugular vein that must cross the thoracic inlet to reach the right atrium was associated with thrombosis in two of three patients. Consideration of placing the conduit within a stented PTFE tube may be a useful adjunct when crossing the thoracic inlet may subject the graft to compression.[20]

This experience with composite spiral saphenous vein grafts for bypass of the obstructed superior vena cava suggests that uniform relief of the signs and symptoms of superior vena cava syndrome may be expected. In patients having benign diseases causing obstruction of the superior vena cava, prolonged relief of superior vena cava is observed and long-term patency of the spiral vein graft has been the rule.[14] Gloviczki and associates[29] use spiral saphenous vein grafts as first choice for superior vena cava replacement. The operation to construct such a bypass graft is not complex and may be performed at low risk. It may be offered with confidence of good early and late results to patients with obstruction of the superior vena cava.

REFERENCES

1. Hunter W. The history of an aneurysm of the aorta with some remarks on aneurysms in general. *Med Obstet Soc Phys Lond.* 1757;1:323.
2. Nieto AF, Doty DB. Superior vena cava obstruction: clinical syndrome, etiology, and treatment. *Curr Probl Cancer.* 1986;10:441.
3. Ahmann FR. A reassessment of the clinical implications of the superior vena caval syndrome. *J Clin Oncol.* 1984;2:961.
4. Lochridge SK, Knibbe WP, Doty DB. Obstruction of the superior vena cava. *Surgery.* 1979;85:14.
5. McIntire FT, Sykes EM Jr. Obstruction of the superior vena cava: a review of the literature and report of two personal cases. *Ann Intern Med.* 1949;30:925.
6. Effler D, Groves L. Superior vena cava obstruction. *J Thorac Cardiovasc Surg.* 1962;43:574.
7. Parish JM, Marschke RF, Dines DE, et al. Etiologic considerations in superior vena cava syndrome. *Mayo Clin Proc.* 1981;56:407.
8. Mahajan V, Strimlan V, Van Ordstran HS, et al. Benign superior vena cava syndrome. *Chest.* 1975;68:32.
9. Dyet JF, Moghissi K. Role of venography in assessing patients with superior caval obstruction caused by bronchial carcinoma for bypass operations. *Thorax.* 1980;35:628.
10. Stanford W, Doty DB. The role of venography and surgery in the management of patients with superior vena cava obstruction. *Ann Thorac Surg.* 1986;41:158.
11. Moncada R, Cardella R, Demos TC, et al. Evaluation of superior vena cava syndrome by axial CT and CT phlebography. *AJR.* 1984;143:731.
12. Levitt RG, Glazer HS, Gutierrez F, et al. Magnetic resonance imaging of spiral vein graft bypass of superior vena cava in fibrosing mediastinitis. *Chest.* 1986;90:676.
13. Doty DB. Bypass of superior vena cava: six years' experience with spiral vein graft for obstruction of superior vena cava due to benign and malignant disease. *J Thorac Cardiovasc Surg.* 1982;83:326.

14. Doty DB, Doty JR, Jones KW. Bypass of superior vena cava: fifteen years' experience with spiral vein graft for obstruction of superior vena cava caused by benign disease. *J Thorac Cardiovasc Surg.* 1990;99:889.
15. Lamberth WC, Doty DB. *Peripheral Vascular Surgery.* Chicago: Mosby-Year Book Medical Publishers; 1987.
16. Haimovici H, Hoffert PW, Zinicola N, et al. An experimental and clinical evaluation of grafts in the venous system. *Surg Gynecol Obstet.* 1970;131:1173.
17. Scherck JP, Kerstein MD, Stansel HC Jr. The current status of vena cava replacement. *Surgery.* 1974;76:209.
18. Hanlon CR, Danis RK. Superior vena cava obstruction: indications for diagnostic thoracotomy. *Ann Surg.* 1965;161:771.
19. Gladstone DJ, Pillai R, Paneth M, et al. Relief of superior vena cava syndrome with autologous femoral vein used as a bypass graft. *J Thorac Cardiovasc Surg.* 1985;89:750.
20. Marshall WG Jr, Kouchoukos NT. Management of recurrent superior vena caval syndrome with an externally supported femoral vein bypass graft. *Ann Thorac Surg.* 1988;46:239.
21. Dartevelle P, Chapelier A, Navajas M, et al. Replacement of the superior vena cava with polytetrafluoroethylene grafts combined with resection of mediastinal-pulmonary malignant tumors: report of thirteen cases. *J Thorac Cardiovasc Surg.* 1987;94:361.
22. Garcia-Rinaldi R, Zamora JL, Torres-Salichs M, et al. Four-year patency of PTFE grafts after replacement of the superior vena cava and the innominate veins. *Tex Heart Inst J.* 1988;15:192.
23. Moore WM Jr, Hollier LH, Pickett TK. Superior vena cava and central venous reconstruction. *Surgery.* 1991;110:35.
24. Semb G, Eie H. Superior cava obstruction: innominate vein to right atrial shunt with a composite vein graft. *Scand J Thorac Cardiovasc Surg.* 1974;8:196.
25. Arai T, Inagaki K, Hata E, et al. Reconstruction of the superior vena cava in a patient with a thymoma. *Chest.* 1978;73:230.
26. Chiu DJ, Tersiz J, MacRae ML. Replacement of superior vena cava with a spiral composite vein graft: a versatile technique. *Ann Thorac Surg.* 1974;17:555.
27. Doty DB, Baker WH. Bypass of superior vena cava with spiral vein graft. *Ann Thorac Surg.* 1976;22:490.
28. Fowl RJ, Martin KD, Sax HC, et al. Use of autologous spiral vein grafts for vascular reconstructions in contaminated fields. *J Vasc Surg.* 1988;8:442.
29. Gloviczki P, Pairolero PC, Cherry KJ, et al. Reconstruction of the vena cava and of its primary tributaries: a preliminary report. *J Vasc Surg.* 1990;11:373.

39

Late Results of Venous Valve Repair

Robert L. Kistner, M D

Surgical treatment of deep vein valve incompetence by valve repair and by valve substitution technique is a development of the past 25 years, and it is only now that we can assess the very long-term results of this more aggressive approach in patients with chronic venous insufficiency. The first valve repair was performed in 1968,[1] and the first series was reported in 1975.[2] The value of this surgical approach has been a matter of investigation and of skepticism from the time of its inception to the present. New approaches to diagnosis and treatment have led to clarification of the importance of reflux in chronic venous insufficiency[3,4] but have not resulted in agreement about the advisability of this type of surgery. The skepticism is based on the known fact that venous disease can be controlled by proper elastic support combined with adjustment of the patient's way of life through rest and elevation.[5] The challenge of surgery is to improve on nonsurgical management by eradicating the swelling, pain, and ulceration of venous insufficiency while keeping the patient at full activity and ultimately to relieve the patient of the need to wear elastic support.

This chapter reviews the results of those who have performed venous valve surgery during 1968 to 1992 and supplements this with results from a current analysis of the very long-term results in my own series that date back 24 years to the beginning of this type of surgery. Because we know that early favorable results in venous disease may be followed by long-term failure, the results of treatment for venous disease should be measured in terms of 10 or more years rather than the conventional 5-year period for arterial disease.

CANDIDATES FOR VALVE RECONSTRUCTIVE SURGERY

Patients selected for deep vein valve surgery in most of the reported series in the literature are those who present with venous ulcers or disabling swelling, pain, or preulcerative changes (grade 3 symptoms in the Classification of the Subcommittee on Reporting Standards in Venous Disease[6]) and who demonstrate severe reflux in the lower extremity veins at the thigh and popliteal levels. In the selection process for valve reconstructive surgery, the most important aspect is a thorough assessment of the patient's clinical state. The cardinal symptoms of venous insufficiency are aching, swelling, stasis change, and ulceration. Each of these can be a major or minor problem, depending on the severity of the symptom and the activity level of the patient. When the leg swells or aches to such a degree that it is too uncomfortable for the patient to remain erect after 2 to 4 hours, the problem is a disabling venous insufficiency to the working individual. If this patient were to assume a sedentary way of life, either by retirement or unrelated illness, the problem would be solved and no longer represent a severe venous insufficiency syndrome. In this same way, ulceration in the leg can be well controlled by a change of life-style, and a person with grade 3 venous insufficiency can be converted to one with compensated venous disease simply because the patient decreases activity and does not stress the extremity. For the patient with a sedentary way of life, it is unlikely that deep vein reconstructive surgery would be worthwhile because the primary purpose of surgery is to keep the patient active and comfortable. For this reason, it is important to analyze the activity level of the patient when the long-term results of chronic venous insufficiency treatment are reviewed.

VENOUS WORKUP

When reconstructive surgery is contemplated, it is necessary to have a thorough knowledge of the veins in that extremity. The surgeon has to know which veins are patent and which are obstructed, and in those that are patent, it is necessary to know where valves are located and whether they are competent. This analysis should encompass the saphenous and perforator veins as well as the deep veins, which include the common, superficial, and deep (profunda) femoral veins, and the popliteal and tibial veins. Assessment of the extremity by physiologic tests for both obstruction and reflux also needs to be a part of the workup by way of plethysmographic or venous pressure data.

An organized approach to this assessment can be achieved as follows:

1. Initial thorough history and physical to establish the clinical grading. The degree of swelling, aching, stasis change, and ulceration are detailed, and the effect of these symptoms on the individual's life-style is determined. When any combination of these problems seriously impairs the individual's work status or life-style, this individual is considered a potential candidate for deep vein reconstruction. The grade 3 clinical severity classification includes all ulcers and patients who are disabled or severely impaired by aching, swelling, and ulceration.

2. A manual Doppler examination of the veins is performed on the first office visit to screen the venous system. This study is frequently correct when its results are compared with the final diagnosis, but it is not sufficiently accurate to replace other tests in the surgical candidate.

3. The patient with a serious venous problem is referred to the vascular laboratory for physiologic and duplex scan testing. The physiologic tests of value include photoplethysmography (PPG), foot volumetry, phleborheography, and venous pressure. All these tests provide qualitative information that reflects overall venous function, but they discriminate poorly between reflux and obstruction and do little to allow analysis of the calf muscle pump function. The physiologic test I prefer now is the air plethysmograph[7] because it provides quantitative data on both obstruction and reflux, and it estimates the calf muscle ability to empty the venous reservoir in the leg.

The color-flow duplex scan is used extensively to study each vein in the leg for patency and reflux. It is an excellent means to study the veins *in situ*. This technology permits real-time analysis of venous flow in the leg and allows observation of the effects of muscle contraction and of Valsalva on the venous flow. The veins of the extremity can be mapped for patency and reflux in about 30 minutes. Incompetent saphenous and perforator veins are readily identified. The various segments of the deep veins, including common femoral vein, superficial femoral vein (SFV), and profunda femoris vein (PFV), and popliteal and tibial veins are separately studied for patency and competence.

With the completion of the vascular laboratory examination, the surgeon has physiologic and anatomic knowledge of the venous function in the leg. The results are analyzed at this point, and the workup is stopped if the diagnosis is complete and the patient is not a candidate for deep vein reconstruction.

Ascending Venography

When further information is needed to plan surgical intervention, an ascending venogram is obtained to map the veins in the extremity and to study the perforator veins in the calf. This study is performed by way of a needle in a dorsal foot vein with the patient semierect at 45 to 60 degrees. With an occluding tourniquet at the ankle to prevent flow in the surface veins, contrast is injected and flow is followed by fluoroscopy as it fills the tibial veins and ascends above the knee. Incompetent perforators are identified by flow from the deep veins to the superficial veins. The usual ascending venogram is then obtained to define the patient tibial, popliteal, superficial, and common femoral veins and to visualize the greater and lesser saphenous veins. In most, the iliac veins are also visualized. The ascending venogram performed in this fashion will diagnose incompetent perforators, obstructed vein segments, and recanalized postthrombotic veins and will provide a map of patent veins in the extremity.

Descending Venography

Descending venograms are performed only on those patients who are probable candidates for valve reconstruction or substitution. It is usually performed by selective technique with a catheter introduced from the other groin.[8] The patient is in the 60-degree erect position, and the vein segments and valves are examined under conditions of both quiet breathing and forced Valsalva, after teaching the patient to do a forced Valsalva maneuver. Individual study of the greater saphenous vein (GSV), SFV, and PFV is important. The valves that are identified are studied for competence with and without Valsalva. When reflux is found, the contrast is followed distally in that segment until it dissipates.

When a valve shows reflux with quiet breathing but becomes competent with Valsalva, it is deemed a competent valve. Conversely, when a valve is competent with quiet breathing and refluxes with Valsalva, it is termed *incompetent.* The Valsalva is important and must be taught to the patient who can be instructed to inflate a balloon or blow a mercury manometer to 40 mm Hg pressure to standardize the force of the Valsalva.

The descending venogram is interpreted in light of the distal extent of reflux. When reflux is limited to the thigh in the deep veins, the patient is not considered to be a candidate for deep valve surgery. When reflux passes through the popliteal vein and into the calf, surgical correction is deemed appropriate. This dependence on the integrity of the popliteal valve has been an arbitrary decision followed throughout my experience with deep vein reconstruction.

Because the descending venogram is a dynamic study, it is necessary that it be performed under fluoroscopy, and it is important that a videotape of the study be made for future analysis.

With the completion of this workup, the surgeon will know the state of patency and of competence in all the veins of the extremity and will be able to compare these findings with the clinical and physiologic data to arrive at a plan for surgery for the individual. In the case of incompetent deep veins, the descending venogram is very accurate in differentiating post-thrombotic secondary valve incompetence (SVI) from nonthrombotic primary incompetence (PVI).

CLASSIFICATION OF DEEP VEIN REFLUX DISEASE

The causes of reflux in the deep veins are PVI, SVI caused by post-thrombotic changes in the veins, and a mixture of proximal PVI in the thigh veins with distal SVI in the calf and popliteal veins. Aplasia is an additional rare cause of reflux.

The occurrence of SVI in the post-thrombotic state is universally recognized. It was described by Homans[9] in 1916 and reported extensively by Bauer[10] in Sweden and Linton[11] in America among many others. This cause of incompetence is due to valve deformity and destruction secondary to the endovenous scarring of the phlebitic process.

Primary valve incompetence was described by Bauer,[10] who was the first to use descending phlebography in the 1940s and found gross leakage of valves in veins that showed no evidence of previous phlebitis. The exact defect of PVI was not understood until this problem was repaired surgically in 1968 by placing reefing sutures on the elongated valve cusp.[1] This development proved the existence of PVI by accurately predicting its presence through descending venography and predictably repairing the defect with surgery on the cusps of the valve. Intraoperative and postoperative studies proved the continued competence of the valve repair.

The existence of combined PVI and SVI has been known since 1968 but not widely discussed. The first patient treated with valve repair was such a patient. Combined PVI/SVI disease is found in the patient who experienced unusually severe venous insufficiency after a relatively localized episode of tibial-popliteal deep vein thrombosis. When this patient was studied, deep vein reflux was found throughout the thigh and calf and not just in the area of the DVT. Descending venography showed that the proximal valves in the thigh were incompetent because of PVI, but the ascending venogram showed that the process in the calf was due to a post-thrombotic disease. The likelihood is that the patient was one with asymptomatic primary valve incompetence in the thigh before the deep vein thrombosis. Because this combination is found in about one-third of my patients with severe reflux disease, I have theorized that the proximal PVI could be a setting in which distal deep vein thrombosis is prone to occur, but convincing evidence has not been published for this possibility.

SURGICAL TECHNIQUES FOR PRIMARY VALVE INCOMPETENCE

The repair of PVI is performed by direct surgery on the valve because the valve is a normal structure with a stretched valve cusp or a dilated vein wall. The original technique of direct valve repair is one of placing interrupted sutures in the valve cusp in such a way that the leading edge of the cusp is progressively shortened (Fig. 39–1) and prolapse of the cusp is prevented.[12] Dilation of the vein is treated by external sutures along the lines of insertion of the valve cusp; these sutures narrow the vein and deepen the cusp, preventing prolapse of the valve cusp margins.

Internal Repair of Valve

The original valvuloplasty operation by the transvalvular approach[12] (Fig. 39–1) was altered by Raju[13] to a supravalvular approach and again by Sottiurai[14] to a supraval-vular approach with a vertical limb into a valve sinus. Both of these modifications have been attempts to make the procedure technically easier, but they retain the same principle of shortening the leading edge of the valve cusp. The results reported from the three techniques are similar, and the choice of procedure is one of individual preference.

External Repair of Valve

A different approach to direct repair is the external approach, which produces narrowing of the vein from outside by either suture or banding techniques. This approach began with a report by Hallberg[15] in Sweden and was followed by sporadic reports of valves that were incompetent by preoperative studies but were found at surgery to be competent when the vein was in a state of constriction, so an external wrap or external sutures were placed to keep the vein at this constricted size. Jessup and Lane[16] then worked out a technique of placing a Silastic cuff around the vein and developed an adjustable appliance called the Venocuff. They experimented with this device in sheep veins extensively and subsequently began human trials with the device in Australia and in the United States. This technique involves placement of a

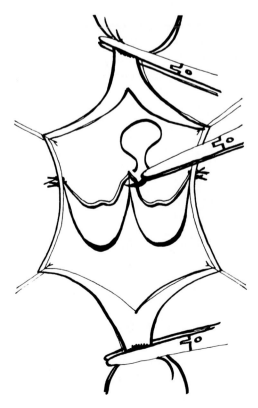

Figure 39–1. Valvuloplasty: one of the steps in valve repair.

Silastic band around the vein at the site of the valve; this band is tightened until all reflux disappears. This approach has the advantage of less dissection and does not require anticoagulation but has the disadvantage that it is not an anatomic precise repair of the valve defect and requires the placement of a foreign body around the vein. Because this procedure is quick and relatively easy to do, it permits multiple valve repairs at different sites such as superficial and profunda femoral veins and popliteal and posterior tibial veins.

A suture technique for external repair was devised in 1987[17] which involves placement of sutures along the lines of insertion of the valve cusp margin from outside the vein. This reliably produces a competent valve at surgery and acts by narrowing and deepening the valve cusp, thereby preventing valve cusp prolapse. Similar to the Venocuff, this technique is simple and quick to perform, but it lacks anatomic precision in that the stretched valve cusp is not shortened. The external suture technique has been modified by Gloviczki et al[18] to a more precise method by use of the angioscope. It is still too early to know the long-term effects of any of these external techniques.

SURGICAL TECHNIQUES FOR SECONDARY VALVE INCOMPETENCE

The techniques for direct valve repair are only useful in the valve of PVI and do not provide a method for restoring competence to patients with post-thrombotic SVI. In SVI, the thrombotic process destroys the valve integrity by scarring of the valve cusps or actual destruction of the valve cusp. Because these valve remnants are essentially nonrepairable, restoration of deep vein competence in these cases requires a new valve from another vein.

Transposition

The first operation used for SVI was the transposition procedure that was introduced in 1978.[19] In this procedure, a proximal competent valve in an adjacent segment is used as the source of proximal competence for the incompetent segment. In the usual

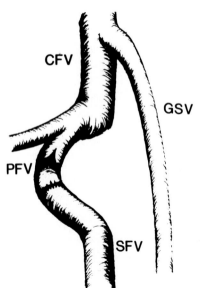

Figure 39–2. Transposition: anastomosis of distal end of divided SFV to proximal divided end of PFV with competent value in PFV.

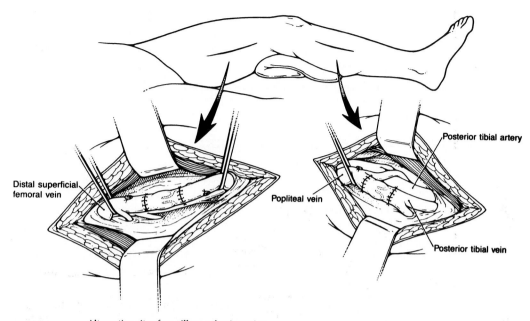

Alternative sites for axillary valve insertion.

Figure 39–3. Transplantation: sites for placement of transplanted vein segment that contains a competent valve *(Reprinted with permission from Raju S. Axillary vein transfer for postphlebotic syndrome. In: Bergman JJ, Kistner RL, eds. Atlas of Venous Surgery. Philadelphia: WB Saunders; 1992:149.)*

instance of a post-thrombotic incompetent SFV–popliteal–tibial system that is adjacent to a competent PFV or greater saphenous vein, the proximal SFV is divided, and the divided distal side is anastomosed to the adjacent competent vein (Fig. 39–2). This may be done by end-to-side or end-to-end technique. There are multiple variations where the incompetent PFV can be anastomosed to the GSV or the SFV, but the principle is that the main source of axial incompetence in the leg is provided with a proximal competent valve.

Transplantation

At about the same time as the transposition operation was introduced, Taheri et al[20] initiated the technique of transplantation of an arm vein containing a competent valve into the incompetent SFV vein, and Raju[21] also experimented with this technique (Fig. 39–3). This approach has the advantage of providing a single competent valve to be placed anywhere in the thigh or popliteal vein that appears most advantageous. After the initial experience with placement of the transplant in the SFV, most surgeons have begun to place this valve in the popliteal vein because they found late dilation of the valve in the SFV with recurrence of valve incompetence during the follow-up period. Raju advocated wrapping the transplanted valve in the SFV with a Dacron sleeve but has not reported the late results of this approach. Taheri et al,[22] Nash,[23] and O'Donnell[24] have all reported improved results up to 4 years with placement of the transplanted vein into the popliteal vein.

EXTERNAL "SUBSTITUTE" VALVE

Another approach to post-thrombotic incompetence at the popliteal level has been that of Psathakis,[25] who introduced the placement of a sling in front of the popliteal vein to act as a valve mechanism during the process of ambulation. This approach has the advantage of great simplicity and has been enthusiastically reported by Psathakis[25] with excellent clinical and physiologic results. The corroborative reports of others are still lacking in the English literature. If this technique could be found effective, it would be a great help because the technique is simple and the location in the popliteal vein seems ideal for the post-thrombotic reflux process.

LITERATURE REPORTS OF SURGICAL RESULTS

Results of surgery after deep vein valve repair can be analyzed by clinical, physiologic, and imaging verification. The most significant of these are the clinical results, because the reason for the operation was to improve the clinical condition. The imaging results are important to confirm that the clinical results are attended by appropriate findings relative to the valve reconstruction. The physiologic results are important as an observation of whether we have learned to measure parameters that are reflective of the clinical state and to see if there are ways to reverse altered physiology in these disease processes.

The reported results from the literature will be classified as clinically good or clinically poor. Good results may have been stratified into good or excellent results by the author, but all these will be regarded as good in this analysis; poor results will comprise everything that is not good in the reports in the literature. When results from different series are organized in this way, the data on the three operations of valvuloplasty, transposition, and transplantation fall into recognizable patterns that appear to be useful.

Valvuloplasty

There are five series of direct valve repair for PVI in the literature that present adequate numbers of cases, comparable follow-up, and similarity of patient selection. They are presented in Table 39–1.

The similarities in these reports are striking in that all show about three-fourths of the cases achieving good results for a minimum of 2 years. There was variability in the management of perforator veins among and between authors,[28–32] but most authors interrupted the perforators at least on a selective basis. In all cases of Eriksson et al,[28] prior perforator surgery had failed to control the patient's symptoms before deep vein reconstruction. This was true in many of the cases of Sottiurai[27] and of Ferris and Kistner[29] as well. In the series of Raju and Fredericks,[26] none of the patients were treated with perforator interruption at the time of valvuloplasty, and we do not know how many of the patients had been treated with perforator surgery before valve surgery. The confusing role of perforator veins in PVI[32] is not clarified by these

TABLE 39–1. VALVULOPLASTY RESULTS IN THE LITERATURE

Author	No. Repaired	Length of Follow-up (mo)	Good Results (%)
Raju & Fredericks[26]	61	24–96	76
Sottiurai[27]	29	56	76
Eriksson et al[28]	27	6–108	70
Ferris and Kistner[29]	32	24–150	80
Perrin et al[31]	22	23	90

reports and their management remains controversial. When the perforators are large (3 mm or greater) incompetent vessels, they should be interrupted.[28,30] When the perforators are small vessels, the necessity of surgical interruption is not clear. When a small incompetent perforator enters an ulcer bed, it should be interrupted to control the clinical problem. In my experience, when small incompetent perforators do not feed an area of induration or ulcer, they can be left in place and are usually not a significant problem in long-term follow-up.

The saphenous veins were ligated or removed by nearly all authors in most of their cases and represent less of a variable than the perforator veins. Raju and Fredericks[26] ligated all the saphenous veins in their cases at the time of valvuloplasty if the veins had not been previously ligated. In the series of Ferris and Kistner,[29] the saphenous vein was only ligated at the time of valvuloplasty when it was shown to be incompetent; there are cases in this series where the saphenous vein was not incompetent and was preserved as a functional part of the venous drainage. In the cases of Eriksson et al,[28] the saphenous vein had been ligated in most instances before valvuloplasty.

The question of what will happen in the very long-term follow-up at 4, 8, and 12 years to the PVI cases is addressed in the report of Ferris and Kistner,[29] where the follow-ups were separated into three groups of 1- to 4-year follow-up, 4- to 8-year follow-up, and 8-years-and-longer follow-up. No difference in results was noted with the passage of time in PVI patients in that report. The SVI patients were too recent to allow analysis. These follow-ups have now been extended to 20 years in my series,[33] and still there are no new cases with recurrent ulcers after 4 years in the PVI cases or beyond 6 years in the SVI cases, indicating that those who are going to have recurrence will usually do so in the first 4 to 6 years after surgery.

Transplantation

This has been a widely practiced approach to post-thrombotic valve reflux problems. The reported results show a wide discrepancy in the six series of cases that dominate the literature as presented in Table 39–2.

The wide discrepancy of reported results is difficult to understand. The experiences of Taheri et al,[22] Nash,[23] and O'Donnell[24] of 75% to 92% good results are strikingly similar and highly enthusiastic. The duration of follow-up in all of these series is comparable, but all are less than 4 years in duration and perhaps longer follow-up will alter these results. The method of follow-up varied; in the report of Taheri et al,[22] much of the follow-up is by a questionnaire, whereas the follow-up of the series of Nash[23] and O'Donnell[24] have been by objective testing with physiologic and imaging methods.

The experiences of Perrin et al,[34] Raju and Fredericks,[26] and Eriksson[35] are

TABLE 39–2. TRANSPLANTATION RESULTS IN THE LITERATURE

Author	No. Repaired	Length of Follow-up (mo)	Good Results (%)
O'Donnell[24]	12	44	92
Raju and Fredericks[26]	24	24–96	44
Taheri et al[22]	48	36	75
Perrin et al[34]	17	28	32
Nash[23]	25	24	80
Eriksson[35]	35	6–60	31

strikingly similar to each other and show a high rate of recurrent disease that is in marked contrast to the experience of Taheri et al,[22] Nash,[23] and O'Donnell.[24] In the experience of Raju and Fredericks[26] and Eriksson[35] there has been a prominent tendency for the transplanted valve to become incompetent coincident with vein segment dilation postoperatively. A cuff of Dacron around the transplant has been placed by Raju, but the results of this modification are not reported to date.

One development over time has been the recommendation of all these investigators to place the valve at the popliteal level rather than the superficial femoral vein level. This has been thought important because there is a better size match between the popliteal and the axillary vein than between the SFV and the axillary vein. An additional and perhaps more cogent reason is that the valve in the popliteal level guards against both SFV and PFV reflux into the calf.

Transposition

The reported experience with transposition surgery has been smaller than that of valvuloplasty and transplantation. In Table 39–3 the reported results of transposition are extracted from multiple series. In each series, except that of Johnson et al,[36] transposition operations were only a small part of the total experience of that author with deep vein reconstruction. Collectively, these cases add up to a total of only 66 reported cases, indicating that the choice of this procedure has been significantly less frequent than the other procedures.

Although there is a marked difference between the lowest and the highest percentages of good results, there appears to be a grouping around the 50% level overall. In my current analysis of the long-term experience in Hawaii, the good results with transposition are 43%, which is in closer agreement to values from the other reported experiences. In the series of Johnson et al,[36] most of the recurrences were edema or pain; only four of 12 (33%) ulcers recurred. The difference in the patients of Johnson et al[36] and the other reports was that the significant perforator and saphenous incompetence states were not treated, so this series is not comparable with the other reports.

There may be a major difference in patient selection for transposition between these series. In the series of Ferris and Kistner,[29] the procedure was performed in conjunction with conventional control of saphenous and perforator problems, and it was only performed when the planned procedure would control all or most of the reflux in the extremity. Because transposition is a proximal procedure, it is only useful when the other segments that are not transposed (i.e., the PFV and GSV do not harbor residual major reflux. In most of the published series, the details of when and why transposition was chosen are not available.

TABLE 39–3. TRANSPOSITION RESULTS IN THE LITERATURE

Author	No. Repaired	Length of Follow-up (mo)	Good Results (%)
Johnson et al[36]	12	24	17
Sottiurai[27]	15	66	20
Ferris and Kistner[29]	14	36	78
Johnson et al[37]	4	48	50
Eriksson[35]	4	12–72	50
Raju[21]	3	24	66
Perrin et al[38]	6	28	50

LATE FOLLOW-UP BEYOND 4 YEARS

We have now reviewed our series of 51 cases, which have been followed for a minimum of 4 years and as long as 21 years: The details of this analysis are submitted for publication.[33] In this analysis, the very long-term good results of valvuloplasty were maintained at more than 70% whereas the results of the transposition procedure fell from the 78% good results reported in 1982 to just more than 40% good results in this latest analysis.

We have now recognized and analyzed three groups of cases in the venous reflux patients, which consist of those with pure PVI, pure SVI, and combined distal SVI with proximal PVI, as discussed earlier in this chapter. The long-term good-to-excellent results reflected in these groups show that in patients with pure PVI there are more than 70% long-term good-to-excellent results, in the PVI/SVI patients there are more than 60% long-term good-to-excellent results, and in those with pure post-thrombotic SVI there are just less than 40% good-to-excellent results. All these categories were followed for longer than 10 years. The specifics of follow-up including clinical, physiologic, and imaging data are detailed in the publication of this series. The overall statistics were that 60% of the cases maintained good-to-excellent results for an average follow-up of 10.5 years.

The operations that were performed for these three groups of valve reflux patients were valvuloplasty for all the PVI and all the PVI/SVI patients. Transposition procedures were performed for all but two of the SVI patients, and these two had transplantation procedures performed. In all three groups, similar numbers of saphenous vein interruptions and perforator procedures were performed.

Results were deemed excellent in this series when the patient was able to return to full activity and remain completely asymptomatic and did not wear elastic support for the duration of the follow-up. Results were classified as good when the patient resumed full activity and remained free of recurrence but did continue to use elastic support.

The 10.5-year results yielded 33% classified as excellent, about 25% classified as good, and 40% classified as poor results because they developed recurrent symptoms. Analysis of the difference between those who had excellent results and those who had poor results showed that the only statistically significant differences were that the valve repair was intact in the excellent group and had failed in most of those in the recurrent group, and the PVI group with more than 70% favorable results fared much better than the SVI group with less than 40% favorable results. The comparison of physiologic data between the excellent and poor groups showed nonsignificant differences as reflected by ambulatory venous pressure (AVP) and PPG data.

The most striking findings in the analysis of very long-term results were that fully one-third of the entire group of patients were classified as excellent. These were cases in whom the individual was able to resume full activity and remain asymptomatic without the need to use elastic support. This represents an essential reversal of the grade 3 CVI syndrome with which the patient presented before surgery. These patients represent the single strongest argument in favor of surgical treatment for chronic venous insufficiency patients.

POSTOPERATIVE PHYSIOLOGIC RESULTS

There is agreement among all the investigators who have written about deep vein reconstruction that there is only partial improvement of the AVP and PPG data between the preoperative and postoperative tests. Many patients do well but have no improvement of the AVP, and other cases show significant improvement of the AVP without an excellent clinical result. The use of these tests to identify the patient with chronic insufficiency is valid, but it does not appear that we can use these tests to predict which patients will do well by comparing preoperative with postoperative data. The fact that these tests remain abnormal after treatment demonstrates that the surgery only partially corrects the problem and the patients are living with clinically compensated but physiologically persistent venous disease.

POSTOPERATIVE PHLEBOGRAPHY STUDIES

Postoperative descending venograms are reported in only about half of those who have had surgery for valve reconstruction in the literature. Of these, postoperative valve competence was maintained in most patients. Significant correlation was found between postoperative valve competence and good results. In the very long-term evaluation of these patients[31] in our series, there was a statistically significant correlation between the presence of a good result and a competent valve, as well as between those who had recurrent ulcers and the occurrence of recurrent valve incompetence. This has also been reported by Sottiurai.[27]

PRESENT STATUS OF VALVE REPAIR

After nearly 25 years of deep vein reconstruction for reflux disease, there are a few lessons learned and many questions to be answered. We know that reflux is a dominant factor in most patients with severe chronic venous insufficiency, and this reflux affects the saphenous, perforator, and deep veins. We have established that reflux in the deep system occurs in a primary form (PVI) as well as in the secondary post-thrombotic state (SVI) and results in similar symptoms regardless of etiology.

We now know that surgery can be performed with predictable safety in the deep veins of patients with severe venous reflux states. We know that PVI can be treated with direct valve repair, and if this is combined with conventional surgical treatment of the perforator and saphenous veins, about three-fourths of these patients will retain good results free of recurrent ulcers and pain for more than 10 years. It appears that about one-third of the patients will be so completely compensated after surgical treatment that they will not even need to wear support stockings over the long term.

Patients who have reflux caused by post-thrombotic SVI have a significantly higher rate of recurrence after surgical treatment with transposition than the PVI patient with the use of valvuloplasty surgery. The final answer is not yet reported for the long-term results with transplantation surgery, but there are a sufficient number of series with high recurrence rates after transplantation surgery that it is doubtful that the present techniques will achieve the long-term good results found with valvuloplasty surgery in PVI disease. The post-thrombotic patient who has a repairable valve in the proximal thigh may have better long-term outlook (60% free of late recurrence) than the patient who has no repairable proximal valve (35% to 50% free of recurrence).

We know that the ambulatory venous pressure and PPG abnormalities only correct to a mild-moderate degree after venous reflux surgery, and the persistence of abnormal values does not statistically relate to a poor clinical result. These studies are qualitative and are accurate in determining patients who have chronic venous insufficiency but are not able to separate clinically compensated deep vein disease from decompensated venous disease.

The quality of the postoperative clinical result is significantly related to the competence of the proximal deep veins. When these valves remain competent, the clinical result tends to be good, and when they are incompetent, poor results are prone to occur.

The widely reported finding of better long-term results after valvuloplasty than after transposition and transplantation surgery may relate more to the fact that valvuloplasty is performed for PVI, whereas the other procedures are performed for post-thrombotic disease. It appears that the post-thrombotic limb is more seriously disadvantaged by its disease process than the limb with PVI.

It appears that patients who have repair of all the venous reflux abnormalities in the extremity have an improved long-term result when compared with those who only have repair of some of the reflux defects.[30] It appears preferable to treat the saphenous, perforator, and deep veins in patients in whom all these systems are significantly abnormal at the time of the initial venous evaluation. Poor results are prone to occur when only the deep veins are repaired and significant disease in the saphenous and perforator veins are left untreated.

We do not know the relative merits of repair of multiple valves versus repair of one valve. We are not certain whether the placement of the valve should be in the popliteal or in the superficial femoral vein, but it seems that wherever the newly competent valve is placed, it needs to control proximal incompetence in both the profunda and the superficial femoral venous branches. We do not yet know the long-term results of external valve repair.

It will not be possible to compare the relative efficacy of nonsurgical versus surgical treatment or the relative merits of treatment by different surgical methods until we establish objective criteria for classification, diagnosis, and postoperative evaluation of all the patients with chronic venous insufficiency.

The time has come to initiate standardized protocols for diagnosis in chronic venous disease and to agree on one classification of chronic venous disease based on clinical, physiologic, and imaging criteria. With these basics in place, it will be possible to conduct comparative treatment trials on a multicenter basis so that answers can be obtained about the validity of various types of management in chronic venous insufficiency.

REFERENCES

1. Kistner RL. Surgical repair of a venous valve. *Straub Clin Proc.* 1968;34:41–43.
2. Kistner RL. Surgical repair of the incompetent femoral valve. *Arch Surg.* 1975;110:1336–1342.
3. Killewich LA, Martin R, Cramer M, et al. An objective assessment of the physiologic changes in the post-thrombotic syndrome. *Arch Surg.* 1985;120:424–426.
4. Wilson NM, Rutt DL, Browse NL. Repair and replacement of deep vein valves in the treatment of venous insufficiency. *Br J Surg.* 1991;78:388–394.
5. Mayberry JC, Moneta GL, Taylor LM, et al. Fifteen year results of ambulatory compression therapy for chronic venous ulcers. *Surgery.* 1991;109:575–581.
6. Porter JM, Rutherford RB, Clagett GP, et al. Reporting standards in venous disease. *J Vasc Surg.* 1988;8:172–181.
7. Christopoulis D, Nicolaides AN, Galloway JMD, et al. Objective non-invasive evaluation of venous surgical results. *J Vasc Surg.* 1988;8:683–687.
8. Kamida CB, Kistner RL. Descending phlebography: the Straub technique. In: Bergan JJ, Kistner RL, eds. *Atlas of Venous Surgery.* Philadelphia: WB Saunders; 1992:105–109.

9. Homans J. Operative treatment of varicose veins and ulcers. *Surg Gynecol Obstet.* 1916;22:143–158.

10. Bauer G. The etiology of leg ulcers and their treatment by resection of the popliteal vein. *J Int Chir.* 1948;8:937–967.

11. Linton RR. Modern concepts in the treatment of the post-phlebitic syndrome with ulceration of the lower extremity. *Angiology.* 1952;3:431–439.

12. Kistner RL. Valve reconstruction for primary valve insufficiency. In: Bergan JS, Kistner RL, eds. *Atlas of Venous Surgery.* Philadelphia: WB Saunders; 1992:105–109.

13. Raju S. Valvuloplasty and valve transfer. *Int Angiol.* 1985;4:419–424.

14. Sottiuari VS. Technique in direct venous valvuloplasty. *J Vasc Surg.* 1988;8:646–648.

15. Hallberg D. A method for repairing incompetent valves in deep veins. *Acta Chir Scand.* 1972;138:143–145.

16. Jessup G, Lane RJ. Repair of incompetent venous valves: a new technique. *J Vasc Surg.* 1988;8:569–575.

17. Kistner R. Surgical technique of external venous valve repair. *Straub Found Proc.* 1990;55:15–16.

18. Gloviczki P, Merrell SW, Bower TC. Femoral vein valve repair under direct vision without venotomy: a modified technique with angioscopy. *J Vasc Surg.* 1991;14:645–648.

19. Kistner RL, Sparkuhl MD. Surgery in acute and chronic venous disease. *Surgery.* 1979;85:31–43.

20. Taheri SA, Lazar L, Elias SM, et al. Vein valve transplant. *Surgery.* 1982;91:28–33.

21. Raju S. Venous insufficiency of the lower limb and stasis ulceration: changing concepts in management. *Ann Surg.* 1983;197:688–697.

22. Taheri SA, Elias SM, Yacogucci MD, et al. Indications and results of vein valve transplant. *J Cardiovasc Surg.* 1986;27:163–168.

23. Nash T. Long term results of vein valve transplants placed in the popliteal vein for intractable post-phlebitic venous ulcers and pre-ulcer skin changes. *J Cardiovasc Surg.* 1988;29:712–716.

24. O'Donnell TF. Popliteal vein valve transplantation for deep venous valvular reflux: rationale, method, and long-term clinical, hemodynamic and anatomic results. In: Bergan JJ, Yao JST, eds. *Venous Disorders.* Philadelphia: WB Saunders; 1991:273–295.

25. Psathakis ND. The substitute valve: operation by technique II in patients with post-thrombotic syndrome. *Surgery.* 1984;95:542–548.

26. Raju S, Fredericks R. Valve reconstruction procedures for non-obstructive venous insufficiency: rationale, techniques, and results in 107 procedures with two-to-eight-year followup. *J Vasc Surg.* 1988;7:301–310.

27. Sottiurai VS. Comparison of surgical modalities in the treatment of recurrent venous ulcer. *Int Angiol.* 1991;9:231–235.

28. Eriksson I, Almgren B, Nordgren L. Late results after venous valve repair. *J Int Angiol.* 1985;4:413–417.

29. Ferris EB, Kistner RL. Femoral vein reconstruction in the management of chronic venous insufficiency: a 14 year experience. *Arch Surg.* 1982;117:1571–1579.

30. DePalma RB. Surgical treatment of chronic venous ulceration. In: Bergan JJ, Yao JST, eds. *Venous Disorders.* Philadelphia: WB Saunders; 1991:396–404.

31. Perrin M, Hiltbrand B, Bergen JM. La reparation valvulaire au niveau du Reseau Veineux Profond sous-inguinal Ganget Technique ou Intervention efficace. *Phlebologie.* 1991;44:649–660.

32. Queral LA, Whitehouse WM, Flinn WR, et al. Surgical correction of chronic deep venous insufficiency by valvular transposition. *Surgery.* 1980;87:688–695.

33. Masuda E, Kistner R. 4–20 Year results of valve surgery. Presented at Society of Vascular Surgery, June 1992, Chicago. Submitted for publication.

34. Perrin M, Bolot JE, Genevoia A, et al. Interposition d'un seqment veineux valvale dans les sequelles de phlebite des frones veineux profonds des membres **inferieurs**. Resultats preliminaires. *Lyon Chir.* 1986;82:211–215.

35. Eriksson I. Reconstructive surgery for deep vein valve incompetence in the lower limb. *Eur J Vasc Surg.* 1990;4:211–218.

36. Johnson ND, Quebal LA, Flinn WR, et al. Late objective assessment of venous valve surgery. *Arch Surg.* 1981;116:1461–1466.
37. Johnson WC, Nagseth DS, Bush HL, et al. Direct venous surgery for venous valvular insufficiency of the lower extremity: updated experience. *Contemp Surg.* 1985;26:35–43.
38. Perrin M, Hiltbrand B, Bolot JE, et al. Resultats de la chirurgie veineuse restauratrice dans les reflux de lu voie veineude profonde au niveau des membres inferieurs. *Proc. 10 eme Congress Mondial Union Internationale de Phlebologie.* Strasbourg:John Libby; 1989:1085–1086.

40

Venous Trauma:

Long-Term Follow-Up of Venous Repair

Timothy J. Nypaver, MD, and James J. Schuler, MD

Because of an increase in urban violence, an increasing number of traumatic venous injuries are being encountered in the civilian setting.[1,2] Although repair of such injuries is now generally favored over ligation, several aspects of the management of venous injuries have remained controversial.[2-4] Although few would argue against lateral venorrhaphy for simple well-localized injuries, the appropriateness of more complex reconstructions such as interposition graft repair has been questioned.[5-7] This controversy of reconstruction versus ligation has persisted, in part, because of the relative paucity of information concerning the long-term clinical, hemodynamic, and patency results of venous repair.

BACKGROUND INFORMATION

It is well recognized that the adverse sequelae of venous injury may not become apparent for years after the initiating traumatic event. Venous injuries can produce and result in significant disability and societal economic burden through the development of chronic venous insufficiency and a postphlebitic extremity. Thus, in any discussion concerning venous repair outcome, the long-term results are of vital and critical importance. Despite this, a large base of information concerning the long-term outcome of venous repair is lacking. The major factors that have precluded this long-term evaluation include (a) the noncompliant and migratory nature of many individuals in the civilian trauma population; (b) the unreliability of clinical examination in determining venous patency at the repair site; and (c) the prior necessity of performing invasive venography to accurately determine repair patency. The advent of high-resolution, real-time ultrasound imaging combined with Doppler signal analysis (duplex scanning) has now provided an accurate and noninvasive means of assessing repair patency in the postoperative period.

This chapter encompasses a review of both the military and civilian trauma experiences in the management of venous injuries, concentrating on the long-term results reported with each. A recent study of 32 patients with extremity venous reconstruction performed for traumatic vascular injury and their long-term (mean follow-up longer than 4 years) follow-up will serve as the basis for this review.

MANAGEMENT OF THE ACUTE VENOUS INJURY

Most traumatic venous injuries are penetrating in nature, often occur in association with a concomitant arterial injury, and most often involve the extremities.[2] Although in the past there had been considerable reluctance to repair injured veins for fear of deep venous thrombosis and pulmonary embolus, subsequent reports, comprising both military[8–10] and civilian experiences,[3,11–14] have consistently verified the inaccuracy of this belief. Thus, a more aggressive approach to the repair of venous injuries was advocated[15,16] and adopted by many major trauma centers.

The objectives of the surgeon in the management of extremity venous trauma are threefold: (a) control hemorrhage; (b) ensure limb salvage; and (c) prevent or reduce the long-term sequelae of venous insufficiency. The rationale for the surgeons approach depends on a multitude of factors, including hemodynamic stability of the patient, location of injury, existence and nature of concomitant injuries, and extent of venous injury. Although repair is preferable, venous ligation, following the basic surgical tenet of "life before limb," remains an indispensable simple method for accomplishing rapid hemostasis, invaluable in the management of the unstable or multiply-injured patient. Ligation of upper extremity venous injuries, because of a reduced hydrostatic pressure, smaller minute volume blood flow, and more collateral pathways in comparison with that of the lower extremity, can generally be performed without consequence.[3,11,14] Even so, reconstruction of large-caliber upper extremity venous injuries, particularly when related to massive injuries in which all venous return has been interrupted, is often warranted. An additional circumstance in which upper extremity venous repair assumes vital importance is in upper extremity replantation after traumatic amputation.[17] Experience with internal jugular venous trauma is limited; however, ligation in the absence of bilateral involvement is well-tolerated. Reconstruction of the internal jugular vein should be considered in bilateral injuries and when simple lateral venorrhaphy can accomplish the repair.

In lower extremity injuries, however, because of an increased hydrostatic pressure and fewer collateral pathways, venous ligation may dispose the patient to the development of venous hypertension and chronic venous insufficiency. Venous valvular insufficiency will result in varying degrees of disability with symptoms of pain, edema, lipodermatosclerosis, hyperpigmentation, and ulceration of the affected extremity. Avoidance of a postphlebitic limb through the reconstruction of axial patency and maintenance of venous competence is the long-term objective of venous trauma reconstruction.

OPERATIVE PRINCIPLES

The types of reconstructions available to the surgeon include, in order of increasing complexity, (a) lateral venorrhaphy (simple repair); (b) end-to-end anastomotic repair; (c) patch repair; and (d) interposition graft repair. In the hemodynamically stable patient, the type of repair performed is primarily dependent on the extent of the venous injury. Lateral venorrhaphy, or simple repair, can be performed expeditiously, controls hemorrhage, and should be applied in all venous injuries in which the luminal diameter will not be significantly reduced. Patch grafts can be used to prevent excessive constriction of the lumen. An end-to-end anastomosis, when performed without sacrificing major collateral vessels and when possible without creating undue tension on the suture line, is also an acceptable repair method.

However, in extensive and complex injuries in which a significant portion of vein is destroyed or damaged, interposition graft repair will be required to restore venous outflow.

Autogenous greater saphenous vein (GSV), usually harvested from the contralateral extremity, is the graft material of choice. Use of ipsilateral GSV should be avoided to not disrupt potential collateral pathways for venous outflow of the traumatized limb. If the GSV is not available, other autogenous sources include the lesser saphenous vein, the cephalic or basilic veins, and the internal jugular vein.[18,19] Prosthetic material, because of low flow and high propensity for thrombosis, is generally not an acceptable conduit for extremity venous repairs. Prosthetic material may be useful in larger-caliber venous reconstruction, such as that of the vena cava; however, its use cannot be recommended in contaminated wounds because of an increased risk of infection. When major size discrepancy between native vein and the autogenous graft is problematic, a composite paneled or spiral graft can be constructed to approximate the adjacent venous luminal diameter (Fig. 40–1). The intention is to allow for preservation of venous endothelium and normalization of venous hemodynamics and flow, thereby reducing the potential for thrombosis.

Other operative principles include meticulous surgical technique, use of monofilament suture, either interrupted or continuous, to loosely approximate tissue edges, and systemic heparinization whenever concomitant injuries do not preclude its use. Manual expression or gentle catheter thrombectomy of proximal or distal thrombus may be required, with care not to disrupt native venous valves. In cases of combined arterial and venous injuries, except in the presence of severe limb ischemia, the venous repair is generally accomplished first to ensure that no proximal or distal

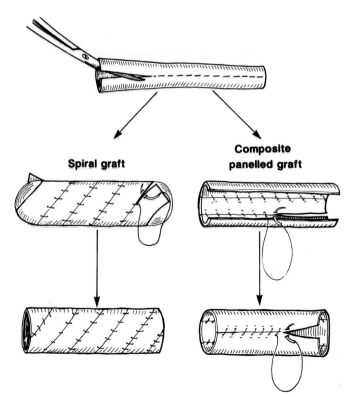

Spiral graft

Composite paneled graft

Figure 40–1. Construction of a large-diameter autogenous interposition conduit from a segment(s) of saphenous vein using a spiral or a composite paneled technique.

propagation of thrombus occurs. Although the results of clinical studies are not conclusive, other adjunctive measures including use of dextran, heparin, and intermittent calf compression may be useful in preventing postreconstructive thrombosis.[12,20,21] The use of a temporary arteriovenous shunt to improve patency rates has been recommended; however, most have limited experience with this technique.[22,23] Liberal use of fasciotomy, either prophylactic or therapeutic, is recommended for injuries in which compartmental hypertension exists or is likely to develop. This is particularly true for combined popliteal arterial and venous injuries. Postoperative limb elevation is routinely practiced and should be strictly enforced for all venous injuries.

EARLY RESULTS OF VENOUS REPAIR

The long-term outcome of venous repair is dependent on the early postoperative results, especially that of patency, achieved by that repair. Venous repairs do exhibit a high propensity to thrombose in the early postoperative period. Factors that contribute to this high incidence of graft failure include low venous pressure and flow, graft-to-host vessel size discrepancy, traumatic disruption of the endothelium, and a hypercoagulable state induced by the trauma itself.[20,24] Military and civilian series of venous trauma, with venography to determine venous repair status, have documented an overall early thrombosis rate between 16% and 58%.[12,25-28] Meyer et al[25] performed venography on postoperative day 7 on 36 venous repairs and found a thrombosis rate of 21% for local venous repair (lateral venorrhaphy, end-to-end anastomotic, and vein patch repair) and 59% for those requiring interposition grafting.[25] The more complex the type of reconstruction, the higher the likelihood of early repair thrombosis. Thrombosis of the repair site, however, did not appear to adversely affect the short-term surgical results.[25] It has been postulated that the initial patency of the venous repair may allow time for the development of collaterals such that when the repair does occlude, collateral pathways have developed and venous hypertension is avoided.[2]

Three primary questions emerge concerning the long-term results of venous repair: (a) What is the overall long-term clinical and hemodynamic outcome of venous reconstruction as compared with that of venous ligation? (b) what is the long-term patency of venous reconstruction? and (c) what is the natural history of early repair thrombosis and how does this thrombosis impact on the long-term clinical and hemodynamic outcome? We attempt to provide answers to these questions through an analysis and review of the data provided by the military experience and the available series of civilian venous trauma.

LONG-TERM RESULTS OF VENOUS REPAIR

Military Experience

Although repair of arterial injuries was accepted practice throughout the Korean War,[29] the significance and morbidity of venous injuries were not completely recognized until the Vietnam conflict. The trauma experience in Vietnam and the late follow-up provided by the Vietnam Vascular Registry at Walter Reed Army Hospital defined the importance of associated venous trauma as a factor in limb salvage, postoperative edema, and the late sequelae of venous insufficiency.[8,27,30,31] In addition, and perhaps more importantly, this work disproved the then-accepted notion that venous reconstruction would result in a higher rate of deep vein thrombosis and pulmonary embolus. There were no clinically recognized cases of pulmonary embolization after vein repair in the initial Vietnam series, which included 124 venous repairs.[31]

In a review of 1,000 cases of arterial injuries suffered during the Vietnam conflict, nearly 38% had a concomitant venous injury. It was duly noted that this number likely represented an underestimation of the actual incidence because of the reluctance of many military surgeons to report venous injuries early in the conflict.[30] A retrospective analysis of 125 popliteal arterial injuries that resulted in amputation found that 80% were associated with a concomitant venous injury; of those with a venous injury, more than 80% were managed by venous ligation. Concomitant venous and arterial injuries had resulted in a higher rate of limb loss than arterial injuries alone.[8-10] An earlier report by Sullivan et al[27] emphasized the significance of popliteal venous injury in terms of limb salvage and prevention of massive postoperative edema. Of 26 patients with popliteal vein injury, 21 were repaired at the time of initial operation, and none of these developed significant edema postoperatively. In contrast, in the four managed by primary ligation, all were complicated by the development of massive edema and compartmental hypertension.[27] More recent military experience, from the Lebanese War, in the management of combined arterial and venous injuries has also emphasized the importance of venous reconstruction in optimizing the short-term surgical results.[32]

Long-term follow-up of these military injuries has been provided through the Vietnam Vascular Registry. In a review of 110 cases of popliteal vein injury at follow-up evaluation, 51% of the patients managed by ligation demonstrated edema in comparison with 13% of those managed by repair.[33] In a complementary study of 51 Vietnam casualties who had interposition vein graft repair for lower extremity injuries at 10-year follow-up, a 12% incidence of residual edema was noted.[34] Rich and Sullivan[35] also demonstrated, through sequential postoperative venograms, the potential for a thrombosed venous repair to undergo recanalization.

Civilian Experience

The military experience in Southeast Asia stimulated interest in the management of civilian traumatic venous injuries. However, the conclusions derived from this military experience, often involving high-velocity injuries with significant soft tissue destruction, may not be applicable in the setting of civilian vascular trauma.

Our series of long-term follow-up of venous repair consists of 32 patients who had undergone venous reconstruction for an extremity vascular injury and who were available for long-term clinical and noninvasive vascular laboratory evaluation. Specifically, we sought to define the long-term physiologic results and patency of extremity venous repair and, by comparison with the immediate postsurgical results, to determine the natural history of venous repair in a civilian trauma population.

Patients and Methods

In January 1981 to December 1990, 83 patients underwent venous reconstruction on the Vascular Surgery services at Cook County Hospital and the University of Illinois Hospital in the management of major extremity venous injury. This was confined to those patients in whom axial reconstruction of the deep venous system was per-

TABLE 40–1. MECHANISM OF INJURY

	No.	%
Gunshot wound	18	56
Laceration/stab wound	10	32
Blunt injury	2	6
Shotgun wound	1	3
Iatrogenic injury	1	3
Total	32	100
Penetrating	30	94
Blunt	2	6

formed and excluded those with primary venous ligation. Thirty-two patients comprised our study group, which consisted of 31 male patients and one female patient. The average age was 29 years, with a range of 15 to 51 years. The time period from operation to follow-up evaluation averaged 49 months and ranged from 6 to 108 months. The noninvasive vascular laboratory assessment consisted of venous Doppler (VD), impedance plethysmography (IPG), photoplethysmography (PPG) (lower extremities only), and color-flow duplex scanning (CFDS). Venous Doppler, IPG, and PPG were performed on both the injured and noninjured contralateral extremity to allow for comparison between the two, whereas CFDS was isolated to the injured limb. Table 40–1 lists the mechanism of injury for these 32 patients; overall 30 (94%) of injuries were penetrating and two (6%) were blunt. Most venous injuries were discovered at the time of initial exploration for a known or suspected arterial injury. There were 26 lower extremity injuries and six involving the upper extremity (Tables 40–2 and 40–3).

The lower extremity venous reconstructions included 16 lateral venorrhaphies (62%), four vein patch repairs (15%), two end-to-end repairs (8%), and four interposition graft repairs (15%). Twenty-two patients (85%) had an associated arterial injury in proximity to the venous injury that required concomitant repair. Fractures or dislocations, requiring orthopedic stabilization, were present in six patients (23%). Only one patient suffered a peripheral nerve injury as a direct result of the inflicting agent. Based on clinical determination, four-compartment calf fasciotomy was performed in 12 patients (46%).

Sixteen of the 26 patients underwent ascending venography in the early postoperative period (mean, 9.4 days; range, 4 to 33 days) for evaluation of venous repair patency. Patients with documented repair thrombosis were placed on an anticoagulation regimen, consisting of initial intravenous heparin followed by conversion to warfarin. Oral anticoagulation was then continued for a period of 3 months.

In contrast, of the six upper extremity venous injuries, repair consisted of two

TABLE 40–2. LOWER EXTREMITY VENOUS INJURIES

	No.	%
External iliac vein	1	4
Common femoral vein	4	15
Superficial femoral vein	16	62
Popliteal vein	5	19
Total	26	100

TABLE 40–3. UPPER EXTREMITY VENOUS INJURIES

	No.	%
Axillary vein	1	17
Brachial vein	5	83
Total	6	100

lateral venorrhaphies (33%), one end-to-end repair (17%), and three interposition grafts (50%). Four of the six injuries involved near-complete neurovascular disruption at the elbow joint incurred as a result of severe lacerations from falls or accidents. Four patients suffered a significant direct peripheral nerve injury and one patient (17%) required a forearm fasciotomy.

Postoperatively, all injured extremities were elevated, wrapped in compressive dressings, and, when possible, had application of intermittent sequential compression devices. No protocol existed for the routine use of either dextran or heparin postoperatively, and in general, these measures were not used.

Results—Lower Extremity

Early postoperative venography was performed on 16 patients and yielded the following results: Eight repairs (50%) were thrombosed whereas repair patency was documented in the remaining eight (50%). The eight thrombosed repairs included three lateral venorrhaphies, three interposition grafts, and two vein patch repairs. All arterial repairs remained patent, and no patient required a secondary vascular operation after their initial reconstruction.

In the early postoperative period, within 3 months from the time of their repair, three patients developed symptomatic extensive deep vein thrombosis (DVT). These DVTs were documented on venography and involved not just the isolated repair site but extended throughout the deep venous system. One of these patients did suffer a nonfatal documented pulmonary embolus. There were no additional or subsequent cases of DVT or pulmonary embolus.

On follow-up clinical evaluation, these three patients were the only ones who exhibited signs and symptoms of chronic venous insufficiency. Three had hyperpigmentation of the involved extremity; two had significant clinical edema requiring the application of support stockings. No patient in follow-up manifested venous ulceration. An additional five patients noted mild asymptomatic swelling of the involved extremity with prolonged dependent positioning of the limb but did not experience discomfort or require elastic support stockings. At the time of their follow-up clinical evaluation, no edema or asymmetric swelling of the extremity could be detected. All arterial repairs were patent and limb salvage was 100%.

Photoplethysmography with measurement of venous refilling times was performed on 25 of the 26 patients with lower extremity venous trauma. The overall venous refilling time of the injured extremity as assessed by PPG (34.9 ± 16.2) did not differ from that of the noninjured contralateral extremity (36.8 ± 16.1) (Fig. 40–2). Table 40–4 represents the overall results of the lower extremity noninvasive tests, the VD, IPG, and PPG, expressed as the percentage of abnormal studies for the injured and noninjured extremity. There were no significant differences in the percentage of abnormal tests between the injured and noninjured extremity with regard to VD or PPG. A higher proportion of patients had an abnormal or borderline IPG study in the limb in which the venous reconstruction was performed in contrast to the contralateral extremity in which all IPG studies were interpreted as normal.

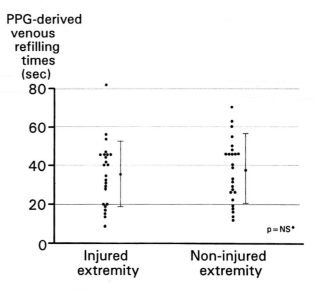

Figure 40–2. Comparison of venous refilling times of injured extremity to contralateral noninjured extremity. Injured extremity (34.9 ± 16.2 second) versus contralateral noninjured extremity (36.8 ± 16.1 second). (*P* = .5 paired Student's *t*-test.)

The results of the CFDS for the lower extremity repairs were as follows: one repair thrombosed, one indeterminate, and 24 patent (Table 40–5). Thus, of the 25 repairs successfully imaged, 96% were determined to be patent. Although classified as patent, four repairs exhibited an abnormality in venous flow or architecture as detected on CFDS. These duplex abnormalities consisted of hemodynamic alterations in flow, increased echogenicity of the venous wall, and an eccentric venous lumen.

Of the eight repairs that were initially determined to be patent, all remained patent on follow-up CFDS. Of the eight repairs that were occluded on postoperative venography, seven were now assessed by CFDS to be patent. Thus, seven patients, with their repair sites previously thrombosed, were now determined by CFDS to have restoration of patency (Table 40–6). The single repair site that remained thrombosed involved a lateral venorrhaphy repair to the superficial femoral vein; this patient had the shortest time interval (6 months) from injury to follow-up evaluation. Within this group of seven patients, two, both of whom had their postoperative course complicated by extension of repair thrombosis to major deep vein thrombosis, demonstrated significant clinical edema on follow-up evaluation. One patient had had an interposition graft repair and was found to have an abnormal venous refilling time on PPG. The other had undergone a lateral venorrhaphy repair of the common femoral vein; although the PPG venous refilling time in this patient was normal, the IPG was abnormal and the CFDS revealed a high-grade stenosis at the repair site. An additional three patients manifested mild asymmetric swelling, which was asymp-

TABLE 40–4. NONINVASIVE LOWER EXTREMITY VENOUS EVALUATION: INJURED EXTREMITY VERSUS NONINJURED EXTREMITY

	Injured Extremity (% Abnormal Test)	Noninjured Extremity (% Abnormal Test)	*P*
Venous Doppler	2/25 (8%)	0/24 (0%)	NS
Impedance plethysmography (IPG)	6/25 (24%)	0/24 (0%)	.029
Photoplethysmography (PPG) (<20 sec)	5/25 (25%)	5/25 (25%)	NS
Venous refilling times (PPG) (*n* = 25) (sec)	34.6 ± 16.2	36.8 ± 16.1	NS

TABLE 40–5. VENOUS PATENCY OF LOCATION OF REPAIR

	Patent	Occluded	Total	% Patent
Common femoral	4		4	100
Superficial femoral	15	1	16	94
Popliteal	5		5	100
Axillary vein	1		1	100
Brachial	3	2	5	60
Total	28	3	31	91
Lower extremity[a]	24	1	25	96
Upper extremity[a]	4	2	6	66

[a] $P > .25$.

tomatic, occurred only with prolonged dependency, and did not limit activity or present any inconvenience to the patient. The venous refilling times in those with early repair thrombosis ($n = 8$) did not differ significantly from the limbs with early repair patency ($n = 7$): 31.00 ± 12.7 versus 34.7 ± 15.2 ($P > .05$) (Fig. 40–3).

Results—Upper Extremity

No patient in the upper extremity venous reconstruction group demonstrated any sign or symptoms related to venous hypertension or insufficiency. Not surprisingly, the major functional disability for these patients was not related to the vascular injury, but to the peripheral nerve injury, with 50% of patients demonstrating some residual neurologic deficit.

Color-flow duplex scanning of the upper extremity injuries revealed the following results: two repairs patent without abnormality, two patent although stenotic, and two occluded (Table 40–5). One injury, that to the axillary vein, underwent probable recanalization, with early postoperative venography revealing repair thrombosis and follow-up CFDS demonstrating a patent albeit stenotic repair site.

Overall, including both the upper and lower extremities, 91% of venous repairs were determined to be patent. There were no differences in the long-term patency achieved between the types of reconstructions performed (Table 40–7).

DISCUSSION

Centers adopting an aggressive approach to venous injuries have cited the superiority of venous reconstruction over ligation in terms of limb salvage and reduction in

TABLE 40–6. COMPARISON OF EARLY VERSUS LATE PATENCY BY TYPE OF REPAIR

Type of repair	Early Patency (Venography)				Late Patency (CFDS)			
	Patent	Occluded	Total	Patent (%)	Patent	Occluded	Total	Patent (%)
Lateral suture	3	3	6	50	5	1	6	83
Vein patch repair	2	2	4	50	4	0	4	100
End-to-end repair	2	0	2	100	2	0	2	100
Interposition vein graft	1	3	4	25	4	0	4	100
Total	8	8	16	50	15	1	16	94

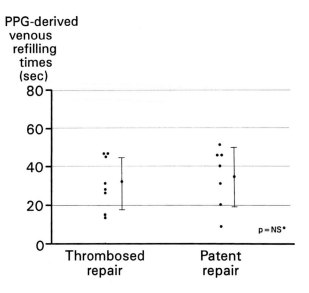

Figure 40–3. Comparison of venous refilling times of extremities with venographically documented early postoperative thrombosis versus those extremities with documented early patency. Extremities with early repair thrombosis (31.0 ± 12.7 second) versus extremities with early repair patency (34.7 ± 15.2 second). (*P* = .6 Student's *t*-test.)

postoperative morbidity.[3,12,22,36,37] In particular, with combined popliteal arterial and venous injuries, ligation has been associated with a higher incidence of limb loss and local complications.[9,10,27,38,39] Thus, unless contraindicated because of hemodynamic instability, reconstruction of the popliteal vein is advocated.[38–41]

Because of the difficulties in obtaining long-term follow-up data of venous repair, most series have been confined to short-term or immediate postsurgical results.[3,11,12,14,22] What long-term follow-up studies are available have generally been limited to clinical results and have been deficient in information concerning the functional hemodynamic condition of the limb or patency status of the repair. Although experimental data have provided considerable insight into the physiologic effect of acute venous interruption and hypertension,[41,42] a model to define the chronic physiologic changes associated with venous interruption has yet to be developed. Thus, conclusions regarding the long-term results of venous repair are often based on a limited number of patients, reflecting a small percentage of the actual number of repairs being performed.

Borman et al[4] by defining repair patency on early postoperative venography, at a mean follow-up of 27 months, determined that 74% of patients with patent repairs had normal limbs compared with 38% of patients with occluded repairs. At latest follow-up, edema was present in 13% of those with patent repairs, 23% of those with occluded repairs, and 42% of those managed by ligation.[4] Other series, at varying lengths of follow-up, have demonstrated an edema rate between 12% to 45% for venous reconstruction (Table 40–8).[4,26,34,43,44] In contrast, Aitken et al[26] demonstrated a

TABLE 40–7. VENOUS PATENCY BY TYPE OF REPAIR

	Patent	Occluded	Total	% Patent
Lateral venorrhaphy	17	1	18	94
Vein patch repair	4		4	100
End-to-end repair	2	1	3	66
Interposition graft	6	1	7	86
Total	29	3	32	91

TABLE 40–8. LONG-TERM FOLLOW-UP OF POST-TRAUMATIC LOWER EXTREMITY VENOUS RECONSTRUCTION

Reference (Year)	No. Patients	Mean Follow-up	Edema/Chronic Venous Insufficiency (%)	Early Patency (%)	Late Patency (%)
Rich et al[10] (1976)	51	10 yr	12		
Phifer et al[44] (1985)	6	6–20 yr	16.6		83
Bormon et al[4] (1987)	36	27 mo	16.6	63	
Aitken et al[26] (1989)	20	19.5 mo	45		55
UIH CCH[a] (1992)	26	47.4 mo	11.5	50[b]	96

[a] University of Illinois Hospital/Cook County Hospital.
[b] Determined for 16 patients.

postoperative clinical edema rate of 83% in those patients undergoing venous ligation. In a review of 169 iliac vein injuries, Burch et al[45] demonstrated a 21% incidence of chronic venous insufficiency in those undergoing ligation compared with 0% for those with reconstruction.

Although this evidence supports an aggressive approach to the reconstruction of venous injuries, other investigators have demonstrated comparable results with ligation. Mullins et al[5] reported a 23% incidence of postoperative edema in follow-up of patients managed by venous ligation. Likewise, Timberlake et al[6] and Hardin et al[7] attained minimal morbidity (3.5% late sequelae) in follow-up of patients managed by ligation. These reports have emphasized the liberal use of fasciotomy and postoperative elevation of the extremity in the prevention of postligation complications. Venous ligation did not predispose to an increased risk of lower extremity amputation in these important studies. However, a noted shortcoming of these studies is their reliance solely on clinical examination, with no information concerning the functional and physiologic status of the affected limb. Although adherence to a protocol of aggressive limb elevation, limb compression, and liberal use of fasciotomy may eliminate or resolve the problems associated with early or transient postoperative edema in the absence of hemodynamic information, it remains possible that these patients have an underlying venous valvular insufficiency that will subsequently become symptomatic. Aitken et al[26] demonstrated that in six patients in whom venous ligation was performed, on follow-up 86% had abnormal venous function of the affected extremity. In addition, those patients who underwent ligation or had a thrombosed repair on follow-up had a shorter venous refilling time compared with those in whom the repair site was patent: 13.4 ± 5.6 versus 21.6 ± 8.7.[26]

The long-term patency rates for venous reconstruction have also been poorly documented. Phifer et al,[44] at follow-up of 6 to 20 years, demonstrated five of six repairs patent with the single occlusion occurring in a prosthetic graft. Aitken et al,[26] on follow-up venography in 11 patients in whom lower extremity venous reconstruction was performed, found that 54% of repairs were patent.

Our series demonstrated, at a mean follow-up of approximately 4 years, the following results in 26 patients with lower extremity venous reconstruction: an 11% rate for clinical evidence of chronic venous insufficiency, a 31% incidence of symptoms including those with mild asymptomatic edema, and an overall 96% crude patency rate. Twenty percent of patients had abnormal venous function of the injured limb as assessed by PPG; however, only two (8%) had a venous refilling time of less than 15 seconds.

Of the five patients with mild asymptomatic swelling, two had hemodynamic evidence (PPG venous refilling time less than 20 seconds) of venous insufficiency. The etiology of the swelling in the remaining patients may be related to calf muscle pump failure secondary to fasciotomy or neurologic injury. This, combined with a possible increased outflow resistance at the venous repair site, may account for the higher incidence of positive or borderline IPG studies obtained in the injured limb in comparison with that of the contralateral extremity.

Although early patency in 16 repairs was 50%, subsequent long-term patency, determined by CFDS, increased to 96%. This improved patency reflects the tendency for thrombosed venous repairs to undergo recanalization with restoration of secondary patency. Although prior investigators have demonstrated that recanalization of a previously thrombosed repair may occur, this finding had been previously limited to isolated case reports.[35,46,47] Our data indicate that the natural history of thrombosed repairs is one of recanalization with restoration of axial patency. Although early repair thrombosis did not appear to alter the early surgical results, does it necessarily dispose to the development of venous insufficiency? The hemodynamic and clinical effects of the thrombosed repairs appear to be primarily related to the extent of the venous thrombosis. In the absence of diffuse DVT, with isolated repair thrombosis, there appears to be preservation of venous competence and unidirectional venous flow. Segmental occlusion of the repair site with preservation of proximal and distal venous valves, followed by recanalization, did not result in serious physiologic impairment in venous function as assessed by PPG. This is in contradistinction to a previous report that revealed a significantly lower PPG venous refilling time in limbs undergoing repair, whether thrombosed or patent, compared with the contralateral noninjured limb.[26]

Reconstruction versus ligation, in the management of venous injuries of the upper extremity, cervical, and thoracic outlet, has not demonstrated any significant difference in acute outcome.[48–51] Ligation of such injuries is generally well tolerated; Rich et al[52] reported that acute or chronic edema of the arm after subclavian vein ligation was unusual. Exceptions to this include massive injuries in which venous return may be compromised and cases of replantation or near-complete neurovascular disruption. Although the optimal management of these injuries remains controversial, many centers have adopted an aggressive approach to the repair of venous injuries in complex upper extremity trauma.[49–51] Our study, on long-term follow-up of a limited number of venous reconstructions of the upper extremity, found an overall lower crude patency rate of 66%. This may represent both an increased disposition to early repair thrombosis or less propensity for thrombosed repairs to undergo recanalization in the upper extremity as compared with that of the lower extremity.

CONCLUSIONS

Long-term results of civilian venous repair after vascular trauma are often limited because of the inability to provide follow-up care for this group of patients. The available long-term data indicate minimal morbidity and physiologic disturbance along with excellent long-term patency associated with venous reconstruction. The natural history of early thrombosed repairs, in the absence of extensive DVT, appears to be one of recanalization with restoration of patency and preservation of proximal and distal valvular competence. Simple repair of venous injury should be accomplished whenever possible because of ease of performance and excellent short- and long-term patency rates. More complex reconstructions, despite a higher likelihood of early repair thrombosis, still retain the potential for recanalization. Although adherence to specific intraoperative and postoperative guidelines consisting of limb elevation and fasciotomy may diminish and eliminate the acute morbidity of venous ligation, the long-term functional outcome for these patients is undetermined at present. Individual injured lower extremity veins can be ligated without immediate serious sequelae; however, the adoption of ligation as the preferred technique when simple lateral repair cannot be performed appears to be a substandard approach. With the major objectives of venous trauma repair being the restoration of axial patency and maintenance of venous competence, reconstruction, despite its complexity, should be attempted whenever time and the patient's condition permit.

REFERENCES

1. Hobson RW, Wright CB, Swan KG, et al. Current status of venous injury and reconstruction in the lower extremities. In: Bergan JJ, Yao JST, eds. *Venous Problems*. Chicago: Yearbook Medical Publishers; 1978:469–484.
2. Rich NM. Management of venous trauma. *Surg Clin North Am*. 1988;68:809–821.
3. Pasch AR, Bishara RA, Schuler JJ, et al. Results of venous reconstruction after civilian vascular trauma. *Arch Surg*. 1986;121:607–611.
4. Borman KR, Jones GH, Snyder WH. A decade of lower extremity venous trauma. *Am J Surg*. 1987;154:608–611.
5. Mullins RJ, Lucas CE, Ledgerwood AM. The natural history following venous ligation for civilian injuries. *J Trauma*. 1980;20:737–743.
6. Timberlake GA, O'Connell RC, Kerstein MD. Venous injuries: to repair or ligate, the dilemma. *J Vasc Surg*. 1986;4:553–558.
7. Hardin WD, Adinolfi MF, O'Connell RC, et al. Management of traumatic peripheral vein injuries—primary repair or vein ligation. *Am J Surg*. 1982;144:235–238.
8. Rich NM, Hughes CW. Vietnam vascular registry: a preliminary report. *Surgery*. 1969;62:218–226.
9. Rich NM, Jarstfer BS, Geer RM. Popliteal artery repair failure: causes and possible prevention. *J Cardiovasc Surg*. 1974;15:340–351.
10. Rich NM, Hobson RW, Collins GJ, et al. The effect of acute popliteal venous interruption. *Ann Surg*. 1976;183:365–368.
11. Gaspar MR, Treiman RL. The management of injuries to major veins. *Am J Surg*. 1960;100:171–175.
12. Hobson RW, Yeager RA, Lynch TG. Femoral venous trauma: techniques for surgical management and early results. *Am J Surg*. 1983;146:220–224.
13. Blumoff RL, Powell T, Johnson G. Femoral venous trauma in a university referral center. *J Trauma*. 1982;22:703–705.
14. Agarwal N, Pravin MS, Clauss MD, et al. Experience with 115 civilian venous injuries. *J Trauma*. 1982;22:827–832.
15. Rich NM, Hobson RW, Wright CB, et al. Repair of lower extremity venous trauma: a more aggressive approach required. *J Trauma*. 1974;14:639–652.
16. Brigham RA, Eddleman WL, Clagett GP, et al. Isolated venous injury produced by penetrating trauma to the lower extremity. *J Trauma*. 1983;23:255–257.
17. Morrison WA, O'Brien BM, MacLeod AM, et al. Major limb replantation. *Orthop Clin North Am*. 1977;8:343–348.
18. Thomas JH, Pierce GE, Iliopoulos JI, et al. Vascular graft selection. *Surg Clin North Am*. 1988;68:865–874.
19. Woodson J, Rodriquez AA, Menzoian JO. The use of internal jugular vein as interposition graft for femoral vein reconstruction following traumatic venous injury: a useful approach in selected cases. *Ann Vasc Surg*. 1990;4:494–497.
20. Haimovici H, Hoffert PW, Zinicola N, et al. An experimental and clinical evaluation of grafts in the venous system. *Surg Gynecol Obstet*. 1970;131:1173–1186.

21. Hobson RW, Croom RD, Rich NM. Influence of heparin and low molecular weight dextran on the patency of autogenous vein grafts in the venous system. *Ann Surg.* 1973;17:773–776.

22. Schramek A, Hashmonal M, Farbstein J, et al. Reconstructive surgery in major vein injuries in the extremities. *J Trauma.* 1975;15:816–822.

23. Richardson JB Jr, Jurkovich GJ, Walker GT, et al. A temporary arteriovenous shunt (Scribner) in the management of traumatic venous injuries of the lower extremities. *J Trauma.* 1986;26:503–509.

24. Barkon JS, Terrazza O, Daignault P, et al. The fate of venous repair after shock and trauma. *J Trauma.* 1988;28:1322–1329.

25. Meyer J, Walsh J, Schuler J, et al. The early fate of venous repair after civilian vascular trauma—a clinical, hemodynamic, and venographic assessment. *Ann Surg.* 1987;206:458–464.

26. Aitken RJ, Matley PJ, Immelman EJ. Lower limb vein trauma: a long-term clinical and physiological assessment. *Br J Surg.* 1989;76:585–588.

27. Sullivan WG, Thorton RN, Baker LN, et al. Early influence of popliteal vein repair in the treatment of popliteal vessel injuries. *Am J Surg.* 1971;121:528–531.

28. Cargile JS, Hunt JL, Perdue GF. Acute trauma of the femoral artery and vein. *J Trauma.* 1992;32:364–369.

29. Hughes CW. Acute vascular trauma in Korean War casualties: an analysis of 180 cases. *Surg Gynecol Obstet.* 1954;99:91.

30. Rich NM, Baugh JH, Hughes CW. Acute arterial injuries in Vietnam: 1,000 cases, *J Trauma.* 1970;10:359–369.

31. Rich NM, Hughes CW, Baugh JJ. Management of venous injuries. *Ann Surg.* 1970;171:724–730.

32. Dajani OM, Haddad FF, Hani AH, et al. Injury to the femoral vessels—the Lebanese war experience. *Eur J Vasc Surg.* 1988;2:293–296.

33. Rich NM. Principles and indications for primary venous repair. *Surgery.* 1982;91:492–496.

34. Rich NM, Collins GJ Jr, Anderson CA, et al. Autogenous venous interposition grafts in repair of major venous injuries. *J Trauma.* 1977;17:512–520.

35. Rich NM, Sullivan WG. Clinical recanalization of an autogenous vein graft in the popliteal vein. *J Trauma.* 1972;12:919–920.

36. Phifer TJ, Gerlock AJ, Vekovius WA, et al. Amputation risk factors in concomitant superficial femoral artery and vein injuries. *Ann Surg.* 1984;199:241–243.

37. Ashworth EM, Dalsing MC, Glover JL, et al. Lower extremity vascular trauma: a comprehensive, aggressive approach. *J Trauma.* 1988;28:329–336.

38. Snyder WH. Vascular injuries near the knee: an updated series and overview of the problem. *Surgery.* 1982;91:502–506.

39. Thomas DD, Wilson RF, Wiencek GR. Vascular injury about the knee. Improved outcome. *Am Surg.* 1989;55:370–377.

40. Wagner WH, Calkins ER, Weaver FA, et al. Blunt popliteal artery trauma: one hundred consecutive injuries. *J Vasc Surg.* 1988;7:736–743.

41. Ross SE, Ransom KJ, Shatney CH. The management of venous injuries in blunt extremity trauma. *J Trauma.* 1985;25:150–152.

42. Wright CB, Hobson RW, Swan KG, et al. Extremity venous ligation: clinical and hemodynamic correlations. *Am Surg.* 1975;20:203–208.

43. Barcia PJ, Nelson TG, Whelan TJ. Importance of venous occlusion in arterial repair failure: an experimental study. *Ann Surg.* 1972;175:223–227.

44. Phifer TJ, Gerlock AJ, Rich NM, et al. Long-term patency of venous repairs demonstrated by venography. *J Trauma.* 1985;25:342–346.

45. Burch JM, Richardson RN, Martin RR, et al. Penetrating iliac vascular injuries: a recent experience with 233 consecutive patients. *J Trauma.* 1990;30:1450–1459.

46. Blumoff RL, Proctor HJ, Johnson G. Recanalization of a saphenous vein interposition venous graft. *J Trauma.* 1981;21:407.

47. Beggs JW. Recanalization of autogenous vein grafts. *South Med J.* 1988;81:1446–1447.

48. Clark GC, Lim RC Jr, Rosenburg JM. Cervicothoracic vascular injuries. Presentation, management, and outcome. *Am Surg.* 1991;57:582–587.
49. Orcutt MB, Levine BA, Gaskill HV, et al. Civilian vascular trauma of the upper extremity. *J Trauma.* 1986;26:63–67.
50. Myers SI, Harward TRS, Maher DP, et al. Complex upper extremity vascular trauma in an urban population. *J Vasc Surg.* 1990;12:305–309.
51. Meyer JP, Goldfaden D, Barrett J, et al. Subclavian and innominate artery trauma: recent experience with nine patients. *Cardiovasc Surg.* 1988;29:283–289.
52. Rich NM, Hobson RW, Jarstfer BS. Subclavian artery trauma. *J Trauma.* 1973;13:485–496.

Index

Abdominal aortic aneurysms. *See also* Aortic aneurysms; Thoracoabdominal aortic aneurysms
  repair of
    aortic tube grafts for, 163–169, 164*t*, 165*f*–168*f*, 165*t*
    modification of long-term survival after, 176–177
    patency after, 3
    prediction of long-term results after, 175–176
ABI. *See* Ankle-brachial index
ACE inhibitors. *See* Angiotensin-converting enzyme inhibitors
Age, treatment of thoracoabdominal aortic aneurysm and, 142, 142*f*
Air plethysmograph, in postoperative surveillance, 38
Ambulatory venous pressure (AVP), 4
Amputations. *See also* Limb salvage
  lower extremity ischemia and, 237*t*, 237–238, 238*f*
  popliteal aneurysm repair and, 290–291, 291*f*
Analog waveform analysis, in upper extremity ischemia, 356
Anastomoses
  in axillofemoral bypass, 397–398, 398*f*
  configuration of, aortofemoral bypass grafts and, 153–154
  in situ saphenous vein bypass and, 263–264
  in pediatric renal revascularization, 335, 336*f*
  primary versus secondary patency and, 5–6
  in upper extremity bypass, 358–359, 359*t*
Anastomotic false aneurysm, with aortofemoral bypass graft, 157–158
Anastomotic neointimal hyperplasia, 22. *See also* Intimal hyperplasia
Aneurysms. *See also specific site*
  false, anastomotic, 157–158
  long-term success and, 3

Angiography. *See also* Arteriogram
  before *in situ* saphenous vein bypass, 260
  before profundaplasty, 280, 281*f*, 282*f*
Angioplasty, transluminal, percutaneous. *See* Percutaneous transluminal angioplasty
Angioscopy, before *in situ* saphenous vein bypass, 261
Angiotensin-converting enzyme (ACE) inhibitors, in intimal hyperplasia control, 25–26
Angiotensin II receptor antagonist, in intimal hyperplasia control, 25
Ankle arteries, as bypass insertion sites, in lower extremity ischemia, 229, 230*f*
Ankle-brachial index (ABI), in peripheral arterial bypass graft surveillance, 35–36, 37*t*
Antegrade aortovisceral bypass, 309, 311, 311*f*
Anticoagulation. *See also specific anticoagulants*
  in upper extremity ischemia, 358
Antiplatelet therapy. *See also specific agents*
  in intimal hyperplasia control, 24
  patency and, 15–16
  of infrainguinal PTFE grafts, 295–296
Aortic aneurysms. *See also* Abdominal aortic aneurysms
  follow-up after repair of, other aneurysms presenting during, 177
  surgical repair of, 171–178
    factors influencing long-term survival after, 173–175, 174*t*
    late complications of, 171–172
    long-term survival after, 172–177, 173*t*, 174*t*
    modification of long-term survival after, 176–177
    prediction of long-term results after, 175–176
Aortic arch, acute tear of, arch replacement in, 129–130, 130*f*, 131*f*
Aortic dissection, 111–132, 113*t*
  acute arch tear and, concomitant arch replacement in, 129–130, 130*f*, 131*f*
  acute type B, medical versus surgical therapy for, 126–129, 128*f*

Page numbers followed by *t* and *f* refer to tables and figures, respectively.

Page numbers followed by *t* and *f* refer to tables
and figures, respectively.

Page numbers followed by *t* and *f* refer to tables and figures, respectively.

Page numbers followed by *t* and *f* refer to tables
and figures, respectively.

Page numbers followed by *t* and *f* refer to tables
and figures, respectively.